PRAISE FOR

Conquering Concussion

This book is impressive for a rare combination of expertise and readability. The historical perspective and excellent illustrations, both light and serious, make this as approachable as a serious medical book can be. Many M.D.s may not know the limits of the MRI, and may not realize the importance of head injury in psychiatry as well as neurology. People acquainted with the term "biofeedback" will gain new understanding here. Our brains need to be in protective custody. Every custodian is different; all can benefit from this fine resource.

—E. James Lieberman, M.D., M.P.H.
Clinical Professor of Psychiatry, Emeritus
George Washington University School of Medicine

Very well written, understandable, comprehensive discussion of a complex and extremely important medical problem. Head (and neck) trauma are common but they continue to be under- and mis-diagnosed. The consequences are immense, causing many thousands of people every year to suffer needlessly. This book indicating etiologies, diagnosis, and potential treatments is a must read for ER physicians, neurologists, neurosurgeons, anyone taking care of people who have suffered trauma with potential for Traumatic Brain Injury.

—Peter Dunne, M.D., Neurologist
College of Medicine, University of South Florida

A fascinating and well-written book on concussion and its aftermath. A complete and interesting history of head injury is followed by a useful, albeit brief, explanation of the brain and its inner workings. Clinical examples help the reader to see the huge impact that biofeedback and neurofeedback therapies have played in alleviating many of the symptoms of TBI.

—John Spencer, Ph.D., Neuropsychologist

Fast-moving and engaging, remarkable for such technical, detailed information. It will be used by professionals and students to expand their perspectives, and by patients and families to gain an understanding of the possibilities.

—Debi Gale, M.S., C.C.C.-S.L.P, C.B.I.S, Speech Pathologist

The historical cases are fascinating, revelatory, and explain an awful lot of bizarre behavior from Henry VIII to Howard Hughes. But these merely set the stage for the detailed discussion that follows on the complex symptomology of head injury, what to look for in sufferers, and how to help their complex and bewildering symptoms. Highly recommended!

—Stephen Larsen, Ph.D.
BCN Psychology, Professor Emeritus
State University of New York (SUNY)

Extensive clinical and research experience provide the basis for this exposition of brain injury symptoms, diagnostics, and treatments. Prevention, symptom identification, and treatment of brain injury are carefully and thoroughly covered. Patients, families, and health care professionals finally have a much needed resource.

—Karen Schultheis, Ph.D., Psychologist

If you've ever suffered a head injury, or worked as a physician or therapist with those who have, you know how important this book really is! The book is not only well-researched, but the writing is accessible, clear, and to the point.

—Thom Hartmann, Author

A wonderful book full of examples, quotes, references to characters in history, books and movies. Educates in an engaging manner, revealing the multiple ways, some subtle but devastating, others bizarre and disconcerting that the symptoms of TBI can manifest in everyday life. With such understanding comes compassion for all those whose ability to think, feel, act, and communicate is impaired and with compassion comes a renewed commitment to continue the search for help for the victims and families affected by TBI.

—Martha Lappin, Ph.D.

A mild traumatic brain injury case presents a far greater challenge in terms of proof and risk than severe traumatic brain injury case. This work gives Plaintiffs' lawyers what they need to meet that challenge "head-on" and dispel the associated myths. A must for Plaintiffs' lawyers.

—Eric Mitchell, Esq.

A compelling book, an important contribution to the field of traumatic brain injury, with riveting stories and case studies. The book highlights how essential it is for clinicians to include a history of head injuries in our intake interviews, something many psychotherapists don't do and many clients don't think to mention. The chapter on war trauma offers renewed hope that emerging tools like neurofeedback can restore quality of life and dignity to our nations' brave troops and veterans suffering the effects of blast injury, post-concussive syndrome, and PTSD.

—Laurie Leitch, Ph.D., Psychologist

Remarkably informative, giving insight into the many facets of brain injury and recovery. In my experience, when patients and loved ones begin to recognize and understand all the issues and symptoms around head injury they can begin to make real steps forward and find the help they need. This book will serve not only TBI recovering community but will be invaluable to the professional community as well. I am so pleased they have undertaken this timely topic and I am sure this will have a tremendous impact on all those who read it and whose lives are touched directly or indirectly by brain injury.

—Marty Wuttke

This book is an unbelievable resource. The history chapter is so interesting, with details of injuries from Henry the 8th to Elvis Presley. Their chapters on concussion symptoms and on case histories creates a one-stop resource about all aspects regarding concussion.

—Gillian Hotz PhD, Director KiDZ Neuroscience Center,
Director, Concussion Program
University of Miami, Miller School of Medicine

Even a "small" concussion can have long-term effects and the symptoms can vary widely. The technology presented in this book abruptly ended our six months of misery and has turned my daughter's life around.

—Patty Whelpley

Informative and inspiring. As a psychotherapist, I have been trained to look at mental health issues through a narrow lens but what I see as depression or attention issues could be more complicated. Now I understand when talk therapy can be helpful and when something more might be going on. I loved the case studies as they made the symptoms more real and memorable. A great job of making complex ideas clear and accessible.

—Katherine Thorn, L.P.C.

When it comes to recognition of Neurotherapy as a valuable treatment for concussion, the medical profession has had a gaping blind spot. Hopefully, Conquering Concussion, by Dr. Esty and C. M. Shifflett, will focus attention on the demonstrated benefits of Neurotherapy in treating concussion and brain injury. Well-written for a broad audience, this book brings together current scientific and clinical information that will benefit consumers and clinicians.

—Richard P. Brown, M.D., Associate Clinical Professor in Psychiatry
Columbia University College of Physicians and Surgeons

Recent revelations about the long-term consequences of concussion show that the traditional medical approach of just *allowing time to heal* is woefully inadequate. Here is a wake-up call to the healthcare professions regarding the need for active treatments — such as Neurotherapy — that improve brain recovery. In presenting the many facets of concussion, this book will contribute to broader discussions regarding the impact of head injury during childhood, sports activities, accidents, and military service. Clearly written with many interesting case examples, *Conquering Concussion* shows how Neurotherapy can help relieve or resolve a wide range of psychological and neurological problems with minimal adverse effects.

—Patricia L. Gerbarg, M.D., Associate Clinical Professor in Psychiatry
New York Medical College

It is only in the last few years that brain injuries are being appreciated for the devastating silent epidemic that they are. This book is an excellent introduction to head injuries--the symptoms and varied presentations, the long history of treatment, and current options available. It is appropriate for anyone wanting a serious, well rounded look at TBI. I wish that a book like this had been part of my education as an emergency room physician during my training.

—David Dubin, M.D.
Former Emergency Room Physician

Conventional medicine is extremely effective handling the acute medical care, TBI included. However, once the acute phase is over and the hard work of rehabilitation and dealing with the chronic aspects of post-concussion syndrome begins, our medical system fails miserably. Explains, at a very readable level, what happens to the brain when injured. More importantly, it explores non-pharmaceutical therapies that are not just a *reasonable* option, they are a *necessity* to battle the growing epidemic we face today. This book should be the primer for anyone wanting to understand the issues surrounding concussion and what could be done if our society really took TBI as seriously as it should.

—Michael Lewis, M.D., M.P.H., M.B.A,. F.A.C.P.M.
Colonel (Retired), US Army Medical Corps

Our son suffered a TBI at age 3, followed by two more concussions. This book gives insight into the aftermath of concussion — far beyond the anticipated headache — that most medical staff fail to acknowledge. This book validates the struggles we had with our son's recovery.

—Katy Hollis

Conquering Concussion

Healing TBI Symptoms

With Neurofeedback
and
Without Drugs

Mary Lee Esty, Ph.D. & C. M. Shifflett

Published by Round Earth Publishing, P. O. Box 157, Sewickley, PA 15143

Distributed by Quality Books.

Printed in the United States of America
Cover illustration: B-A-C-O/Shutterstock
Cover design: design-savvy.com
Text illustrations copyright © 2014 by C. M. Shifflett
Other copyrights retained by their respective copyright holders.

DOONESBURY reprinted with permission of UNIVERSAL UCLICK. All rights reserved.

Sherman's Lagoon used with the permission of the Jim Toomey, King Features Syndicate and the Cartoonist Group. All rights reserved.

Conquering Concussion

Healing TBI Symptoms with Neurofeedback and Without Drugs

MEDICAL DISCLAIMER: The following information is intended for general information purposes only. Individuals should always see their health care provider before administering any suggestions made in this book. Any application of the material set forth in the following pages is at the reader's discretion and is his or her sole responsibility.

Publisher's Cataloging-in-Publication
(Provided by Quality Books, Inc.)
    Esty, Mary Lee.
      Conquering concussion : healing TBI symptoms with
    neurofeedback and without drugs / by Mary Lee Esty, Ph.D. and C.M. Shifflett.
    -- First edition.
     280 pages cm
     Includes bibliographical references and index.
     ISBN 978-0-9653425-0-6

     1. Brain--Concussion--Treatment. 2. Neural
transmission--Regulation. I. Shifflett, C. M.
II. Title.

    RC394.C7E88 2013   617.4'810443
                 QBI13-600161

Contents

LIST OF FIGURES

LIST OF TABLES

COLOR SECTION

FOREWORD BY MARY LEE ESTY

This book began as a simple informational brochure for my clients with concussions. Making the long list of post-concussion symptoms and the many treatments that may be needed brought the full impact of concussion and its aftermath into extreme focus.

Fueling my resolve to finish this ever expanding project was the frustration I had experienced in early years as clients shared their experiences and looked to me for explanations. As I learned more about the consequences of concussion, it became clear that a lack of understanding was creating extra barriers for those struggling. I became determined to share what I have learned from my courageous clients in the hope of making life after concussion easier for others.

This book touches on the importance of integrating other therapies synergistic with neurofeedback. The case histories given here are with the neurofeedback type that I use, but there are other forms widely available and I recommend them to anyone searching for help; no one has a monopoly on positive outcomes.

For those of you searching for help for yourself, or someone else, it is my sincere hope that you will find this information useful and share it with others. —MLE

FOREWORD BY C. M. SHIFFLETT

Regardless of previous function, no matter how intelligent a person may be, injury changes the brain. If you or someone you know has had a concussion, you may notice some or many frightening and baffling symptoms. In this book, we will tell you why you have those symptoms. We will also present a new way of treating them, called *neurofeedback*.

In children and adults, some with injuries so severe that it was believed nothing else could be done, neurofeedback not only helped, it triggered remarkable improvements years, sometimes even decades, after the original injury. Case histories are from actual clients. Names and personal details have been changed to protect privacy, but their stories are real. They are not made up, they are not exaggerations. They are not composites — with two exceptions.

One is "Chris Pratt," from the 2007 movie, *The Lookout*. To date, it is the best media portrayal of the aftermath of traumatic brain injury, but not even Chris is entirely fictional. Writer / director Scott Frank based him on a friend with TBI. Leading man Joseph Gordon-Levitt developed his character from what he learned by attending a year of brain injury support meetings. This tale combines TBI with a fairly standard bank heist story, but the TBI symptoms shown in the movie are painfully real.

Another fictional character is Doonesbury character "B.D." by Gary Trudeau, whose panels tell the story of veterans and their families far better than I ever could.

If you have suffered a TBI, you may recognize them all too well. If you have family members or friends with TBI, you may better understand their symptoms through Chris and B.D. and through the Real Life stories of our own cast of characters. —CMS

ACKNOWLEDGEMENTS

The creation of this book is rooted in the work of many people whose work and insights over decades have culminated in a rapidly growing body of knowledge about an effective therapy for symptoms of central nervous system problems.

We are indebted to our clients. Their experiences laid the foundation of this book and their courage and determination led them to persevere in their search for a better life.

Reviewers who have given of their time and expertise to shape and build credibility to the final product are enthusiastically thanked for their invaluable contributions.

Dr. Erin Bigler guided us to invaluable sources illuminating the discrepancies between current neuropsychological findings and clinical evidence.

Dr. Angelo Bolea provided insight on neuropsychological testing.

Dr. Peter Dunne, neurologist, brought his vast experience to bear, helping to clarify medical material and adding personal clinical observations.

Dr. Edward T. Esty provided a keen eye, tireless review, and ongoing encouragement.

Dr. Richard Feely provided comments on cranial motions and distortions after trauma. His knowledge of structural problems related to concussion helped clarify the importance of hands-on therapies.

Debi Gale, speech-language pathologist and cognitive rehabilitation specialist at Brain Matters, Springfield, VA, a special thanks for recognizing the potential of neurofeedback for her TBI clients and her contribution to the overall message.

Rick Jaffe, J.D., provided legal insight.

Neera Kapoor, Ph.D., for invaluable insights on the visual symptoms of TBI.

Dr. Robert Kohn, neurologist and neuropsychiatrist explained functional neural relationships.

Laurie Leitch, Ph.D., provided clinical details on neurofeedback and PTSD.

Harriet Lesser, Fine Art Curator at the Strathmore Mansion, contributed her artistic eye.

Dr. James E. Lieberman, psychiatrist and author, provided medical commentary.

Tammy Liller, president and co-founder of The National Fibromyalgia Partnership plied her skills as clarifier-in-chief for making material accessible.

Eric Mitchell, J.D., Washington D.C., recognizes the value of new treatments as he fights through the legal system for his clients struggling with life after concussion.

Elizabeth Mubarek, M.S., assisted with historical research.

Emily Perlman, MS, LGPC, BCB, SMC-C, provided descriptions of muscle biofeedback for posttraumatic pain. Her clinical expertise continues to aid recovery of clients treated at The Brain Wellness and Biofeedback Center of Washington.

Dr. Elizabeth Stuller, psychiatrist, reviewed the neurological nd neurochemical issues.

Dr. Forest Tennant provided detailed forensic data directly from the medical records of Howard Hughes and Elvis Presley.

For their enthusiasm, time, and support thanks to Diane Badger, Trudy Barnum, Line Bouthilette, Linda Braverman, Wendy Jane Carrell, Dr. David Dubin, Dale and Franklyn Gorell, Katy Hollis, author Jim Robbins, Karen Schultheis, Ph.D., Corey Snook, John Spencer, Ph.D., graphic artist Jessica Stevens, neurologist Jonathan Walker, Andrea Weisman, Ph.D., Lisa Weiss, MSW, Patty Whelpley, and historian David Zeih.

We would also like to express fond memories of neurosurgeon Dr. Ayub Ommaya, an internationally known expert on brain injuries, a man of many interests and creative curiosity. A Rhodes Scholar, a champion swimmer and debater, and a trained opera singer, he was famous for his ability to think outside individual boxes. As Chief of Neurosurgery at the National Institutes of Health, his research on brain injury and interest in preventing it led him to serve as Chief Medical Advisor to the National Highway Traffic Safety Administration (1980-1985). There he helped to establish systematic data collection and study of traffic accidents to improve highway and vehicle design in hopes of reducing injuries.

Having seen the potential of biofeedback for rehabilitation after TBI, Dr. Ommaya supported and frequently presented at the Mid-Atlantic Society for Biofeedback and Behavioral Medicine. He referred his private TBI patients to Dr. Esty for FNS treatment because he had seen the rapid changes in their symptoms. In 1997, after watching Dr. Esty treat several clients for post-concussion symptoms, he volunteered to help recruit participants and wrote a supportive recruiting letter for the NIH-funded study of Mild to Moderate TBI done with the Kessler Rehabilitation Hospital.

Many of the stories told here are based on that research. And new research continues.

For those who are about to read our thoughts, thank you for your interest and we look forward to your comments and any concerns. This is a broad topic and we have been able to touch only briefly on difficult subjects. Many things, from omega-3 fish oil to hyperbaric oxygen chambers have helped many patients. Some professionals may feel that their fields have been slighted but the constraints of space and time rule; we too have been frustrated by those factors. Please enjoy as suits you, and please know that we are trying to provide glimpses of wonderful possibilities for every reader.

Main characters in our story are presented with their injury and pre-treatment symptoms. Bolded text indicates those with full case histories. To follow them through the book, see "Cast of Characters" in the Index. Historical figures are indexed under People and Quotes.

Cast of Characters	
Historical Figures (in order of appearance)	
Phineas Gage	Construction accident. Iron tamping rod blown through skull. Extreme changes in personality, temperament, and executive skills.
Henry VIII	Sports injuries (jousting). Migraines, depression (melancholia), weight changes, emotional lability, paranoia, spending and hoarding, possible Obsessive Compulsive Disorder (OCD).
Admiral Lord Nelson	Blast injuries and infections. Confusion and depression. Blind in one eye, possibly due to blast-induced detached retina.
Edweard Muybridge	Vehicle crash. Headaches, loss of executive function; risky behavior, impulsivity, murder, obsessions.
Mary Lincoln	Vehicle crashes (car and airplane). Headaches, obsessions, impulsivity, paranoia, spending and hoarding.
Howard Hughes	Vehicle crashes and assaults. Severe OCD, headache, light sensitivity, sexual obsessions, spending and hoarding, impulsivity, paranoia.
Elvis Presley	Multiple concussions from fights and falls. Possible additional injuries from motorcycles, horses, skating, football and martial arts. Headaches and body pain, impulsivity, obsessions, paranoia, eventual drug addiction.
Children	
Archie	Sports injuries (soccer). Auditory hallucinations; AD(H)D.
Bridgett	Sports injuries (soccer). Severe headaches, cognitive problems, muscle spasms and weakness, light and sound sensitivity.
Bruce	Sports injuries (lacrosse). Headaches, extreme fatigue and excessive sleep, poor concentration.
Jake	Fall from diving board onto concrete. Severe TBI with loss of muscle control, including speech and swallowing. History of AD(H)D and sensory integration.
Adults (Civilian)	
Ben	Vehicle crash. Recovered enough to drive, but with memory problems; could not remember if another car was at 4-way stop.
Bill	Vehicle crash. Organization / sequencing problems, couldn't remember faces or people, lost 1/4 field of vision. Halting speech, dysautonomia. Unable to stay awake for more than a couple hours at a time. Low body temperature.
Bobbie	Vehicle crash. Severe memory loss, spatial disorientation, visual problems, migraine headaches. fatigue and dysautonomia. Low body temperature.
Brian	Sports injuries (martial arts, diving). AD(H)D, fibromyalgia, sensitivity to light and sound, migraines, memory loss, fatigue, excessive sleep, flat affect. Low body temperature.

Carol	Sports injuries and fall on ice with basal skull fracture. Migraines, body pain, poor executive function, memory loss. Sound and light sensitivity, loss of sense of smell and direction, low body temperature.
Charlotte	Fall on playground. Slowed thoughts, memory problems, difficulty finding words, high IQ but poor academic performance.
Gregory	Hit in head with a thrown rock. Daily migraines, with twice-monthly trip to ER.
Honor	Vehicle crash (severe whiplash). Migraines, neck and back pain, fatigue, dizziness/severe balance problems, light and noise sensitivity.
Jenna	Dropped on head at a fraternity party. Could not stay awake in class or work.
Katherine	Multiple TBIs from domestic abuse. Headaches, severe depression, body pain. Body temperature around 95 F.
Louise	Frontal and left temporal cysts. Poor executive function, violent rages.
Marie	T-boned on her side at 35 m.p.h. Memory problems and unable to make lists.
Morgan	Fall down stairs. Severe Diffuse Axonal Injury (DAI).
Nick	Fall 50 feet from window. Fractured skull, broken ribs, collapsed lungs, 27-day coma. Lost long-term memory.
Phyllis	Sports injury, skied off 1,500-foot cliff. Severe dysautonomia. Low body temperature. Required hot tub to maintain normal temperature.
Robin	Vehicle crash and falls. Multiple whiplash injuries. Headaches, fibromyalgia, reading difficulties, noise sensitivity, depression, short-term memory loss.
Sam	Vehicle crash (motorcycle). Migraines, sleep disturbances, severe AD(H)D.
Sophia	Vehicle crash (whiplash). Fibromyalgia and loss of cervical curve.
Steve	Vehicle crash (bicycle). Memory loss, PTSD, impulsivity, fatigue, insomnia.
Thea	Vehicle crash (severe whiplash). Headache, fatigue, vertigo, anxiety, partial vision loss, irritability insomnia. Extreme sensitivity to light, sound, and motion. Loss of depth perception, speech comprehension, math skills. *MRI "normal."*

Military TBI / PTSD Study Subjects (Iraq / Afghanistan)

David	Migraines, PTSD, explosiveness, loss of executive function, insomnia, pain, drug abuse, depression. Suicidal.
Jay	Severe headaches, memory loss, fatigue, body pain, depression, explosiveness, sleep apnea, night sweats, severe PTSD. Suicidal.
Kevin	Severe cognitive and memory problems, seizures, PTSD, nightmares, pain, numbness, drug abuse, malnutrition, poor handwriting. Suicidal.
Kyle	Headaches, crushed vertebrae, back pain, loss of executive function, memory. Insomnia, inability to read, poor balance.
Mike	War correspondent (civilian) in the thick of the Afghanistan / Iraqi wars.
Paul	Migraines, PTSD, insomnia, poor concentration, back pain.

AD(H)D	Attention Deficit (Hyperactivity) Disorder
ANS	Autonomic Nervous System
BWB	Brain Wellness and Biofeedback Center
CN	Cranial Nerve
CSF	Cerebro-Spinal Fluid
CT	Computerized Tomography; a computer-driven X-ray
CTE	Chronic Traumatic Encephalopathy
DAI	Diffuse Axonal Injury
DSM	Diagnostic and Statistical Manual
DTI	Diffuse Tensor Imaging
EEG	Electroencephalogram
fMRI	Functional MRI
FNS	Flexyx Neurotherapy System
GSR	Galvanic Skin Response
HRV	Heart Rate Variability
IED	Improvised Explosive Device
MTBI	Mild Traumatic Brain Injury
OCD	Obsessive Compulsive Disorder
OEF/OIF	Operation Enduring Freedom / Operation Iraqi Freedom
PCS	Post-Concussion Syndrome
PTSD	Post-Traumatic Stress Disorder (also Post-Traumatic Stress, PTS)
QEEG	Quantitative EEG
sEMG	Surface or Surficial Electromyography
SPECT	Single-Photon Emission Computed Tomography, an imaging technique.
TBI	Traumatic Brain Injury
TSH	Thyroid Stimulating Hormone
TMJ	Temporo-Mandibular Joint; TMJD, TMJ Dysfunction
VBIED	Vehicle-Borne Improvised Explosive Device
USUHS	Uniformed Services University of the Health Sciences.
VA	Veterans Affairs
WRAMC	Walter Reed Army Medical Center
WWE	World Wrestling Entertainment; (World Wrestling Federation (WWF)

HISTORICAL MONEY CONVERSIONS

Incomes and expenses for historical figures were converted to modern equivalents using the calculator at: **www.measuringworth.com.**

Part 1

The Story of What Happens

Introduction

HEAD INJURIES IN HISTORY, FROM PHINEAS GAGE, KING HENRY VIII, LORD NELSON, EDWEARD MUYBRIDGE, TO MARY LINCOLN, HOWARD HUGHES AND ELVIS PRESLEY.

C oncussion is a common but poorly understood affliction. By general definition, it is an injury to the brain that happens at or after birth and comes from an outside mechanical force (such as a blow) that impairs brain function.

When this happens (especially with loss of consciousness or body functions), one has been *concussed*, but the words commonly used to describe it sound trivial: you've "had your bell rung" or suffered a "ding."

In reality, a concussion and its aftermath can be far more serious than these silly words can convey. We may fail to realize that anything meaningful has happened at all and we have no popular model for what actually happens.

What we *think* we know comes largely from the Fantasy World of film and comic books. Legions of superheroes and "normal" characters are regularly knocked unconscious, but within seconds the James Bonds and Mike Hammers (knocked out by the usual Bad Guys), or a Spiderman (knocked out by The Incredible Hulk) are on their feet and fully functional with nothing more than a brief groan and a colorful comment.

They are never blinded by the blow to the visual cortex in back of the head. They do not lose memory, mental or physical skills or their sleek super-hero figures. They will not suffer headaches or relentless pain for the rest of their lives. They are never downgraded or let go from their jobs. And . . . they will do it all again next week.

That is fantasy.

In the Real World, things don't work that way.

Head Injuries in History

There are obviously problems with putting historical figures on the psychiatrist's couch . . .
Yet, we do have many contemporary reports of the king's behaviour and speech . . . some of
Henry's letters and the theological treatises he worked on and we possess a whole panoply
of state papers, royal proclamations and Acts of Parliament. Together, such evidence allows
us to make cautious judgements about Henry VIII's character.

—Suzannah Lipscomb (2009b)

There are many famous persons whose traumatic and well-documented head injuries were followed by sudden changes in behavior and personality. The list includes the once beloved then terrifying Henry VIII, the heroic and half-blinded Admiral Lord Nelson, the despised Mary Lincoln, the photographic genius and murderer Edweard J. Muybridge, aviation pioneer Howard Hughes, and singer Elvis Presley.

You may wonder: How much of their behavior should be attributed to concussion?

They were not imaged by MRI and we can't put these people on the couch at this late date. Nevertheless, their behaviors after very public injuries were seen and commented on by friends, family, and the general public, and documented by the physicians and neurologists of their day. Today their symptoms of concussion tend to be attributed to psychological issues. That said, it is an odd, if long-held belief, that psychology and behavior are somehow separate from the brain itself.

After Henry's two *best known* accidents (for such an avid sportsman, there were certainly more), his life bore little resemblance to romantic TV portrayals. How and why Henry changed from a gallant Prince Charming to a murderous Bluebeard comes from Suzannah Lipscomb's book, *1536: The Year that Changed Henry VIII* (2009a). After Henry's 1536 fall *and two hours of unconsciousness* it was said (and is still widely believed) that Henry sustained no injury. Many historians ignore his obvious brain damage in favor of unrelated depression or mid-life crisis. In contrast, Lipscomb (who is Research Curator at Henry's Hampton Court Palace), lays out the before and after evidence of his post-traumatic downward spiral with devastating clarity.

Mary Lincoln had an extensive education and excellent financial and organizational skills. She was an important power behind her husband's political career, but her abilities ended with a carriage accident.

Elvis Presley's difficulties can be attributed to many things besides head injury, for example, drugs and depression. Both are understandable in context. He was using drugs by high school, then lived his entire adult life under virtual house arrest by his manager and fans. But his precipitous decline and early death corresponds closely to a traumatic head injury in 1976.

The death of icons such as Elvis Presley or Howard Hughes often inspires claims, counter claims and wild speculation. So how is the information here any different from any other material on Hughes or Presley? It is based on actual medical records and autopsy reports compiled by Dr. Forest Tennant for legal hearings and trials, and includes information that was not recognized or understood at the time of their deaths.

These people were presented in this chapter because they were *extreme examples of serious, sometimes multiple injuries*. You may recognize at least some of the symptoms. But just as their symptoms are the same ones experienced by others today, so were their underlying injuries largely ignored, unrecognized, or denied, as still happens with many concussions today.

The one outstanding exception is also the most famous: Phineas Gage.

Despite the millions of people over thousands of years whose lives were changed by head trauma[1], the case of Phineas Gage is widely considered to be the first medically documented case of brain damage impacting personality and behavior.

---

1. It may also include "The Red Baron" (Manfred von Richthofen, the WWI fighter pilot), a long list of madmen and murderers such as H. H. Holmes (the serial killer who may also have been Jack the Ripper), Ted Bundy, Richard Speck, and others who were severely abused or suffered accidental head injuries as children. For more historical examples, see Masferrer R and Others (2000).

Phineas Gage

PERSONALITY CHANGES, LOSS OF EXECUTIVE SKILLS, EXPLOSIVENESS, AND SEIZURES.

In 1848, Phineas Gage, a railroad construction foreman, was tamping blasting powder into a hole. It sparked, blowing the 14-pound, 3-foot 7-inch tamping rod up under his left cheekbone and out the top of his head (Figure 1-1). The rod landed 80 feet away, smeared with blood and globs of brains.

Witnesses disagreed on whether Gage lost consciousness. Some said he never did. Others thought he might have been unconscious (or merely dazed) for a few minutes. But all agreed that he was fully conscious, and sitting up in the wagon when carted to a nearby hotel where he joked with the doctor. Amazingly, his terrible wounds healed. But all was not well. Far from it.

Before the accident, his employers had considered Gage to be their most capable and efficient foreman. Afterwards, they found the change in his mind, behavior, and personality, so marked that they could not give him his job again.

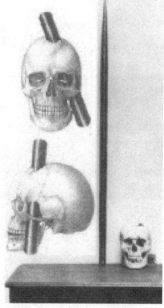

FIGURE 1-1. Gage's Skull

He is fitful, irreverent, indulging at times in the grossest profanity (which was not previously his custom), manifesting but little deference for his fellows, impatient of restraint or advice when it conflicts with his desires, at times pertinaciously obstinate, yet capricious and vacillating, devising many plans of future operation, which are no sooner arranged than they are abandoned in turn for others appearing more feasible. In this regard, his mind was radically changed, so decidedly that his friends and acquaintances said he was "no longer Gage."

—Dr. John Martyn Harlow (1848)

The Gage who was no longer Gage survived for another 12 years, struggling through a series of odd jobs, wandering from New England to Chile to California. In 1860, he died in San Francisco of a massive seizure.

The injuries of others throughout the ages have also been documented, but their clear symptoms long remained unrecognized as a result of brain injury. Gage's injury was outstanding because of its visible severity, far beyond simple concussion, and the fact that he survived to be observed by many people who knew him well and who experienced his extreme changes in skills and personality. There are other documented cases that also resulted in extreme personality changes.

One of the most tragic (and unrecognized) examples is that of King Henry VIII of England.

King Henry VIII

MIGRAINES AND LOSS OF EXECUTIVE SKILLS. PERSONALITY CHANGES, EMOTIONAL LABILITY, OBSESSIONS, SPENDING AND HOARDING, AND SEVERE OBESITY

Young Henry was a true Prince Charming, tall, handsome and robustly athletic, with an excellent mind. By all accounts, he was a healthy and happy teenage boy who became the Merry King Hal, admired and beloved by all.

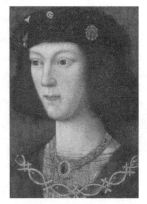

FIGURE 1-2. Henry 1509

Envoys from other countries, even rival courts, consistently described him as warm and affable, gracious and benevolent, "a man who harmed no one."Erasmus, the great Renaissance humanist, saw "a man of gentle friendliness, and gentle in debate; he acts more like a companion than a king."

Henry excelled in music, mathematics, languages (he spoke four) and sports, including fencing, hunting, wrestling, and tennis. He was especially fond of jousting. His grandmother had forbidden it as too dangerous, but, at 18, when she was dead and he was King, he jousted.

At a match in March of 1524, Henry *forgot to lower his visor*, an error that should never have happened, that was immediately seen by the horrified onlookers, who screamed a warning that Henry, galloping forward on his powerful warhorse, did not hear or heed. And then . . .

> . . . The Duke [of Suffolk] struck the king on the brow right under the guard of the headpiece [and] when the spear landed on that place there was great danger of death since the face was bare, for the duke's spear broke into splinters and pushed the king's visor or barbette so far back with the counter blow that all the King's head piece was full of splinters.
>
> —George Cavendish (1524)

Taking all blame for the foolish mistake, Henry picked himself up saying that all was well. But all was *not* well, and all manner of things would never be well again. From that day on, Henry's downward spiral would bring tragedy and grief to him, his family, and thousands of his subjects. The most obvious symptom was severe migraine headaches that would plague him for the rest of his life. When in severe pain and unable to exercise as before, most people lose their appetites, but Henry ate, drank, and *spent*, without restraint. Soon he was clinically obese and thanks to lavish and impulsive expenditures for clothes, feasts, toys and entertainments, the massive fortune left to him by his frugal father was nearly gone. It was during this same period that Henry became obsessed with Anne Boleyn.

By 1533 he had broken from the Catholic Church, divorced Queen Catherine, and married Anne, but their marriage was short-lived, due in part to radical changes in Henry's personality and behavior. He was no longer the affectionate warm-hearted man he had once been. Many blamed Anne, but no one was more shocked by Henry's behavior than Anne herself, who would soon die from the emotional and cognitive effects of her husband's brain injury.

A final joust on January 24, 1536 was a turning point in both their lives. The severely obese Henry fell from his horse in full armor. The horse, also in full armor, fell on Henry. For two hours he lay unconscious, and arose from his bed a different man. Desperate for money after years of overspending, Henry seized monastery lands and assets. This was also the year when inconvenient persons, regardless of rank, began to be charged with high treason on flimsy (or no) evidence, then executed without trial (Lipscomb S, 2009a).

On May 2, 1536, Henry had his wife arrested on wild charges of adultery with no fewer than five men (including her brother); he also pushed a bill through parliament declaring that adultery by the queen was now (for the first time in the history of England), high treason. On May 19, Queen Anne, once the King's "own darling," was beheaded by order of her husband, once her "loyal servant and friend." Just 11 days later, Henry married the quiet Jane Seymour, as different from Anne as anyone could be. Henry passed his time in painting and embroidery and Jane produced a son (Edward VI) but the child was sickly and by October of 1538, Jane was dead from complications of childbirth.

Henry began looking for his next queen but Anne's execution horrified the noble families of Europe and their daughters. (One young lady of interest, 16-year old Christina of Denmark, is famously said to have remarked that she *might* consider the marriage "*if I had two heads.*") He married Anne of Cleves, as a political alliance with Germany against Spain, divorcing her as soon as her parents were dead. His next marriage to the flighty young Catherine Howard (just 17) ended in her execution.

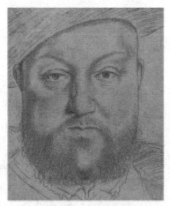

FIGURE 1-3. Henry in 1540

Henry terrified his court with his volatile and violent moods. He would have one opinion at breakfast, an entirely different one by dinner. He would rage at his counselors, then dissolve into tears. Now there were no good words for Henry.

In 1540, the French ambassador described him as fearful, inconstant and "so covetous that all the riches in the world would not satisfy him."

Morbidly obese, depressed, paranoid, and in horrific pain, Henry continued to deteriorate. When he died at age 56, he weighed nearly 400 pounds and was riddled with infections, rotting flesh, and severe debt.

Historians have long struggled with the mystery of how the beautiful fairy-tale prince became a murderous monster.

It would be almost 500 years before we understood the reasons why.

Lord Horatio Nelson

BLINDNESS, CONFUSION, DEPRESSION, NIGHT SWEATS AND PARANOIA.

Lord Horatio Nelson (1758-1805) was the man who saved England from invasion by Napoleon Bonaparte.

As a child, he was delicate. As an adult he suffered malaria and typhoid; as a soldier, a string of severe battle injuries.

In 1794, at the Siege of Calvi, a shot slammed into the battery beside him. An explosion of stone and sand and splintered wood struck him in the chest and face. It was . . .

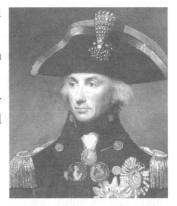

FIGURE 1-4. Admiral Nelson

> . . . [A] blow so severe as to occasion a great flow of blood from my head, yet I most fortunately escaped, having only my right eye nearly deprived of its sight, although the wound there was a very slight scratch towards my right eye.

He reassured his wife that "the blemish is nothing; not to be perceived, unless told." He could still tell light from dark[1]. If injury had been from a foreign body ripping into the eyeball, medical practice of the day would have dictated immediate removal of the eye rather than leave it intact and run the greater risk of infection. As it was not removed and the surgeon predicted return of sight, a more likely possibility was that Nelson suffered a detached retina or internal damage to the optic nerve. When the minor superficial cuts healed, there was no disfigurement, except that the pupil was dilated, "nearly the size of the blue part," said Nelson. Sight never returned. A blast powerful enough to produce all these symptoms could easily have also caused concussion and other injuries.

In July 1797, under heavy fire at Teneriffe, Nelson lost his right arm. In August of 1798, at the Battle of the Nile, he was struck so hard on the left forehead by a piece of langridge[2], that he was knocked unconscious. He awoke to headaches and confusion as revealed in his various letters.

> [To the Governor of Bombay]: If my letter is not so correct as might be expected, I trust your excuse, when I tell you, my brain is so shaken with the wound in my head, that I am sensible I am not always as clear as could be wished.

> [To the Earl of St. Vincent]: My head is ready to split, and I am always so sick: in short, if there be no fracture my head is severely shaken. My head is so wrong that I cannot write that I wish in such a manner as to please myself.

1. Nelson's health records are online at www.aboutnelson.co.uk/health.htm.
2. *Langridge* was a crude form of ordnance — scrap metal, nails, broken tiles, bricks, gravel — loaded loose into guns.

Shortly after, he fell severely ill with a fever. "For eighteen hours," he wrote, "my life was thought to be past hope; I am now up, but very weak both in body and mind."

He was nursed back to health by the beautiful Emma, wife of Sir William Hamilton, the English envoy to Naples. Emma and the married Nelson fell in love. Two years later, in the throes of deep depression, he returned to England. He asked to be relieved of command, broke off all relations with his wife, and lived with Emma and her elderly husband.

Society was horrified, not at Nelson's having a mistress, but for his complete lack of discretion or concern for social proprieties, and for abandoning his wife in the process. The scandal deepened when Lady Hamilton bore a child, Horatia, in 1801. Belatedly concerned about public opinion, Nelson and Emma swore that Horatia was adopted. Meanwhile, Nelson descended into paranoia and jealousy, imagining that the Prince of Wales was sneaking into Emma's bed (McGrath C, 2006).

In 1804, six years after his 1798 head injury, Nelson wrote to a Dr. Baird of continuing symptoms including "night sweats, with heat in the evening and feeling quite flushed[1]." He never recovered. In 1805, he was killed shortly before the victory over Napoleon's fleet at the Battle of Trafalgar. Nelson was deeply mourned by his men and his country, but accolades were mixed with confusion and bewilderment.

Brain injury has always been suspected as the cause of Nelson's odd behavior, clearly even by Nelson himself, but the idea apparently has been resisted as too disturbing, or even insulting to the memory of a hero.

Sir Arthur Conan Doyle's Regency novel, *Rodney Stone,* published in 1896, sketches a scene in which Rodney and his father encounter Nelson and Lady Hamilton. Writing long after Nelson's death, Doyle recreated the bewildered sorrow of decades before, foreshadowing our own confusion and shock at the mysteriously altered behavior of the best and bravest of men damaged in war.

---

1. Sweating is a common in soldiers who have had blast injuries. After Nelson's many encounters with cannon fire, he may well have suffered this autonomic symptom. It may also have been a lingering symptom of malaria.

Mary Todd Lincoln

MIGRAINES, EMOTIONAL LABILITY, SPENDING AND HOARDING, DRUG ADDICTION, HALLUCINATIONS, PHOTOPHOBIA.

"Whatever of awkwardness may be ascribed to her husband, there is none of it in her," a journalist from the New York Evening Post wrote. "She converses with freedom and grace, and is thoroughly *au fait* in all the little amenities of society." Frequent mention was made of her distinguished Kentucky relatives, her sophisticated education, her ladylike courtesy, her ability to speak French fluently.

—Doris Kearns Goodwin, *Team of Rivals* (2005, p. 265)

The daughter of a wealthy Kentucky family, Mary Todd received an education far superior to most girls (or boys) of that day. For four years she studied languages and literature at a school run by an aristocratic French couple. Later she studied mathematics.

Young Mary was described as "sunning all over with laughter one moment, the next crying as though her heart would break" (Goodwin DK, 2005, p. 96). Nevertheless, she was a very popular young lady, courted by the most eligible young men of her day. When she fell in love with poor and homely Abraham Lincoln, her wealthy family was sure she could do better. Mary disagreed and they married.

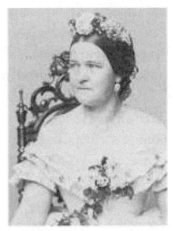

FIGURE 1-5. Mary Lincoln (1861)

Beautiful, social, and passionately interested in politics, Mrs. Lincoln was intimately involved in her husband's career. During his long absences as a circuit lawyer, she managed home, children, finances and building renovations. When he ran for President, Republican papers had nothing but praise for her abilities. A few years later she was the most despised woman in America. This was due, in part, to the political suspicion and intrigue of the Civil War[1]. And due, in part, to the lingering effects of traumatic brain injury.

On July 2, 1863, as the Battle of Gettysburg raged 80 miles away, the Lincolns were returning to the White House from the Soldier's Home (where they stayed in summer), Mr. Lincoln on horseback, his wife in the carriage. As the road turned downhill, the carriage seat tore loose, hurling the driver to the ground. The horses bolted, and Mary (in hoop skirts) leapt from the runaway carriage. When she slammed into the rocky ground, she almost certainly rolled. We don't know how far, but we do know that she suffered multiple

---

1. A Southerner by birth, Mary fiercely opposed slavery. The South saw her as a traitor. Northerners saw her as a spy, while criticizing her clothes, her "frontier" manners, and even the amount of time she spent with wounded soldiers, bringing them food baskets and writing their letters home.

lacerations to head and face. A deep gash at the back of her head developed a life-threatening infection. Eventually the superficial wounds healed, but the concussion that she certainly suffered triggered changes in personality, abilities, and health and behavior. Her life-long migraines worsened and the once-capable Mary suffered delusions and hallucinations.

After her son Willie died, in February of 1862, Mary sought out spiritualists and mediums, but not until *after* her 1863 injury did she report actually *seeing* Willie's ghost and *hearing* him speak to her. Meanwhile, she shopped compulsively, in a style far beyond mere extravagance. In just four months, she ordered 300 pairs of kid gloves, spent $3,000 for earrings and a pin, $5,000 for a shawl, thousands more for gayly colored silks and ribbons for which she could never pay and would never wear because after Willie's death she wore only black. By 1864, she was a serious campaign liability. Republicans feared that public knowledge of her massive debt (probably well over $30,000), would harm Mr. Lincoln's chances of re-election.

After her husband's assassination, Mary continued to deteriorate. She complained of a ghostly Indian putting wires in her eyes, a thief who had stolen her purse but promised to return it, a waiter who tried to murder her with poisoned coffee. Although she had plenty of income, Mary was terrified of poverty and starvation, and despite these fears, she continued her lavish spending and hoarding.

In 1875, suddenly and inexplicably certain that her last son was dying, she hurried to Chicago. There, Robert (quite healthy) found her wandering the hotel in her nightgown, carrying on whispered conversations with "people in the walls" and terrified that Chicago was burning (as it had in 1871). Fearing for his mother's mental state and personal safety, Robert had her committed, through a jury trial, to an asylum (actually a luxurious minimum security home). She remained there for just four months; on release she fled to Europe.

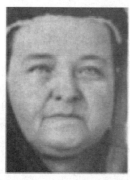

Years later, she returned to Illinois with a massive hoard of possessions. She lived behind shades and heavy drapes, allowing only candles, complaining that the bright gaslight was the work of the Devil. She also bought a gun and threatened to murder her son for his "betrayal."

Mary died in 1882 at 63. Those who remembered her strengths and kindnesses of earlier years explained her oddities by pointing to all she had endured, including the deaths of her brothers, sons and husband. Yet the same tragedies, and worse, were suffered by countless others throughout the terrible years of civil war.

FIGURE 1-6. Mary c. 1871

In his testimony at Mary's infamous insanity trial, her son did not dwell on her losses (Goodwin DK, 2005, p. 535). Instead, Robert, weeping, stated his firm belief that his mother had "never quite recovered *from the effects of her fall*."

Edweard J. Muybridge
HEADACHES AND LOSS OF EXECUTIVE FUNCTION. OBSESSIONS, RISKY BEHAVIOR, IRRITABILITY AND MURDER

One of the baffling symptoms of brain injury is that it does not necessarily impact intelligence, although it may have powerful impact on everything else.

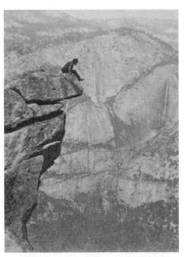

Edweard Muybridge, born near London in 1830, came to America in 1852, at the height of the California gold rush. He settled in San Francisco as a bookseller and an agent for the London Printing and Publishing Company. He also developed an interest in photography. His first famous photo series proved that during a gallop, a horse has all four feet off the ground. This seemingly simple investigation required many years of work and vast improvements in the primitive photographic techniques of the day.

FIGURE 1-7. Muybridge in Yosemite

In 1860, he set off for a month in the wildly beautiful Yosemite, to evaluate the potential for sales of photographs of scenery. On return, he planned to sail to London (via New York) for a book-buying tour. He started east by stage coach.

North of Fort Worth, Texas, the coach's "six wild mustang horses" broke into a dead run. On cresting a mountain they hurtled downhill, running so madly that the crude wooden brakes were useless. The coach careened off the road, slammed into a tree, and shattered to pieces. One passenger was killed when he attempted to jump (as Mary Lincoln had done) from the runaway vehicle. Muybridge, thrown free, flew headfirst into a boulder and knocked unconscious. He may have remained so for hours or even days; his first memory was waking up in bed, 150 miles (by horse-drawn rescue wagon) from the crash in Fort Smith, Arkansas. He had a fractured skull, severe headache, deafness, double vision, no sense of taste or smell and no memory of the accident. He was unable to travel for three months.

When he finally arrived in New York, a prominent physician warned that his injuries were permanent. In England, Queen Victoria's personal physician could do no more than suggest healthful outdoor exercise and encourage his photographic excursions.

At the end of the Civil War, Muybridge returned to San Francisco and began working with an old friend, Silas Selleck. His photographs of Yosemite were wildly popular, making him the Ansel Adams of his day. He married pretty young Flora Stone who bore a son but six months later Muybridge discovered that Flora had a lover, a Major Harry Larkyns, and that she considered the boy to be his.

Muybridge immediately sought out Larkyns and shot him dead.

His trial, the celebrity murder case of its day, addressed the 1860 head injury. Muybridge himself reported only that he woke to find a small wound on the top of his head and that since then he had suffered headaches. Friends and business colleagues reported far more. They said that since the accident Muybridge's formerly pleasant nature had changed dramatically with "eccentricities of speech, manner, and action" to one that was irritable and subject to emotional outbursts. Based on 26 years of acquaintance, his friend, Silas Selleck testified that:

> After his return from Europe he was very eccentric and so very unlike his way before going; the change in his appearance was such that I could scarcely recognize him after his return.
>
> —*Sacramento Union*, 5 February 1875

Business skills had also suffered. An associate reported that, while Muybridge was strictly honest, he would "make a bargain or contract at night and next morning go back on it *in toto* and make a new contract." He was also horrified by the risky behavior shown in a photograph of Muybridge perched on a steep cliff edge (Figure 1-7). The drop below his idly swinging legs plunged over 3,000 feet (Clegg B, 2007, p. 94).

The jury dismissed the insanity plea (to which Muybridge himself had fiercely objected) but acquitted him on grounds of "justifiable homicide" (the last such verdict in California). An insanity defense was nothing new, but this one was based on a 14-year-old head injury and the trial held in the same city where Phineas Gage had died, just four years after Dr. Harlow published the medical report of damage to Gage's skull, brain, and behavior.

Friends may have emphasized Muybridge's oddities in an attempt to save his life, but for the rest of that life, long *after* the trial, he was always described as extremely eccentric, with profound emotional swings. He was known for remote and risky projects and complete disinterest in personal appearance. When hired by the University of Pennsylvania to do photographic research, he was told he would have to dress better. He was apparently bewildered by the request, but an assistant mentioned seeing him wearing pants "so decrepit that it was not safe for him to go outside the studio" (Clegg B, 2007, pp.192, 201).

In spite of his injuries, Muybridge revolutionized photography—and art. Thanks to his single-minded obsession, his tens of thousands of photos, the very idea of moving pictures spun from light and motion, changed the world. His books, still in print, are wonderful resources for artists and to students of kinesiology and body mechanics.

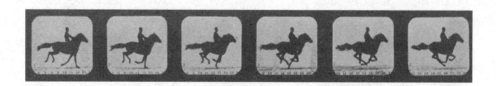

Howard Hughes
HEADACHES, POOR EXECUTIVE SKILLS, OBSESSIONS AND PHOBIAS, PAIN, PARANOIA, AND SENSITIVITY TO LIGHT

Howard Robard Hughes was an American industrialist with three youthful goals: to become the world's greatest golfer, greatest film producer, and greatest aviator. He also became a mystery: How did such a brilliant and enthusiastic young man end as a paranoid, reclusive madman?

Hughes loved movies, speed, and fast living. As a boy, he had a horse and a motorbike, both classic causes of head injury. As an adult he survived multiple car and plane crashes and a series of physical assaults by angry women, their husbands or lovers.

His mother died when he was 16, his father two years later. A millionaire at 18, Howard immediately quit school. Besides plenty of money, he had excellent mechanical skills, a superb memory, an eye for detail, and a fascination with Hollywood.

In 1925, at age 20, Hughes went to Hollywood. His first production was too terrible to release. The second earned a modest profit, the third won an Academy award for director Lewis Milestone.

In 1927, he began his best-remembered movie: *Hell's Angels*. Rather than keep experienced and capable directors, Hughes took over, shooting and re-shooting scenes. For the famous aerial scenes, he hired experienced WWI combat pilots, but ignored their warnings about a shot calling for a vertical dive, pulling up at an altitude of 1,000 feet. Hughes flew the scene himself but, as the pilots had predicted, he crashed. He was pulled unconscious from the wreck with extensive injuries, including a shattered cheekbone and chin.

Symptoms typical of TBI began to appear and would worsen with additional injuries.

- Impulsiveness and even more risky behavior,
- Poor self-awareness, poor grooming and self-care,
- Severe Obsessive-Compulsive Disorder (OCD), manifesting most famously as germ phobia and compulsions such as sorting and counting the peas on his plate,
- Extreme paranoia and controlling behavior; he kept an entire staff of spies,
- Extreme and indiscreet sexual behavior.
- Insomnia.
- Extreme sensitivity to light.

During the 1930s, Hughes founded Hughes Aircraft and set multiple aviation records. World War II brought millions in contracts (most famously for the huge Flying Boat, the "Spruce Goose"), but Hughes remained heavily involved in movie production. With these conflicting demands, Hughes became infamous for working non-stop for two to three days at a time.

Many believed Hughes' primary interest in Hollywood was women, as many as possible. Women of interest (and potential rivals) were followed and spied on. Sometimes the women, their husbands or lovers struck back.

- While out with Ava Gardner, Hughes' car was broadsided by his jealous 16-year-old fiance.
- On learning that Hughes had been out with his wife, budding fashion designer Oleg Cassini hit him with a 2x4.
- A 1940 car crash (while engaged to Ginger Rogers) threw him head-first through the windshield.

On learning that her supposed fiance had been out with someone else, Rogers stormed into his hospital room and hurled her emerald engagement ring at his bandaged body.

Ava Gardner was more forceful. Hughes had long pursued Gardner, who steadfastly rejected his proposals. Why?

Because you smell, Howard. Your collar is dirty and you stink. Like a goddamn canary died under your shirt and . . . you left it there (Hack R, 2001).

In 1943, when Ava objected to Hughes' continued spying, he flew into a violent rage and gave her a black eye. She, in turn, grabbed a heavy bronze bell (in other accounts, an ashtray) and smashed him so hard between temple and cheekbone that she knocked out two of his molar teeth and caused a gash that required 22 stitches to close (Hack R, 2001; Gardner A, 1992, p. 90).

In 1944, while he was landing a sea plane on a quiet lake under perfect conditions, the plane tipped, spun, and split apart. Hughes slammed into the ceiling instrument panel, gashing the top of his head (Barlett DL and Steele B, 1979; Gardner A, 1992). Soon after, the man with the superb memory began giving dozens of repetitions of the same orders he had given seconds before. He was said to be suffering from a" nervous breakdown," not an actual medical term or diagnosis, but a general term for an inability to function normally due to overwhelming stress. For Hughes, it was most likely a symptom of multiple concussions compounded by impossible levels of stress and severe chronic pain. And there would be more.

In 1946 Hughes crashed while testing his XF-11 reconnaissance plane. He was pulled from the wreckage with extensive third-degree burns, multiple fractures, and a punctured lung. For the rest of his life he would suffer migraines, intractable chronic pain and extreme sensitivity to light (photophobia), a common symptom of both migraine and TBI. Windows were blocked with plywood and heavy curtains. Hughes retreated into the dark.

In 1947, he locked himself inside a dark screening room for four months, naked and alone, living only on milk, chocolate, and pecans, watching movies over and over. Later, from other darkened rooms, Hughes ran his business affairs with a steady stream of memos scrawled on yellow legal pads. These included absurdly detailed instructions such as a 9-step essay on the correct procedures for opening a can of fruit. But even more injuries were to come. In 1951, a pummeling from an ex-football star over a woman re-broke his ribs and chin.

In 1976, at age 71, Howard Hughes died of kidney failure and neglect in his darkened luxury penthouse. His left shoulder was dislocated and his once athletic 6′4″ frame so wasted by malnutrition that he weighed just 93 pounds. The probable cause of his years of deterioration in health and behavior is most likely to have been multiple brain injuries compounded by extreme stress.

His most passionate dream was to be a leader in aeronautics and defense, but he could neither manage well nor allow others to manage for him. He hired excellent staff, but many left upon realizing they had no real authority. With $40 million in military contracts he delivered just one X-11. Hughes might eventually have learned critical skills, but a classic TBI symptom is *inability* to change behavior. In a rare confession (that sounds remarkably like bragging), Hughes said that trying to make *Hell's Angels* "by himself" had been a huge mistake, learning "by bitter experience that no one man can know everything."

> At twenty-six, Hughes had apparently learned the rule of all successful executives: leaders must delegate authority. Yet in the years ahead, he would routinely disregard the lesson, making it a custom to interfere with, second-guess, and deny authority to his managers. If, as he claimed, he "went to school" making *Hell's Angels*, he promptly forgot what he had learned.
>
> — Barlett DL & Steele B (1979, p. 69).

The near-fatal X-11 crash occurred because Hughes ignored all standard test protocols. Instead of using the Army Test Flight Base in the barren Mojave desert, he flew from his Culver City headquarters. With the plane overloaded with fuel and at 30 minutes beyond prescribed flight time, the propellers malfunctioned *due to a known oil leak*. He tried to land on the Los Angeles Country Club golf course but, unable to clear houses in Beverly Hills, he crashed and burned. This may have been due to over-confidence or to one of the worst symptoms of TBI: remembering what you *used* to be able to do but can no longer do— from good organization to good judgment calls.

Howard Hughes made many real contributions to aviation. His speed records were the last set by non-military designs, his record-breaking flight around the world set the stage for world-wide air travel. After TBI, his gift for meticulous planning and exquisite detail, the root of his greatest successes, became a tar pit of confusion, indecision, and failure.

After a series of brain injuries that no one could survive unchanged, a once fine mind descended into madness.

Elvis Presley
HEADACHES, BODY PAIN, DEPRESSION, INSOMNIA, IMPULSIVITY, OBSESSIONS, DRUG ADDICTIONS, PARANOIA, AND POOR JUDGMENT

Elvis Presley was born at the height of the Great Depression on January 8, 1935, in Tupelo, Mississippi. At 13, his family moved to Memphis, Tennessee, where he was exposed to country, gospel and African-American jazz, rhythm and blues which he melded into his own musical style. Presley grew up to be one of the greatest recording artists of all time, "The King of Rock and Roll."[1] He graduated from high school in 1953. In 1954, the $35 per week truck driver landed a recording contract with Sun Records; he celebrated by buying a motorcycle. Within a year, his contract was bought out by RCA and Presley was one of the most famous and highest paid performers in the world. His fees and sales were a string of financial firsts. By the end of 1956, Elvis Presley merchandise had brought in $22 million (roughly $400 million today) above record sales (Austen J, 2005). So much money and fame, too much too soon, is the long-time explanation for his descent into drugs and ill-health. But as for another young king, there was also a long series of head injuries.

Head trauma may have begun with his rough-and-tumble youth, growing up poor and male in Memphis, with bar fights, and football. But with growing fame, Presley also became a target. In 1956 he pulled into a gas station and was recognized by other customers who asked for autographs. Station owner Ed Hopper asked him to move on, but when Presley continued to sign, Hopper shoved, Presley punched. An employee coming to the aid of his boss hit Presley in the back of the head. All three were arrested for assault and battery.

Boys in general targeted Presley. As recalled by Bob Neal, an early manager,

> So many of them, through some sort of jealousy, would practically hate him. There were occasions in some towns in Texas when we'd have to be sure to have a police guard because somebody'd always try to take a crack at him. They'd get a gang and try to waylay him or something (Rogers D, 1982).

While sitting with band mates in the bar of Toledo's Commodore Perry Hotel, Presley was confronted by 19-year-old sheet-metal worker Louis Balint, who shouted, "My wife carries *your* picture but doesn't carry mine!" (Gilmore G, 1956). Balint slugged Presley in the face.

Was he injured by Balint's blow? We don't know, but at his concert the next day, Presley (who rarely touched alcohol[2]) was said to "stagger" onto the stage.

---

1. He had more hits and sold more records than any other recording artist to this day, including the Beatles.
2. Not only did alcohol turn him into a "mean drunk," but several family members, including his mother, died from alcoholism, a fate he hoped to avoid.

In 1958, before entering the Army, Presley rented a rink and threw a week-long skating party featuring "war games" on skates. Play was rough and painful. Presley was reported to have been tackled and knocked down; he was also reported to have handed out pain-killing Percodan (oxycodone/aspirin) to his teammates and took four himself (Tennant F, 2013).

In the Army, Presley was assigned to the 3rd Armored Division in Friedberg, Germany. There he is said to have used amphetamines extensively, to stay alert. There he was also exposed to karate which he studied intensely. Sergeant Presley was honorably discharged in 1960.

Back in the U.S., he returned to TV and movies. On beginning work on *Flaming Star*, he was afraid of horses (one ran away with him during filming), but he soon bought an entire stable of horses and a riding ranch, constantly riding and camping with friends[1]. He also earned his first black belt in karate[2] and in 1964, after begging to be allowed to do his own fight scenes for the movie *Roustabout*, he received a nasty blow requiring stitches, above his left eye.

In March 1967, filming began for *Clambake*. One night Presley tripped over a television cord in the dark, hitting the front of his head on the bathtub. He lay unconscious for some unknown period of time and in the morning he was too woozy to work.

The first assumption seems to have been drugs, but when his manager, Colonel Tom Parker, went to the bedroom to check on him, he emerged looking grim, then arranged for a physician, radiologist, and portable X-ray equipment. Presley was diagnosed with a "slight" concussion (Guralnick P, 1999, p. 257). The incident was widely reported, always dismissed as trivial or harmless. Yet filming was delayed for nearly two weeks and this "slight" injury marks the start of a downward spiral into increasingly odd behavior and poor health.

On the set, Presley played an album by French actor Charles Boyer over and over and over, giving copies to cast and crew (Guralnick P, 1999, p. 258). There were wild mood swings and depression. Back at home, he retreated to his room for days at a time and there were startling sessions when his language, normally marked by courtesy and deference, became uncharacteristically crude and foul. By November of 1967, Presley had lost interest in his beloved horses and the social interaction of riding. Ranch and horses were sold; only a few favorites returned to Graceland. In their place he became obsessed with government and police badges.

As an honorary deputy of Memphis, he used his badge to pull over cars on the street, just to chat with the drivers. A $7,000 donation to the Los Angeles Police Department won him a Commissioner's badge. In 1970, when the Bureau of Narcotics and Dangerous Drugs failed to respond to his requests for a badge, he flew to Washington and met with a bemused

---

1. http://www.cowboysindians.com/Cowboys-Indians/July-2012/All-The-Kings-Horses/
2. Awarded by Hank Slomanski. An account of Slomanski's demands and approach to training is available here: http://www.tracyskarate.com/Stories/was_elvis_really_a_black_belt.htm

President Nixon who gave it to him. (He got no response from the dour J. Edgar Hoover who was apparently not amused at the idea of making Presley an honorary FBI agent.)

By 1973, Presley was increasingly and obviously unwell. Twice that year he overdosed on barbiturates. The first incident sent him into a three day coma, the second one left him semi-comatose; both brought the risk of anoxia, inadequate blood supply to the brain. And yet 1973 was his busiest year ever, a grueling schedule of 168 concerts (Keogh PC, 2004, p. 238).

By 1974 (age 39), Presley was forgetting words and slurring lyrics so badly he was barely understandable. He was morbidly obese, with chronic high blood pressure, a damaged liver, and an enlarged colon (*megacolon*). His dark glasses were not mere costume; he now had glaucoma in both eyes. When not performing, he retreated to his room and books. His reclusive behavior and paranoid obsessions (including terror of germs and assassins), reminded a cousin of Howard Hughes who had died the year before (Guralnick, Peter, 1999, p. 489, 642). In 1976 Presley recorded *Hurt*. "If he felt the way he sounded," noted music historian Dave Hurt, "the wonder isn't that he had only a year left to live but that he managed to survive that long."

On August 16, 1977, the day he was scheduled to leave on yet another tour, Presley was found dead on the bathroom floor. His death at 42 caused widespread shock and disbelief. "Sightings of Elvis" have continued to this day. Some speculate that he simply wished to retire quietly, away from the crush of fans and crowds. Others claim conspiracy and assassination, but he died of a massive heart attack with drugs as a powerful contributing factor. Why Presley's health failed so precipitously in the 10 years after 1967, and why his drug use progressed as it did, was debated for years. Dr. Forest Tennant (because of his earlier investigation of Howard Hughes' death done for the U.S. government) was called as an expert witness in the malpractice suit against Presley's physician[1]. In a 2013 article Tennant wrote:

> Elvis' myriad medical problems and early death has mystified me ever since. Elvis Presley was quite well until approximately the last 10 years of his life. In the last 3 years [he] was so ill and disabled he required around-the-clock nursing care. After Dr. Nick's trial, I carefully stored all of my records knowing that someday science would pony-up enough information to permit an understanding of Elvis' medical and pain problems. . . . After piecing the evidence together, it is quite clear to me that Elvis' major disabling medical problems stemmed from multiple head injuries that led to an autoimmune inflammatory disorder with subsequent central pain. His terminal event was cardiac arrhythmia, underpinned by drug abuse, genetic defects, and hastened along by an atrocious diet.

That is, *many of Presley's problems began with concussion.*

---

1. Although widely blamed for his death, Presley's physician, Dr. George Nichopolous, prescribed only two of the 10 drugs found at autopsy. See Dr. Tennant's forensic article online at: www.practicalpainmanagement.com/elvis-presley-head-trauma-autoimmunity-pain-early-death.

Concussion 101

CONCUSSION IN CHILDREN AND ADULTS, IN SPORTS AND DAILY LIFE.
THE HOLLYWOOD HEAD INJURY AND WHY MOST OF WHAT WE THINK WE
KNOW ABOUT CONCUSSION IS WRONG.

F ew of us are clear on the meaning of *concussion*[1]. When concussions are trivialized as mere "dings," it is difficult to recognize and understand what they really are and how serious they can be. So here it is: *A concussion is a brain injury.*

Both terms often trigger denial. *Brain injury?* Surely not. Many people think that *real* brain injury victims look funny, talk funny, and they drool. In reality, they look like everyone else because they *are* everyone else. They are teachers and coaches, sales people and lawyers, truck drivers, computer programmers, doctors and athletes. They are military officers and soldiers who can no longer function. They are CEOs who are terrified because they can no longer read or make sense of a spreadsheet. They are mothers now unable to protect their children. They are the neighbors that you never see, the commuter afraid of driving, the "lazy" or clumsy kid who just isn't living up to his potential.

Adding to the problem are the different words used for the same injury. "Traumatic brain injury" (TBI) sounds even worse than "concussion," but they are often the same. Media reports on war and sports injuries have made TBI increasingly familiar, but every TBI has some element of concussion or *sub*concussion (a word now used by brain injury researchers for the hit that doesn't produce immediate symptoms — but will eventually).

A concussion is much like dropping a hammer onto the *motherboard* (the "brain") of your computer. But unlike damage to a computer brain, damage to a human brain can trigger a domino effect of progressive injury. Affected tissues release a flood of chemicals that kill brain cells and destroy their connections. The chemical cascade can involve anything from blood

---

1. From Middle English *concussioun*, a bruise, from Latin *concutere*, to strike together. In this book you will see TBI and concussion used interchangeably.

(toxic to brain tissue) to imbalances of electrolytes and hormones[1]. These may continue for hours or days, months or years developing into endocrine and autoimmune diseases. The resulting physical and behavioral changes can be temporary or last for a lifetime.

The human computer is a truly wonderful computer as it is self-healing. However, it does not heal in the ways that we often think it should. Healing isn't helped by getting back on the horse or bike, the ice, mat, mound, or field after a brain injury. Trying to "work through" dizziness, nausea, or pain does *not* work because damage to the computer is not repaired by hitting it again with more or better hammers. Pushing a brain to do more while injured is extremely dangerous — to the point of equipment dysfunction, or to the point of fatal error[2].

In the everyday world, we do not smash our laptops together or hurl our SmartPhones through windshields and then be surprised that they don't work well afterwards. In contrast, we are strangely willing to believe that inflicting the same abuse on a massively complex computer with the consistency of Jello will do no harm. Then, when harm has clearly been done, its symptoms are misunderstood, ignored, or treated with disdain and hilarity.

> "Too many hits to the head!" Hee-hee-hee!
> "Punch drunk!" Hee-hee-hee!
> "Did your mother drop you on your head as a baby?" Hee-hee-hee!

To those who have suffered concussions — or the loss of friends and relationships, skills and abilities— it's no joke. Even seemingly minor TBI can cause weeks of emotional upheavals, waves of sadness or impulsive anger. It may be difficult or impossible to organize, prioritize, sequence events, or multi-task. There may be extreme sensitivity to light and sound, and sleep problems despite crushing fatigue. There may be memory loss, sudden problems with reading, speaking or reasoning coherently, problems understanding what is being said, learning new things, or dealing with old familiar things like time, numbers, or money. Watching TV or sports may be physically and mentally painful. Being in public places can be hideously exhausting or painful because of the noise, the light, and the cognitive demands.

Problems with focus and eye coordination can damage reading ability; problems with memory and concentration can impair the ability to absorb and then store information in long-term memory. TBI can also trigger hormone disruptions resulting in low body temperature, weight gain, sexual problems and infertility. Loss of interest in former activities and friends are also common.

---

1. It may seem odd that blood is toxic to brain tissue, but this is roughly equivalent to the driver of a car being doused with antifreeze and gasoline when hoses break in an accident.
2. Only forensics-oriented shows suggest the possibility of real damage, but even there it is rarely shown and seldom with real accuracy.

Children

A concussion is an academic injury, in the sense that it affects the capacity for learning. There are rarely times in school when these concussion issues do not have some potential effect on a kid's grades and academic pursuits.

—Gerard Gioia, Ph.D.
Pediatric neuropsychologist
Children's National Medical Center, Washington DC

When children are injured, normal physical and sexual growth, mental abilities and social skills may fail to develop at all. Problems often begin in the delivery room, at birth, with oxygen deprivation or other trauma, then continue through childhood.

Toddlers are top heavy, like ungrounded bobble-heads. While learning to walk, they trip, they fall, they tumble down stairs. Older children have leapt out of windows and trees because they were trying to fly, or played "bullfighter" by running headfirst into walls (or boards, or other hockey or football players). They fall off bicycles, crash into trees and cars, or play contact sports long before bones and brains and bodies are up to the task. Snoring and sleep apnea deprive their brains of oxygen (anoxia), critical for development.

Some children are physically abused, but even emotional stress and abuse or seeing abuse of others, can damage the limbic (emotional) system and development of the organizational left brain (Teicher MH, 2002).

We expect children to heal quickly, but their brains are more delicate, and injury can be more damaging than in adults. Even seemingly minor head bumps before age five can harm normal brain development. After injury, a young child may be fussy, but unable to explain what's wrong. It may seem as though all is well, but that may be only because they do not go to the office the next day and apply high-level skills. Problems may go unnoticed until the child starts school and has difficulty learning to read, write, or concentrate. Even then they may go unrecognized for what they truly are.

One problem with concussion is understanding what a concussion really is. An article in *Pediatrics* magazine presented the problem very neatly.

My child doesn't have a brain injury, he only has a concussion.

The disturbing title comes from the startling discovery that many parents who had taken their children to the ER were *relieved* on being told that the injury was *merely a concussion*. The diagnosis was strongly associated with quick release from the hospital and return to school and activities (Dematteo CA and Others, 2010). There was poor recognition by parents *and physicians* that a *concussion is a brain injury*. Returning a child regular to regular school and activities, in the false belief that a concussion is trivial, leads to more problems.

A 2014 study found that children prematurely returned to the highest levels of "brain work" and activities took the longest to recover from their symptoms. They averaged 100 days to recover from symptoms compared to 20 to 50 days for those allowed to rest (Brown NJ and Others, 2014).

Damage that does not heal can continue — and worsen. A study of 87 children (ages 5-14) admitted to trauma centers with mild TBI were tested for neurocognitive problems and appearance of new psychiatric disorders. The rate of new disorders six months after injury was disturbingly high. Damage to tissue in the front of the brain significantly predicted new disorders and was associated with slower processing speed, lower intelligence and language skills (Max JE and Others, 2013). Later, these children showed *increased* rates of hyperactivity / inattention and conduct disorder, especially if the concussion occurred before age five.

When injuries occur during elementary school years, basic pathways should already have developed. Only *some* skills, not all, are likely to be impeded. This is great news for eventual recovery but it can also be a source of conflict and frustration. "How can you be so good at [X] but failing [Y]? You do only the things you like to do."

Injuries just before or during puberty can disrupt hormones critical to future growth and maturation. Meanwhile, the mental effort of school work while the brain is trying to heal can worsen concussion symptoms. This is a problem under the best of circumstances, but worse when the concussion remains unrecognized or unacknowledged; the harder the student tries, the more severe symptoms may become. He may earn a diagnosis of Attention Deficit (Hyperactive) Disorder, AD(H)D. She may be scolded for "day-dreaming." They may be punished for being impulsive or disruptive and drugged into a placid chemical calm, further damaging self-esteem, mind and body. Meanwhile, poor grades drive educational choices and opportunities, and often the rest of life.

Nancy was a good student age 15. In a hockey game, she was hit so hard in the face by a slapshot that the stick shattered; ER physicians had to remove wood splinters from her face and eye. It was an obvious and dramatic injury, but no one realized that it might be the reason that her grades began to fall. Years later, all of her siblings went straight to college. Nancy never made it and as an adult was limited to a series of menial jobs.

Adults

When childhood injuries continue into and through adulthood, they are typically attributed to "your age." The childhood incident is long forgotten or seen as too far in the remote past to matter.

Many adults, even with severe symptoms, deny ever having had a concussion at all. With careful questioning, they often recall amazingly traumatic injuries — including falls from second story windows and monkey bars, car crashes and multiple blackouts from playground or sports injuries — with shocked surprise that these *do* matter after all. Even though symptoms began soon after the event, these incidents were dismissed because they seem small or not intuitively connected.

There is a long tradition of evaluating the likelihood of brain injury based on loss of consciousness and the long-held (but false) notion that without loss of consciousness, no harm was done. Nevertheless, we are so resistant to the idea of brain injury that we often trivialize it even when unconsciousness *does* occur and even when there are obvious physical and cognitive post-injury symptoms. A spectacular example of this was the person who insisted that the auto injury couldn't have been serious because he couldn't have been unconscious for *very* long. He "knew" this because "When I woke up, the police and ambulance *were already there*."

Were those brain injuries? Do they count? They do[1].

Adults may be painfully aware of what they once could do but no longer can, but no idea why this is so. They may call the strange feelings "burnout." Others may call it "laziness" or "lack of motivation." Loss of interests and long hours spent sleeping may be called *depression* although they deny feeling sad: "I just feel *empty*," they say, and the visible symptoms may go unnoticed and misunderstood.

Bobbie, a Licensed Social Worker, was a busy and effective supervisor. After her car crash, she had no memory, got lost trying to walk two blocks in a familiar area, and reading became "crazy difficult," in part because of light sensitivity.

> I can't begin to tell you the shame, embarrassment, and frustration this caused me. People's lives were in my hands — but I had no sense of time, bills went unpaid, I couldn't fill out paperwork without major help.

Bobbie, whose business was helping, could no longer help herself — or others.

When skills and abilities suffer, households and children suffer, society suffers.

---

1. Far less obvious trauma can ruin lives, from seemingly harmless thrill rides and roller coasters to blood pressure too high (causing tears and lesions) or too low (starving the brain of nutrients).

Concussion and Crime

One year at Princeton University: $37,000.
One year at a New Jersey State prison: $44,000.

—Brian Resnick (2011)

We met no Jimmy Cagneys or Robert Mitchums among the inmates in the prisons we visited.
We found ourselves rather, in the company of a pathetic crew of intellectually limited,
dysfunctional, half-mad, occasionally explosive losers. Long before these men wound up on
death row, their similarly limited, primitive, impulsive parents had raised them in the only
fashion they knew . . . . had set the stage on which our condemned subjects now found
themselves playing out the final act. It was a drama generations in the making.

—Dorothy Otnow Lewis, Ph.D., *Guilty By Reason of Insanity*

. . . visiting the iniquity of the fathers upon the children, and upon the children's children, unto
the third and to the fourth generation.

—Exodus 34:6-7

The behaviors and symptoms of Post-Concussion Syndrome (PCS) are strongly associated with violent behaviors and substance abuse, entry into juvenile detention and later the adult prison system. In England, a study of 197 youth offenders (boys aged 11 to 19), found that they were three times as likely to have had a TBI than their non-offending counterparts. About 50 percent of them reported a brain injury; those with multiple brain injuries were more likely to have committed more violent crimes (Williams WH and Others, 2010). Among 61 male juvenile offenders, over 70 percent reported at least one head injury; over 40 percent reported having had a head injury with loss of consciousness. Their post-concussion symptoms reliably increased with the frequency and severity of TBI (Davies RC and Others, 2012).

One notorious example of TBI and violence is that of Joseph C. Palczynski. After years of violent and abusive behavior towards others (primarily girlfriends) he killed four people and took a family hostage. What is rarely mentioned is that he was once a perfectly normal child, remembered by his father (who left when he was 8) as charming and generous.

In September 1983, 14-year-old "Joby" was standing on the bus[1] when it slammed into another in the school parking lot. He was hurled into a window then thrown to the floor. Six days later, he collapsed onto the kitchen floor, screaming, biting and scratching. Diagnosis: a "post-traumatic psychotic episode" from the earlier TBI (Mishra R and Kunkle F, 2000).

---

1. Joby's absent father was unaware of the bus accident until told about it by a reporter, but had begun to notice difficulties, including sudden anger, a year later when Joby was 15.

Joby graduated high school in 1987, but that summer he assaulted a girl, punching her and threatening her with a razor blade. Over the next 12 years, from that summer until the day he died in a hail of bullets, he would spend all but 10 months in prison, mental institutions or on probation.

When psychiatrist Dorothy Lewis and neurologist Jonathan H. Pincus did psychological and neurological evaluations of Death Row murderers, they made a stunning discovery. Every inmate they examined had a three-part history of horrific child abuse, paranoia, and *brain injury* (Lewis DO, 1998; Pincus J, 2002). It didn't matter that abuse was denied by inmates and families. Both had reason to deny that it had ever happened. Nevertheless, abuse was revealed in hospital and school records and in the testimony of more distant relatives with less to hide. Or, abuse might not be seen as abuse. Many little boys are treated with special physical harshness with the idea that they must be "toughened up." In her 1998 book, *Guilty By Reason of Insanity,* Dr. Lewis tells of a mother who apologized for not having punished her son *enough*, and yet there was a switch in every room, every hallway of the house.

This pattern is sadly common in domestic violence. The spouse or child who "won't pay attention" or "just won't learn" gets hit again and again. Oddly enough, adding brain injury to the abuse doesn't toughen anyone up – it simply makes them less functional, more impulsive, with poorer reality testing skills. It also trains the notion that this is the way to treat others, planting the seeds of future violence.

Not everyone who is concussed as a child becomes a violent offender. Most children with head injuries simply grow up unable to understand why they can't understand, why they are so slow to make words, why getting thoughts out feels like wading through fog and molasses.

Charlotte was knocked unconscious after a fall from the monkey bars in elementary school. Until then, school had been easy and fun, and she had been an excellent student. After that incident, school became increasingly difficult. "The only explanation I could think of," she recalls, "was that I was actually very stupid." But then, after comprehensive testing in high school, Students were given their IQ scores. On seeing hers, said Charlotte,

> I had a physical reaction, a visceral shock, because the number was so high. All day I asked myself how that could possibly be correct when, despite all my efforts, I was such a poor student? How could I be so dumb (based on my grades) if (based on my test scores) I was actually so *smart*?

Few of us understand what is actually involved in concussion, how damaging it can be, or why or how it really happens. For many years, the best known model for concussions has come from Hollywood and that model is *wrong*.

The Hollywood Head Injury

> I never said it was always *wrong* to enter fairyland.
> I only said it was always *dangerous*.
> — G. K. Chesterton, *The Sins of Prince Saradine* (1911)

We often confuse fantasy with reality. For decades, the estates of composers Rodgers and Hammerstein have had to defend copyright of *Edelweiss*, their original composition, against those who innocently believe it to be a traditional Austrian folksong because it was presented as such in *The Sound of Music*. Visitors to the (real) bridges featured in the novel *The Bridges of Madison County* have burst into tears on realizing for the first time that star-crossed lovers Francesca and Kinkaid were *fictional*. Fans still search for the haunts of the *Blair Witch* (completely made up) and Dan Brown's *Da Vinci Code* (ditto), and there has never been a red phone in the White House (that came from *Dr. Strangelove* and *Fail Safe*[1]).

Most film fantasies do no harm. Others do. Besides super-heroes who are never injured, Hollywood presents *ordinary* humans who are also never injured, despite severe trauma.

In *The Wedding Planner*, a hyper-organized young woman is "saved" from a runaway dumpster by a young doctor who shoves her out of the way with a flying tackle, smashing the back of her head to the pavement. When she awakens in his hospital, she is told that her X-rays and MRI "are clear" and therefore she does not have a concussion (despite having remained unconscious throughout all these tests). In the Real World, she would probably find that she could no longer organize, read or sleep well, nor continue to work as a planner. She would find that she had suffered a very real and damaging brain injury.

A *more accurate* film portrayal is Frankenstein's monster. After death and brain surgery, he was jolted with thousands of volts of electricity. He probably awoke with a massive migraine in addition to his obvious symptoms of poor impulse control, violent outbursts, balance and gait problems. The monster may be fictional, but his depiction is more true-to-life than that of a concussed wedding planner, unconscious for hours, but *with no post-injury symptoms at all*.

The *most accurate* example appears in Frank Scott's film, *The Lookout*. "Chris Pratt, high-school hockey star and golden boy, caused a prom-night car crash that killed two friends but left him alive with "moderate" TBI. He is impulsive, prone to verbal outbursts, and his severe inability to sequence causes overwhelming difficulties with simple daily routines. He has lost the basic skills that healthy brains handle on autopilot.

---

1. National Geographic had to hire extra operators to deal with requests for the fictional issue of the magazine featuring photos by the fictional Kinkaid. Burkittsville, MD, where some of the *Blair Witch* footage was shot, had to redesign the town sign because the original was repeatedly stolen.

Chris looks fine (his scars are visible only in a shower scene), but his symptoms inspire disdain and impatience. They also inspire attention from a group of strangers who appear to appreciate him. In truth, what they *really* appreciate is only his job as night janitor at the bank they plan to rob.

All the gang members have problems suggesting TBI injuries of their own. The silent and flatly expressionless "Bone" never removes his dark glasses, even at night. "Luvlee" is good-hearted but dim. Then there is the notion of bank robbery as a viable career; behind their swagger, these characters give the impression that there is simply nothing else they *can* do.

Writer / director Frank Scott based Chris on a friend with TBI, and leading man Joseph Gordon-Levitt observed brain injury support meetings for nearly a year. The resulting movie is a tiny but brilliant drop of reality in an ocean of misinformation.

Besides misrepresenting injures, Hollywood also *inspires* injuries. In the 1980s, a restaurant owner (who was also a martial arts instructor) reported that fights between intoxicated patrons *always* involved a John Wayne right hook to the jaw. Having seen that in the movies they thought it was how to fight. As a rule, little serious damage occurred aside from broken hands (jaws are harder than finger bones). Far worse is the current movie fight fad: head butts. Even in helmets, these are a really bad idea[1], *so* bad (for the butt-*er*, not just the butt-*ee*) that they are forbidden in all martial arts competitions, including the supposedly no-holds-barred Ultimate Fighting Championship.

By extension to fights, falls, and car crashes during filming, Hollywood *causes* injuries. Victims include stunt actors and camera operators, but also stars who perform dangerous stunts out of pride or from a director's demand for continuity and fewer cuts (McCann M, 1988). Behind-the-scenes footage showing actors diving off buildings and jerked to a sudden stop by their safety harnesses may explain much odd behavior by A-listers and others.

It may be surprising, but in the Real World, brain injuries have real consequences. They are probably more common now than they have ever been in the history of the world. We have bigger bodies, faster cars and sports, and bigger explosions in war zones. While these offer greater opportunities for damage, the symptoms remain the same.

You may recognize some of the same signs and symptoms suffered by Henry, Mary, Howard and others. Over the last few years, we have begun to recognize them in soldiers and sports figures, who in turn have helped many of us recognize the problem — and therefore the potential for treatment and healing — in ourselves.

---

1. In the 2012 *Avengers* movie, Thor head-butts Iron Man. Of course, Thor is a god, and Iron Man is protected by iron. Natasha, a small delicately boned female, head-butts her large, thick-boned male interrogator, then strolls away unharmed. *All* fantasy.

Sports Injuries

We define chronic traumatic encephalopathy (CTE) as a progressive neurodegenerative syndrome caused by single, episodic, or repetitive blunt force impacts to the head and transfer of acceleration-deceleration forces to the brain.

—Omalu B, Bailes J and Others (2011)

It has long been known that repetitive brain trauma causes problems. Back in 1928, the neurological deterioration seen in "punch drunk" boxers was dubbed *dementia pugilistica*, the "madness of fighters." Today it is called Chronic Traumatic Encephalopathy (CTE). It features degeneration of brain tissue and accumulation of an abnormal protein designated as *tau*. On thin slices of brain tissue, the tau proteins look like coffee stains (Figure 2-1).

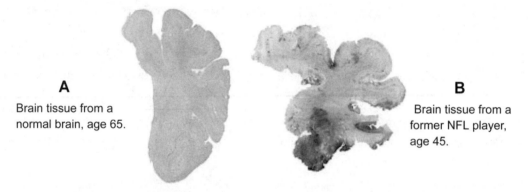

A
Brain tissue from a normal brain, age 65.

B
Brain tissue from a former NFL player, age 45.

Photo by Ann C McKee, MD, VA Boston/Boston University School of Medicine.

FIGURE 2-1. Tau Staining in CTE: John Grimsley

Symptoms may appear quickly or over many years. One of the first is memory problems. Victims often fear Alzheimer's. The two diseases are similar — but different. Alzheimer's starts in the hippocampus, the part of the brain responsible for processing new memories. Autopsy shows starchy bodies (beta amyloid) but not tau staining, and brains may shrivel. CTE features tau staining (Figure 2-1B) with no (or much less) beta amyloid. Autoimmune bodies also appear (See Color Section), yet on the surface, the brain may look perfectly normal.

Because CTE diagnosis has required actual slices of brain tissue, currently the condition has been verified only on autopsy, often after years of symptoms and behavior confusing and terrifying to both victim and family. In the living, CTE is suspected from signs and symptoms including headaches, vertigo, memory problems, erratic behavior, aggression and an explosive temper. Muscular speed, reflexes, and coordination fall; speech and gait abnormalities appear (McKee A and Others, 2009). These may progress to tremors and symptoms of Parkinson's Disease, as famously suffered by boxer Muhammad Ali.

Boxing

> I never had no frontal lobe. I don't even know what it is.
> That was just my lawyers trying to keep me out of jail.
>
> — Former heavyweight boxing champion Riddick Bowe[1]

The sport best known for traumatic brain injury is boxing. Its goal is a knockout, loss of consciousness, the one symptom universally considered to indicate a serious brain injury — unless there is a win and/or money at stake.

Boxing was originally done bare-knuckled. Boxing gloves ("muffles") were introduced in the mid-1700's to protect hands and faces of aristocratic aficionados[2]. Old-style bare-knuckle matches were limited by damage to hands; throughout the 19th century bare-knuckle boxers might fight for decades, into their fifties and beyond. Modern matches appear "cleaner" because most damage is *internal*. Today, a pro boxer who lasts for more than 100 fights is rare, and brain damage is the rule rather than the exception.

"Punch drunk" is the old term for chronic symptoms of head injury, including memory loss and problems with sequencing so terribly common in boxers. An example appears in the first *Rocky* movie, in which the apparently has-been, mumbling boxer tries desperately to remember the sequence of numbers he has used for years to open his gym locker.

In real life, after a brutal beating by Andrew Golota, Riddick Bowe's speech was so badly slurred that he was barely understandable. Besides impaired speech, neurologist Margaret Goodman[3] observed impaired balance, reflexes and ability to take and throw a punch, "symptoms of classic chronic brain injury," said Goodman. "It doesn't go away completely with rest" (Dahlberg T, 2004).

For Bowe, there would be no glorious comeback. His attempt to reconcile with his ex-wife (by kidnapping her at knife point) landed him in prison for 17 months. His lawyer, the late Johnny Cochrane, based his defense on Bowe's head injuries, specifically frontal lobe damage.

CTE has been verified in the brains of athletes from all fields of combat — football, hockey, soccer, wrestling, and soldiers with blast injuries — yet as a society, we still seem surprised that this condition fails to limit itself to boxers.

---

1. Quoted in Dahlberg T (2004).
2. An innovation explained by Henry Fielding in his 1749 novel *Tom Jones*.
3. Chief ringside physician for the Nevada Athletic Commission.

Football

In 2002, former Pittsburgh Steeler "Iron" Mike Webster died at age 50. Cause of death appeared to be heart attack, but it followed years of physical and cognitive decline, severe depression, dementia, drug and alcohol use. Severe insomnia drove him to drink multiple bottles of "night-time" cold formula. Eventually he resorted to shocking himself with a taser to win a few hours of unconsciousness (Garber G, 2005).

During autopsy, Dr. Bennet Omalu examined Webster's brain[1]. On the surface, it looked perfectly normal, but what he found that What he found would change forever how we see concussions. In Webster's brain and in the brains taken from the next eight NFL players he tested, Omalu saw the same thing: damage previously seen only in punch drunk boxers and in the elderly with dementia[2]. His findings were pointedly ignored by the NFL until the death of another Pittsburgh Steeler.

Justin Strzelczyk was an offensive linebacker from 1990-1998. After retirement, divorce and drugs, he complained of depression and of hearing voices from "the evil ones." On the morning of Sept. 30, 2004, he snapped. During a high-speed police chase, Strzelczyk crashed into the fuel tank of a tractor-trailer. He was killed instantly in the explosion. His behavior was attributed to bipolar disorder, but autopsy showed a brain severely damaged by CTE.

Omalu's autopsy data (published in 2005 and 2006) linked the symptoms and deaths of four star NFL players — Webster and Strzelczyk, Terry Long and Andre Waters. All four had shown the same ominous pattern: repetitive concussions and extensive brain damage similar to that seen in boxers, with clinical depression, bizarre behaviors, and early death.

Suddenly the evidence was impossible to ignore. This horrific fiery death jump-started a very public discussion of concussion in sports. Dr. Robert Stern[3] estimates that linemen hit their heads about 1,000 times a season. Not all hits result in concussions, but repetitive trauma from lesser injuries ("subconcussions") is also associated with CTE. Clearly, professional players were taking terrible risks for their paychecks.

With at least a theoretical interest in concussion, in 1994 the NFL formed a Committee on *Mild* Traumatic Brain Injury. In 2007, the NFL held a Summit Meeting on concussion but Dr. Omalu was pointedly *not* invited. On realizing this, Dr. Julian Bailes presented Omalu's data in his place, but it was dismissed by Committee co-chair, Dr. Ira Casson, as "unacceptable and unscientific." Casson insisted that CTE had been "scientifically, validly documented" *only* in

---

1. Forensic neuropathologist and assistant medical examiner for the city of Pittsburgh.
2. Age is not necessarily an issue. College lineman Owen Thomas (age 21), and high-school full-back and linebacker Austin Trenum (17) committed suicide. High-school football star Nathan Stiles (17) died of second-impact syndrome. On autopsy, all three were found to have CTE.
3. Co-Director of the Center for the Study of Traumatic Encephalopathy.

boxers and steeplechase riders (Milhoces G, 2007), never in any other athletes. Casson (an NFL employee) ignored not only Dr. Omalu's extensive scientific credentials, but also the fact that his papers *did* document CTE in former NFL players.

Players who died before awareness of CTE showed troubling symptoms years earlier.

- TERRY LONG. NFL 8 seasons. Over the years he became increasingly irrational, impulsive, paranoid and suicidal. He survived suicide attempts involving sleeping pills and rat poison but died, at 45, from drinking anti-freeze.

- CURTIS WHITLEY. NFL 6 seasons, bouncing among 6 teams, thanks to his alcohol and drug use. In 2008, he was found dead of a drug overdose on the bathroom floor of his trailer home. He was 39.

- FORREST BLUE. NFL 11 seasons. He died at 65, but symptoms of paranoia and dementia began to appear in his 40s. Blue spent his last two years in an assisted living facility where, as Mary Lincoln had done over a century before, he heard voices and complained of "people who lived in the walls" (Branch E, 2011).

In 2012, within the space of two weeks, two retired NFL players committed suicide. One was Ray Easterling who began showing signs of dementia 20 years before his death at age 62. Like so many other players, he suffered from depression and insomnia. His was the first NFL concussion lawsuit filed in federal court.

The second suicide was former linebacker Junior Seau (43). In 2010, Seau was arrested on a complaint of domestic violence. Later that day he drove his SUV off a 100-foot cliff. Some suspected a suicide attempt; Seau said he had simply fallen asleep. Injuries were described as minor, and he wept with relief at being alive[1]. Over a 20-year NFL career (and a 100-foot fall), Seau never reported a concussion, but was known to have suffered severe insomnia for at least seven years. Friends and family reported his use of the sleep aid Ambien®, which can produce suicidal behaviors in depressed patients; it should never be mixed with alcohol, but Seau continued to drink. In 2012, as Dave Duerson had done a year before, Seau shot himself in the chest. CTE was verified in January 2013.

Meanwhile, Ann McKee and colleagues continue to collect the brains of deceased former NFL players. As of March 2014, 74 brains have been obtained. Of these, 55 have been analyzed and 54 found to have CTE[2].

---

1. Bishop G and Davis R (2012); Moore DL and Brady E (2012). It seems likely that a 100-foot fall produced injuries other than the "minor" superficial ones reported.
2. Personal communication, March 10, 2014, Anne McKee, Boston University.

Hockey

> Four deceased players – Reggie Fleming, Bob Probert, Rick Martin, Derek Boogaard. Four dissected brains. Four cases of degenerative brain disease, according to Boston University researchers. They have sounded the alarm about the potential consequences of concussions and repetitive brain trauma in the NHL, while sparking a debate about what we know, what we don't know and what we need to do.
>
> —Nicholas J. Cotsonika (2012)

What matters in brain injury isn't the uniform, it's the brain and it's the injury. Too often, hockey is boxing and armed assault on ice. Skates allow high speeds, and collisions produce falls on ice that is as hard as concrete.

2011 saw the deaths of three hockey players within a space of four months. Rick Rypien (age 27, with 6 NHL seasons) and Wade Belak (age 35, with 17 AHL/NHL seasons) died as suicides, both after years of depression. In 2011, Derek Boogaard (age 28,with 9 seasons ECHL/AHL/NHL) died from an apparently accidental but lethal combination of pain-killing alcohol and oxycodone. All three were "enforcers," players whose specialty is fighting and are particularly likely to suffer concussions[1].

Within four months of Boogaard's death, two more players died. Bob Probert (age 45, 18 seasons AHL / NHL) another enforcer, had extensive legal problems with alcohol, drugs, and assaults. Rick Martin (age 59, 12 seasons NHL). He was not an enforcer, but played without a helmet until a 1978 game when his head hit the ice hard enough to cause seizures.

Both men died of apparent heart attack.On autopsy, both were found to have had CTE.

Wrestling

Professional wrestling is an oddity, more performance art than contest. "Winners" and "losers" are scripted, as are their running soap-opera story lines of heroes and villains, victory and revenge. It is drama and illusion; it is acting as a team sport, where no one is really supposed to get hurt. The most seemingly brutal throws are carefully stage-managed by the apparent opponents to protect their fellow performers. This cartoon fantasy world of spandex and guys in tights has provided some of the most spectacular examples of TBI. Amazingly, it has also provided some of the best first steps towards its recognition and prevention.

Chris Nowinski played defensive tackle for Harvard University and was a member of the 1997 Ivy League Championship football team. In 2000, he graduated *cum laude* with a degree in sociology but went to World Wrestling Entertainment (WWE). His wrestling career ended

---

1. To improve his "hockey" skills, Derek Boogaard was sent to boxing lessons. His story is detailed in a series of feature articles in *The New York Times*. See Branch J (2011).

in 2003 with a kick in the head, "mild TBI," and severe Post-Concussion Syndrome (PCS), a collection of frightening symptoms. Trying to get help, or even information about his mysterious symptoms, Nowinski saw doctor after doctor; his eighth was neurologist Robert Cantu. In 2006, Nowinski published a book, *Head Games*, on his career-ending injury and subsequent research into TBI. He was also instrumental in obtaining family permission to evaluate brains of other athletes[1].

In June 2007, Nowinski's fellow WWE wrestler, Chris Benoit, murdered his wife and their young son, then killed himself. The double-murder / suicide was horrifying but also baffling to those who knew Benoit off-stage as a devoted husband and father. Toxicology tests found therapeutic levels of painkillers, but failed to support suspicions of "'roid rage" from anabolic steroids. Somehow this made it worse. If it wasn't the madness of drugs and steroids, then it was cool-headed purposeful death and destruction.

Benoit had two signature moves: *delivering* flying head butts (by launching himself from the ropes) and *receiving* shots to the back of his head with steel folding chairs. Nowinski and Benoit had discussed concussions over the course of their careers. How many concussions had Benoit had? "More than he could count," Nowinski recalled later.

But what if it wasn't *him*? What if it was his damaged brain?

Nowinski persuaded Benoit's grief-stricken father to contact neurologist Julian E. Bailes[2] of the Brain Injury Research Institute. Tests quickly revealed a brain so severely damaged that it resembled an 85-year-old Alzheimer's patient *and* the brains of the dead NFL players.

---

1. His book also presents a vivid contrast between the NFL and the WWF in their treatment of TBI. For advice on brain injury, the NFL long relied on *rheumatologist* Elliot Pellman, infamous (as "Doctor Yes") for sending concussed players back into the same game. The WWF attempted to keep injured performers off the mat.
2. Bailes is the former team physician of the Pittsburgh Steelers. For details on athletes with CTE, see www.SportsLegacy.org.

In Daily Life

[In 1926] Automobiles and their often-drunken drivers remained the city's greatest killers, taking 1,272 lives in a year. There had also been 984 suicides, 356 murders (mostly shootings), and 585 alcohol-related deaths. 87 people had died in elevator accidents . . . 47 falls into open shafts, 36 crushed by the doors, three killed when cables broke and the machines fell. Then six people had been killed playing baseball, six people had died in sleighing accidents, football had killed one, three had died in fistfights, and eight people had lost their lives in diving accidents.

—Deborah Blum, *The Poisoner's Handbook* (2011)
on New York City deaths in 1926

It was a stupid, fluke accident: I was standing up, and I slammed my head straight into a cabinet door I didn't realize was still open. I was dizzy, saw stars, and felt sick to my stomach. When my husband asked me who the president was, I drew a blank.

—Jane McGonigal (2009)

Some of the worst injuries happen in the course of daily life but we worry about all the wrong things. The biggest is motor vehicle accidents, some 200 a year involving collisions with deer. We panic when the elevator lurches, but yearly deaths from elevator accidents are now around 6 and deaths from shark bites about 1-2, a tiny fraction compared to deaths from falls (6,000)[1]. We tumble from ladders, trip over curbs and cords, slip on ice and in bathtubs.

In April 2003, Dr. Robert Atkins, 72, creator of the "Atkins Diet," slipped on icy pavement outside his office building. Rather than dying of heart disease, as detractors had long hoped, he died of his head injury; officially "blunt force trauma followed by hematoma" (New York City DHMH, 2003).

But the numbers of deaths pale in comparison to the vastly larger numbers of survivors. Some endure a few days or weeks of mild discomfort. Others face months or long difficult years of pain and dysfunction. In 1967, Elvis Presley tripped and hit his head on the bathtub. Publicly, the injury was dismissed as "slight," but it delayed rehearsals for almost two weeks and may have been a critical turning point in his life and health.

In the U.K., thousands of injuries severe enough to require hospital admission are caused by tea cosies, vegetables, and sofas; false teeth were responsible for 933, toilet-roll holders for 329. Over 10,000 were hospitalized by socks. Due to patient confidentiality, details cannot be revealed. It is, therefore, impossible to know precisely how 750 people were injured by household sponges, but chances are good that it had to do with falls[2].

Sometimes something simply falls out of the sky.

---

1. Strangely, we have "Shark Week" but no "White Tail Deer Week," and when falls and crashes with obvious head and neck injuries are shown on "funny video" programs, viewers laugh.
2. UK Department of Trade and Industry (1999 and 2001 data), reported in Chrisafis A (2001).

- FOUR-YEAR-OLD SALLY WAS HIT IN THE HEAD BY A BASEBALL BATTED OUT OF THE PARK. For the rest of her life she had hearing problems, no sense of direction and was unable to recognize faces. This extremely intelligent woman assumed she was stupid.

- JENNA WAS FLIPPED UPSIDE DOWN AND DROPPED ON HER HEAD AT A FRATERNITY PARTY. For years after this "pile-driver" injury, she was unable to stay awake for more than a few hours at a time. She finished her coursework and graduated from college partly because her professors enjoyed throwing erasers at her in class to keep her awake.

- NICK, AN HONOR STUDENT AT A MAJOR UNIVERSITY, FELL 50 FEET FROM A WINDOW. He suffered a fractured skull, broken ribs, a collapsed lung, kidney failure, and lay in a coma for 27 days, so near death that he was given last rites. He survived, but after 2-1/2 years of rehab programs, he still had no memory of anything before the fall. His family taught him about his history from old photos but he could only remember part of it. He could recall only the first few words of a sentence. Speech and social skills were poor. Spatial and navigation skills lost.

- GREGORY WAS HIT IN THE HEAD BY A RANDOMLY THROWN ROCK. The result was 14 years of blinding migraine headaches. Literally. Attacks caused sudden loss of vision.

Military injuries are often add-ons to previous hurts from sports and daily life. Couch potatoes rarely volunteer for military service where fitness is required. Service is most attractive to people who are already fit and active, who run and wrestle, who have played football or other sports. Stories of military personnel in Chapter 8 reveal histories of all the usual childhood falls bangs and scrapes, the memorable goose-eggs, sports injuries and often loss of consciousness.

The same is true of professional ball players. Professional careers do not begin fully formed. They begin in high school or even earlier. The Pop Warner football program begins with children as young as five. See their website at: http://www.popwarner.com/.

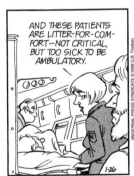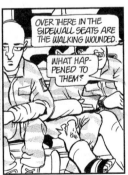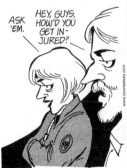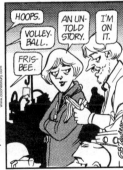

FIGURE 2-2. The Walking Wounded

Far worse injuries occur on the battlefield. In 2008, researchers from the Walter Reed Army Institute of Research found a strong link between TBI and Post-Traumatic Stress Disorder (PTSD). PTSD was far higher in TBI patients who had lost consciousness compared to those with injuries believed to involve only the body, not the head. Exactly how TBI contributes is unknown, but PTSD always involves danger, combined with damage to the hypothalamic-pituitary-adrenal (HPA) axis (Hoge CW and Others, 2004).

Patients with PTSD show brain abnormalities in areas (such as the amygdala) associated with extreme vigilance. Hypervigilance is key to staying alive in deadly situations, but when the actual threat is gone, that once-protective mechanism doesn't necessarily turn off. In combat zones, genetics, stress (both physical and emotional) and TBI combine with deadly consequences.

Policy changes have made potential for injury far worse. During the Vietnam war, draftees did one tour. Subsequent tours were volunteer only, or carried out by career soldiers. One of the problems of trying to run today's army with volunteers is the low number of volunteers. Now troops are sent on repeated tours — even when unfit for duty. From 1998 to 2000, David served with ground forces in Bosnia then Kosovo and suffered multiple TBIs and PTSD so severe that his medical record clearly stated that he should never be deployed again (Nelson DV and Esty ML, 2012). Nevertheless, in 2002, he was sent to Afghanistan then on to Iraq for two more tours. He returned violent and suicidal.

Another example is Army Staff Sgt. Robert Bales, charged with having shot and killed 17 Afghan civilians — mostly children — while they slept in their homes. Problems may have started with high school football. In 2001, Bales joined the army and was trained as a sniper. In 2002, he was charged with misdemeanor assault after a drunken fight with two casino security guards. There were further arrests for DUI, and a fight at a bowling alley where police described Bales as "extremely intoxicated."

In combat, in 2010, his vehicle was hit and rolled by an IED.

In March 2012, during his *fourth* tour of combat duty and after a night of drinking, Bales snapped. "*Suddenly,*" they said. Bales remembers little or nothing of the massacre, but reports severe nightmares, night sweats, flashbacks, and persistent headaches. In August 2013, he was sentenced to life in prison.

There are far better ways to treat our people, military and civilian, to prevent further pain and tragedy.

CHAPTER 3 # Symptoms of Concussion

POST-CONCUSSION SYMPTOMS OF MIND AND BODY, THE CONTAGION OF
CONCUSSION, AND WHEN "MILD" MEANS SOMETHING VERY DIFFERENT
FROM WHAT WE THINK IT MEANS.

C oncussion symptoms are divided into *primary* and *secondary*. In the aftermath of
TBI, there are also *acute* symptoms, the emotions and behaviors that appear within
the first 48 hours of injury. These include:

- UNCONSCIOUSNESS. May be momentary or lingering. Victims should be watched through the night and awakened regularly to ensure that they *can* be awakened.

- HEADACHE AND NAUSEA. One of the most common side effects, but aspirin and ibuprofen must be avoided as these increase clotting time and could increase bleeding in the brain.

- FATIGUE. Victims often become very sleepy.

- ACUTE MEMORY PROBLEMS. These are so common that they are used as a *test* for TBI. The inability to remember zip codes or long-held phone numbers is different from long-term problems of being unable to remember how to get to the office or how to get home.

- EMOTIONAL LABILITY. "Roller coaster" emotions, which may range from hilarity to panic or fear, sadness or anger in the blink of an eye.

- REPEATED DEMANDS OR ACTIONS (PERSEVERATION). Asking the same question over and over, forgetting that they have asked (and been answered) already.

- OBSESSIVE TALKING. Often appears as non-stop chattering, especially on a particular topic.

In very mild TBI, these symptoms may fade away within days or weeks. With more severe injuries, symptoms may persist or worsen.

Table 3-1 on page 38 lists primary symptoms that *may* occur. Not all will be present in any one individual. Given time, initial symptoms may progress into even more debilitating secondary conditions.

Table 3-1. Primary Symptoms of Concussion / TBI
Cognitive (Page 39)
Memory problems, especially short-term
Perserveration (repeated requests or demands)
Slowed thoughts, difficulty finding words
Decreased focus / concentration
Problems with organization, sequencing, and decision-making
Spatial disorientation, loss of sense of direction
Loss of old, familiar skills
Loss of ability to remember dreams
Physical and Sensory (Page 45)
Headache, nausea, and body pain
Visual problems: light sensitivity, gritty eyes, difficulty reading
Severe fatigue and apathy
Physical weakness
Gastro-intestinal problems, especially constipation
Sensory dysfunction and overload by light, sound, motion
Autonomic dysfunction including abnormal cold or sweating
Hallucinations: auditory, visual, olfactory, or tactile.
Changes in food preferences
Slowed reaction time and poor balance
Altered speech
Sleep disruptions from insomnia to inability to stay awake
Movement disorders and muscle spasms
Seizures, from "blanking out" to grand mal
[On blowing nose] Tear ducts that squirt fluid
Emotional (Page 53)
Loss of a complex (or adult) sense of humor
Emotional lability / "roller-coaster" emotions
Impulsiveness and risky behavior
Anger, explosiveness, rage, despair
Flat affect
Loss of social skills
Obsessive talking or writing
Poor hygiene and grooming
Depression, apathy, and detachment
Anxiety and panic attacks
Paranoia

Primary Symptoms

If I can't think, who am I?

—Jane McGonigal (2009)

Cognitive

Cognitive problems can be terrifying. People often fail to report them for fear of being thought crazy, or that they are developing Alzheimer's disease and dementia.

MEMORY PROBLEMS

Some form of memory loss is a common symptom. Profound and long-term amnesia is rare. But short-term memory loss is so common that it is used as a test for TBI on the field of injury and in the ER. With continuing impairment, it may be impossible to remember a telephone number long enough to dial it, to retain memory of *words* long enough to read to the end of a sentence, or to drive complex routes.

Ben recovered from a TBI, apparently well enough to drive, but for 12 years, he was halted in his tracks by a four-way stop sign. He would stop and look to the left, but when he looked to the right he could not remember if there was a car on the left. In the end, after several minutes of this, he could only enter the intersection hoping that all was clear, or that he would be spotted in time by any oncoming vehicles.

A less dangerous example appears in Computer Solitaire. This seemingly simple game requires matching and sequencing, focus, hand-eye coordination and *memory*. If you can't recall the cards you have, or even see the cards on either end of the screen, scores suffer. The slower the game, the lower the score. A score of 6,000 requires that the game be finished in 120 seconds or less; 7000 or higher, 110 seconds or less; 8000 or higher, 95 seconds or less. High scores are impossible for the player who must check each stack individually for a match, who can't remember if there's a matching card on the end or if it is black or red.

Things get worse if you can't remember to pick up the children from school, how to get to the store or what work needs to be done.

Marie, with "mild" TBI, could not remember what she needed to do once the thing was no longer visible. Out of sight, out of mind.

At night, as I added to the laundry basket, I would see that it was full and tell myself that I needed to do laundry. The next the day I would completely forget until I saw it again before bed. After a very long time I recognized the pattern and corrected it by moving the full basket to the bedroom doorway so I couldn't miss seeing it in the morning when I could do the wash.

—Marie

PERSERVERATION AND REPETITION

TBI victims may ask the same questions, say the same things, perform the same actions over and over. Reassurance or advice may go unheeded because the injured person cannot comprehend, absorb what is being said.

In 1944, Howard Hughes suffered his fourth plane crash. Two of his passengers died and Hughes suffered additional head injuries. Soon after he began repeating himself. He was persuaded to see a doctor only after his concerned business manager logged, on a note-pad, over 30 repetitions of the same sentence (Barlett DL and Steele B, 1979).

SLOWED THOUGHTS AND SPEECH

Injured drivers may fail to notice red lights, stop signs, or oncoming traffic. Processing speed may drop to such low levels that a person is essentially sleepwalking — with about the same functionality that one would expect of a person in that state. To the patient, life may feel like a dream or a very slow-motion movie.

It may also be extremely difficult to find words. There may be a 10-15 second delay in forming a simple *Yes* or *No* answer. The difficulty of producing actual thoughts in the form of sentences may be worse.

As an adult, Charlotte, injured in elementary school, reported that, disappointed as she was in her academic and professional abilities, the most distressing problem was her very slow ability to find words to express feelings or ideas.

> It would take me 15 minutes or more to find the words that I wanted to say. By then the entire situation would have changed and anything I wanted to say seemed strange or brought puzzled looks because the conversation had moved on. So most of the time I said nothing. In personal relationships my silence was naturally taken as either indifference or rejection.
>
> — Charlotte

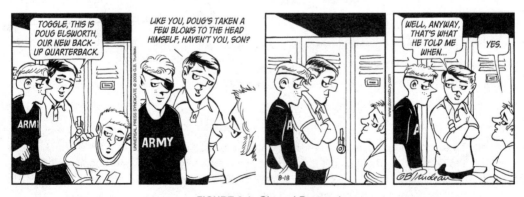

FIGURE 3-1. Slowed Processing

DECREASED FOCUS AND CONCENTRATION

He made a during-dinner speech something like this: "I like this fine. I never camped out before; but I had a pet 'possum once, and I was nine last birthday. I hate to go to school. Rats ate up sixteen of Jimmy Talbot's aunt's speckled hen's eggs. Are there any real Indians in these woods? I want some more gravy. Does the trees moving make the wind blow? We had five puppies. What makes your nose so red, Hank? My father has lots of money. Are the stars hot? I whipped Ed Walker twice, Saturday. I don't like girls. Why are oranges round? Have you got beds to sleep on in this cave? Amos Murray has got six toes. A parrot can talk, but a monkey or a fish can't. How many does it take to make twelve?"

—O. Henry, *The Ransom of Red Chief* (1910)

Attention Deficit Disorder (ADD), alone or combined with hyperactivity, AD(H)D, is a common diagnosis in today's children. Many wonder if it is real; it often correlates all too well with overcrowded, understaffed classrooms and funding cuts. It isn't reasonable to expect a child to sit quietly in his seat all day after eliminating recess, gym, art and music classes. Add caffeine, TV in the bedroom with resulting poor sleep, and the results may be misinterpreted by harried parents and teachers. Nevertheless, AD(H)D is very real and it is not new[1].

In both children and adults, symptoms of Post-Concussion Syndrome (PCS) overlap with symptoms of AD(H)D which in turn, can be associated with brain trauma[2]. Many AD(H)D children have had diagnosed head injuries before age five; many therapists look

Table 3-2. Overlap of AD(H)D and Post-Concussion Syndrome[a]	
AD(H)D	**PCS**
Attention/Fogginess	Yes
Failure to hear or follow through	Yes
Easily fatigued, poor sleep	Yes
Inability to multi-task	Yes
Careless mistakes	Yes
Losing items	Yes
Poor organization	Yes
Problems starting / finishing tasks	Yes
Impulsivity	Yes
Compulsive speech	Yes
Lack of motivation	Yes
Irritability and aggression	Yes
Inappropriate social behavior	Yes
Personality changes	Yes

a. *Diagnostic and Statistical Manual of Mental Disorders*, 4th Edition (DSM-IV-TR).

for that in their histories (Freeman J, 2003)[3]. These children may also have histories of trauma that make it difficult to know whether they have both AD(H)D and PTSD (Leitch L, personal communication, September 2013). The overlap has also been seen in veterans (Adler LA and Others, 2004).

1. The condition first appeared in the medical literature in the 1930s as Minimal Brain Dysfunction (MBD), considered to be the result of the flu pandemic of 1918.
2. Post Concussion Syndrome is in the DSM while TBI itself is in the ICD (*International Classification of Diseases*) published by the World Health Organization.
3. Director of the Johns Hopkins Pediatric Epilepsy Center, Baltimore, Maryland.

DISORGANIZATION AND LOSS OF EXECUTIVE FUNCTION

Executive functions involve organizing, sequencing and ranking things in order of importance, and making the decisions required to deal with them. In *The Lookout*, Chris can barely make a list, but without one, he can't organize even the most basic tasks. He puts a pan on the stove, flame on high, but forgets to put anything in it. He starts the coffee maker, but forgets to grind the beans. The movie doesn't say, but bills might have been a problem too.

Bills may be unpaid because there is no money, or, if money is available, because of confusion and disorganization. Before his TBI, Edweard Muybridge (see page 11) was an excellent businessman. After, he was strikingly unable to deal with bills or paperwork that seemed simple and obvious to others, such as *collecting* money for work he had done. When a client who owed $700 (around $14,000 today) objected to paying, Muybridge "at once proposed to send him a *receipted* bill; and so with others" (Clegg B, 2007, p. 93). He may have been equally casual about *paying* his bills. He stumbled across the photograph of his wife's infant son, labeled "Little Harry" in his wife's handwriting, at her midwife's house. He was there to settle the account *6 months after the birth*. This discovery, perhaps in association with Muybridge's damaged frontal lobes, led to the immediate murder of Harry Larkyns, his wife's lover.

SPATIAL DISORIENTATION

One of the most frightening symptoms is loss of sense of direction, where you are and how to get to where you need to be.

Nick (an honors student in graduate school) was a skilled orienteer, spending weekends navigating over tough terrain with map and compass. After his TBI, those skills were completely lost. He was unable to reliably choose the right Metro train, often getting on the one headed in the wrong direction, recognizing a problem only at the end of the line and then arriving an hour or more late to appointments.

For the injured brain, it may be difficult or impossible to find a way around a building; it may be necessary to rehearse the process with a friend or family member[1]. Looking for landmarks and *naming them aloud* helps to transfer visual imagery into verbal memory. For example, how do we get out of the building?

1. "Go to elevator. Press button to go down. Hit 1 for First Floor. Now what happens?"
   "The elevator is going down."
   "Good. Now what?"
2. "Go to the door."
   "OK, what next? Right? Or left?
3. "Go left, walk straight . . . ."

---

1. Neera Kapoor, O.D., Chief, Vision Rehabilitation Services, SUNY College of Optometry, New York. Personal communication (2012).

LOSS OF OLD SKILLS

After my TBI, I stared at my computer screen for hours. I couldn't remember how to start the program. When I finally did, I couldn't remember how to use the program I had designed and written. I couldn't read or make sense of the computer code.

—A Programmer

One of the most frightening effects of TBI is the loss of long-held skills. Victims *remember* being able to do things, but things have changed. We remember being able to run a business and a life, but now we can't. We remember being smart and capable, but that is gone. This is rarely shown in the media. It may be mentioned on the more reality-based forensic shows, but even there, the depiction may be wildly inaccurate.

On the forensics-based drama, *Bones*, Agent Seeley Booth has been shot, blown up, and knocked out repeatedly, both in Iraq and in the course of his duties at the FBI. After a three-week coma following brain surgery, his once-excellent marksmanship skills are gone. They miraculously reappear at the end of the episode; the previous difficulty is explained away as *psychological*, due to "confusion" over a personal romantic relationship.

In Real Life, skills of brain and body may stay lost, and this can be terrifying. Many TBI victims report feeling like "Charlie" in *Flowers for Algernon*[1]. The story begins with intelligence-enhancing experiments on a lab mouse (Algernon). The mentally disabled Charlie, who can barely function as a janitor, becomes the first human subject. Within months, his IQ zooms to genius levels and he begins a tender love affair. But Algernon begins losing his enhanced intelligence, then dies. Charlie realizes that he faces the same fate. Even as his mind slips away, Charlie can remember what he once was. Unable to face the pity or contempt of friends and co-workers, he orders his lover to leave, asks that flowers be left on Algernon's grave, then retreats to a State mental institution, where no one will know him.

Watching former abilities slip away is made worse when others continue to insist that Nothing Is Wrong (*except* that you are lazy and need to get a grip). Loss of skills is dangerous, especially when one is unaware of deficits due to lack of insight and memory. Thanks to cognitive slowing and decreased reaction time, every concussion increases the likelihood of another. There may be falls around the house or crashes on the street. Drivers do not lose their licenses just because they've had a TBI. Many continue to drive, accumulating accidents and tickets. As pedestrians, they may stroll in front of an unnoticed car or bus, ignore or fail to recognize other dangerous situations.

Manfred von Richthofen, "The Red Baron," was a skilled WWI fighter pilot, credited with 80 air combat victories. After a crash, he was never again the careful and effective pilot he was

---

1. Published as a short story in 1958, then as a novel in 1966, by Daniel Keyes.

before. His final error was obsessively chasing an enemy plane (a British Sopwith Camel) at low altitude, an extremely foolish tactical error. He was shot through heart and lungs by a single .303 bullet fired from the ground.

Death "while cleaning his guns" is often a euphemism for suicide, softened for the sake of the family. Anyone who accidentally shoots himself while cleaning guns, as John Grimsley did, had no business cleaning guns. But sometimes it is a forgotten skill.

Grimsley was an avid hunter and was very familiar with guns — or was once. After eight seasons as an NFL linebacker, eight or nine concussions (as reported to his wife), and four or five years before his death at 45, Grimsley began showing irritability and short-term memory problems typical of CTE. "I would tell him what to get at the store two miles away, and he'd forget and have to call me from there to ask," said Grimsley's widow (Schwarz A, 2008). Just as many others forget how to drive, dress, or cook, it is possible that Grimsley simply forgot how to clean his guns safely, because that part of his brain was gone. (See Figure 2-1 on page 28).

Consider loss of driving skills, dangerous for the impaired driver and for others. Reviews of *The Lookout* on Amazon.com share a common thread: If Chris was so badly injured, how can he still be *driving*? Short of seizures, licenses are not lost for having a TBI, "if," notes Chris, "you can afford to pay more for your insurance than for your rent." And if you look Fine.

Notice how many people in this book were driving after injury. But driving through traffic is the ultimate in multitasking, especially when processing speed is slowed. Ben was challenged by a four-way stop sign. Marie was unable to process highway signs fast enough to act on them. Morgan had to guided in by phone — a block at a time. Many others pray for red lights so they can figure out where they are. But all are *driving*.

Better to bring them in. People with symptoms of memory loss, disorientation, who have problems with multi-tasking are *not* Fine. They should not be left to wander about on their own, a risk to themselves and others.

LOSS OF MEMORIES OF DREAMS

Dreams may disappear. They may be there, but the sleeper is unable to remember them. This is a terrible loss to persons with an active dream life.

For seven years after her TBI Carol had no dreams. "That," said another dreamer (who lost hers for three years), "is the saddest thing I have ever heard."

One of the first signs of a healing brain is the return of a memory of dreams.

Physical

HEADACHES AND BODY PAIN

> Three days of each week, almost, I am incapable of any exertion, on account of my severe headaches.

> —Mary Todd Lincoln (1865)[1]

Chronic pain is often attributed to "getting older," or to arthritis or fibromyalgia. Regardless of what it is called (some call it "malingering") it often comes after TBI. Every historical example presented in the Introduction, from Henry VIII to Elvis Presley, suffered headaches or migraines for years after their injuries. After concussion and whiplash, one of the earliest, most common and long-lasting symptoms is headache. Injury strains pain-sensitive nerves, muscles, and connective tissue. Tissue in the neck, commonly injured in whiplash, sends pain directly to the head.

VISUAL PROBLEMS

> One does not see with the eyes, one sees with the brain, which has dozens of different systems for analyzing the input from the eyes.

> —Oliver Sacks (2012)

Vision doesn't come from the eyes only. It also comes from the brain. Half of the 12 cranial nerves are involved with vision, and visual problems — especially problems with reading — are extremely common after brain injury. After a concussion, it may suddenly be impossible to read at all, either because the words no longer make sense, or because the strain of reading triggers a headache.

TBI victims may have sudden problems with walking or driving in the dark. Because of increased sensitivity to light, they may prefer the dim and the dark, but see no better there than Normals. Movement (whether seen through car windows, on TV, or in the faces and bodies of other speakers) can be too much to bear. There may be nothing wrong with the eyes, but the brain can't process their information. Overload triggers nausea, vertigo, and balance problems as the brain struggles to adapt. Vision is highly specialized in a specific area of the brain (Figure 3-2). Symptoms of TBI can include any or all of the problems below (Suchoff IB, Ciuffreda KJ and Kapoor N, 2001).

- Sensitivity to light or light/dark changes. May include problems with color perception.
- Difficulty focusing. May be mistaken for presbyopia.
- Blurriness or dry/gritty sensations. May vary with blinking.

---

1. Turner JG and Turner LL (1972).

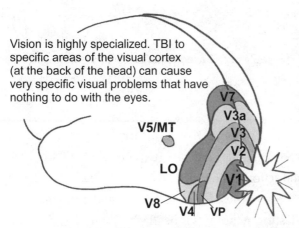

Vision is highly specialized. TBI to specific areas of the visual cortex (at the back of the head) can cause very specific visual problems that have nothing to do with the eyes.

V1 is the Primary visual cortex. It receives all visual input. Processing of motion, shape, and color starts here.

VP, V1 and V3 continue processing. V3a is especially sensitive to motion and texture.

V4 Color and form.

V5 / MT Motion detection.

V6 (not shown) spatial processing.

V7 visual memory.

V8 Color vision.

LO perceives Large Objects.

FIGURE 3-2. Areas of Visual Processing

- Difficulty shifting or sustaining gaze.
- Eyestrain or double vision eliminated by covering one eye.
- Poor balance, dizziness or vertigo in visually "busy" environments.
- Missing a portion of the vision field.
- Failure to perceive information on one side of the body.
- Slowed visual and spatial processing, impaired visual memory.

Light and Dark, Contrast and Color

Photosensitivity (sensitivity to light) is common after concussion. Slowed pupil response makes it difficult to adapt to changing light levels. Light can be blinding, painful, and even disorienting due to inability to filter or process information including color, contrast, and movement (including the flicker of fluorescent lights). Driving at night may be impossible or dangerous because the injured driver is blinded by oncoming headlights and unable to adapt to the following darkness.

Howard Hughes famously blocked the windows in his living areas with plywood and heavy curtains, a behavior that seems to have begun after his 1946 X-11 plane crash. As with Mary Lincoln, this was attributed to a desire for privacy, even though his rooms were in penthouse apartments on top floors of hotels, far from any public scrutiny. It is more likely that by then light was painful, even nauseating, and dark was necessary for comfort.

Problems with Focus, Dry or Gritty Eyes

Focus (*accommodation*) is the ability to change the shape of the eye. This ability (especially when looking at close items) decreases with age, but brain injury can speed the process. The primary symptom is blurred vision, constant or intermittent. Focus can also be impaired by dry eyes. Normally, a film of tears washes over the eye with every blink. If not, blurred vision may clear with blinking, but a gritty sensation, like sand, may remain.

Tracking Movements and Convergence

To follow targets, their positions or motions, eyes must move and work together in three dimensions. When nerves or muscles that control these movements are shocked or damaged, eyes may shift too far, not far enough, or with poor coordination producing double vision and eye strain. Reading becomes slow, fatiguing, and may trigger ferocious headaches. Test by covering one eye. If double vision goes away, the problem is convergence. If double vision persists, it is a problem with processing of visual information.

Visual-Vestibular Interaction

Balance depends on our eyes and inner ears. Concussion can damage both, causing dizziness, vertigo, and balance problems. Clues to which is most heavily involved can be found in the environment. If symptoms are worse in visually stimulating environments (such as the grocery or mall, while riding in a moving vehicle, scrolling on the computer, watching sports or movies), vision is suspect. If equally bad with eyes open or closed, the problem may be vestibular. But vestibular trauma can cause vision problems because the visual system strives desperately to compensate (Suchoff IB and Others, 2001).

Visual Field Loss

Brain injury can damage vision in several ways. One possibility is damage to the optic nerve, a cranial nerve (CN I) which supplies the eye. But information critical to vision is scattered throughout the brain; most of it in the *back* of the head. Figure 3-3 shows areas of damage and vision loss with damage to specific brain areas.

Damage to the parietal lobe (just behind the crown of the head) can result in inattention ("neglect") to an entire side of the body, common after stroke. Problems usually appear on the *left* side of the body. In most humans, scanning of body space (both sides) is done by the parietal section of the *right* brain[1]. If this area is damaged, the left brain monitors only its own territory (the right side of the body) never noticing what is going on with the left. A person may paint on only the right side of the canvas, fail to comb hair on the left side of the head, to apply makeup on the left side of the face, or notice food on the left side of the plate. In about 10 percent of humans, this pattern is reversed. Hair, makeup, food, or other items remain unnoticed on the *right* side. They may consistently lose at Solitaire because they fail to see cards on one side.

---

1. Right and left halves of the brain control opposite sides of the body. That is, the right brain controls the left body and eye, the left brain controls the right body and eye.

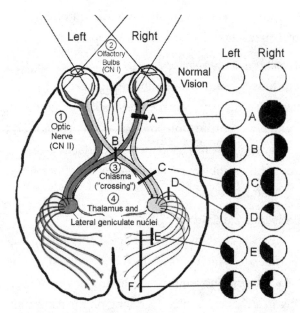

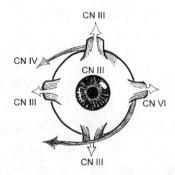

Most of the *Left* visual field goes to the *Right* visual cortex. Most of the *Right* visual field goes to the *Left* visual cortex, thus damage to connections on one side can produce blind spots on one or both sides.

Specific patterns of visual field loss (shown in black) come from problems at points A, B, C, D, E, and F. These can arise from tumors, inflammation, infections, ischemia, or direct trauma.

TBI causes so many visual problems because vision requires so much of the brain. Of the 12 cranial nerves, 6 are involved in vision or eye movements.

CN II (the optic nerve) senses light. CN III, CN IV, and CN VI control eye muscles critical to reading. CN III opens eyelids and controls pupil size.

CN V (the trigeminal nerve) provides sensation to eyes and tear glands.

CN VII (the facial nerve) closes eyelids and controls the tear film that normally washes over the eye with every blink; damage can result in dry gritty eyes. Jaw and facial muscles controlled by CN V and CN VII also lurk behind many painful headaches and migraines.

FIGURE 3-3. Visual Wiring of the Brain and Loss of Field of Vision

Visual Processing and Memory

After TBI, visual processing may slow to the point of virtual blindness. In *The Lookout*, Chris, unable to recognize the can opener in the kitchen drawer (after "moderate" TBI), attempts to open a can of tomato sauce with a hammer. Lewis returns home to find the can on the floor, battered but intact, and Chris sitting huddled and defeated, in the corner. Lewis picks up the can, pops it into the under-cabinet electric can opener, and cheerfully continues fixing dinner. "When I first saw this scene," said Carol (after "mild" TBI), "I cried."

> Like Chris, I was unable to see the can opener in a drawer of utensils. I too tried to open a can of tomato sauce with a hammer. It seemed reasonable at the time, but it didn't work. Just like Chris, I ended up huddled on the floor, weeping in confusion, fear and frustration.

Visual agnosia can range from failure to recognize a can-opener, keys or road signs to inability to recognize faces of friends and family ("face-blindness"). Sally, hit in the head by a batted baseball at age four, has extreme difficulty recognizing faces. Instead, she must rely

rely on body language, movement patterns, the sound of a voice. She cannot recognize her husband in old photographs, *because he no longer has that face.*

There may even be problems recognizing other life-forms. When another TBI patient, lost and confused, stopped to ask directions, there was no response because what she thought was a *person* was actually a *tree.* She realized this only when a concerned passerby stopped to ask if she was OK (Neera Kapoor, personal communication, 2012).

Visual Hallucinations

Different aspects of visual perception (such as recognizing faces, colors, movement) come from specific areas of the brain. If a person is blinded with eye patches or left in the dark, the result may be visual hallucinations using the same visual areas and pathways as sight itself. It often receives an undeserved assumption of schizophrenia or dementia, but more often the reasons are neurological (Sacks O, 2012, p. 24, 164).

SEVERE FATIGUE AND APATHY

> "I did my laundry today," said Bill.
> "Oh. That's nice."
> "No, you don't understand. I did my laundry *today*."

After even a supposedly *mild* brain injury, fatigue can be overwhelming, to a degree that the uninjured simply cannot understand, cannot believe possible. Because of fatigue, combined with confusion and noise of the laundry room, Bill needed five days to do laundry.

- A day to gather it up, perhaps followed by many days of working up the energy to drag it down to the laundry room and put it in the washer.
- A day to transfer the washed clothes to the dryer.
- And maybe another to pull it, now wadded and wrinkled, from dryer to hamper and home.

More time is needed to sort because sorting requires memory and many decisions. Clean or dirty? Light or dark? Even making pairs of things, such as matching socks is mentally fatiguing. So is organizing the means to iron the wrinkles out of wadded unwearable clothes. Easier to put wrinkled or souring clothes back in the hamper to wash them again. TBI fatigue is like the heavy, leaden feeling of climbing out of a swimming pool where once you floated effortlessly. The mere act of getting up and walking into another room can be a major hurdle — or victory.

"For years," reported Carol, I had what I called *One Days*, meaning that if I could do just *one* thing, the day was a success. It might be something as simple as washing *one* dish, paying *one* bill, or picking up the *one* pencil that had fallen on the floor weeks ago.

PHYSICAL WEAKNESS

When motor areas of the brain are damaged, muscles are uncoordinated or simply weak. It may not be an issue of working or "strengthening" the muscles, but of healing the brain, because signals simply don't get through to muscles.

GASTRO-INTESTINAL PROBLEMS

In a review of 126 TBI patients injured in various crashes and falls, gastro-intestinal (GI) problems were seen in 41 percent. Some involved diarrhea, but the most common problem was constipation (Expósito-Tirado JA and Others, 2003).

Constipation may be the natural result of post-injury changes in diet, dehydration, lack of exercise, or pain-killing drugs (especially opiates). It can also be a direct symptom of TBI. GI problems do not require spinal injury; TBI alone can do the job if messages between the GI tract and brain are interrupted, such as those controlling muscular movements in the colon or sphincters. Constipation can also be a symptom of endocrine disruption, including deficiencies of thyroid and human growth hormone (DCoE, 2012). The most severe and potentially deadly variety is *impaction*, one of Elvis Presley's most damaging health problems.

SENSORY OVERLOAD AND DYSFUNCTION

I could drive in the dark, but not if it was dark *and raining* because the noise of the rain was too much. I had to pull over until the rain stopped.

—Marie

Sensory dysfunction, after TBI, can involve changes in any of the senses. Using any of them too much or all of them just a little can be completely overwhelming. While recovering from even "mild" TBI, it is shocking to realize that attempting to pass the time on the computer or with video games or movies won't work; it's too much mental stimulation. Problems may appear with:

- VISION: including double vision, or vision loss. (See page 45).

- HEARING: especially fluctuating or variable deafness, sounds in the ears (ringing, squealing, or rushing noises). Damage to the tiny structures of the ear can result in vertigo and eventually vision problems. (See page 194).

- HEARING COMPREHENSION: When this symptom appears, people often pretend they hear to avoid the embarrassment of admitting that they have no idea what was just said, but this only makes a bad situation worse. Others tend to assume that they are being purposely ignored.

- AUDITORY HALLUCINATIONS: "Hearing voices" has long earned a diagnosis of schizophrenia or bipolar disorder, even in the absence of supporting clinical symptoms or history. In 1875, Robert Lincoln found his mother carrying on conversations with "people in the walls" just as retired football player Forrest Blue did a century later.

- TOUCH: includes numb fingers or the feel of being touched by a hair, a breeze, a ghostly hand, of bugs crawling on or under the skin, or skin being painfully pulled and stretched.
- OLFACTORY DISORDERS: includes loss of sense of smell (*anosmia*) or extreme acuity of smell. Anosmia is common after head injury. The long olfactory (CN I) nerves are easily sheared off in basal skull fracture or even a mild TBI; victims cannot smell smoke, gas, spoiled food — or good smells and good food. Smell may be so distorted that once-favorite foods smell or taste terrible. Or, phantom odors may be "sensed" that really aren't there at all[1].

Sensory messages may exist but fail to reach the level of awareness or action. As reported by the profoundly damaged Mike Webster: "I'm cold and I don't realize I can fix that by putting a jacket on" (Fainaru-Wada M and Fainaru S, 2013). Many other TBI victims become malnourished or severely dehydrated despite hunger pangs or burning thirst.

In contrast, senses can be so raw that interactions with other humans are impossible. The lights, the noise, or the mere effort of social activities (whether at home or requiring travel to other places) may be stupefyingly overwhelming. A movie or TV show filled with noise and fast movement is too much. Plot twists and strong emotions are exhausting.

In *The Lookout*, Lewis is kidnapped by bank robbers. Chris, who has gone to rescue him, waits and watches from his car as the suspense builds and then . . . *he falls asleep*. But this is not normal *sleep*. It is loss of consciousness, the shutdown of a system overwhelmed.

SLOWED REACTION TIME AND MOVEMENT DISORDERS

Reflexes slow when connections are damaged or broken. One of the most important connections is the *corpus callosum*, the "cable" that connects the two halves of the brain. The right brain controls the left side of the body; the left brain controls the right. For the two halves of the body to function effectively together most effectively, connections must be intact.

With dysfunctional sensory systems, bodies become "accident-prone" or "klutzy." The combination of confusion, dizziness, poor balance, slowed reflexes and impaired judgment sets the stage for additional injury and a downward spiral into dysfunction and disability. There may also be tremors, uncoordinated movements (*ataxia*), and intense contractions (*myoclonus*) of muscles of arms, legs, and other body parts. It may even include inability to close eyelids and keep them quiet. A person may think his eyes are closed but the whites of the eyes are still visible below the quivering lids (another reason for dry eyes after TBI).

Another movement disorder is bad handwriting. Like everything else, writing (good or bad), comes from the brain. Changing the brain may change the handwriting. For this very reason, many clinicians track handwriting over the course of treatment.

1. In his book *Hallucinations*, migraineur Oliver Sacks reports an interesting prodrome: a phantom smell of French toast before an attack.

Slurred, Difficult, or Altered Speech

> It was as if a complete stranger had taken over her husband's body, one who sometimes bizarrely spoke in a southern drawl that Brian had never used before the blast.
>
> —Carroll L and Rosner D (2011, p. 79).

Speech may be slow, slurred, or disjointed, either because of damage to areas that control the muscles of speech, or to the areas that store or retrieve the words. There may be a 10- to 15-second delay in response to a question. Or there may be *pressured speech* in which the speaker fails to inhale, and consistently runs out of breath. This can change the body's balance of oxygen and carbon dioxide, leading to anxiety and panic attacks.

One of the most bizarre changes is known as Foreign Accent Syndrome. The causes are still unclear, but the result is that victims pronounce words differently than before the injury, a trait that listeners interpret as a foreign accent or, at best, an annoying affectation. There are also examples of brain injury (including stroke) in which a native language is lost but a second or third, learned in adulthood, remains (Aglioti S and Others, 1996; García-Caballero A and Others, 2007; Martinell-Gispert-Saúch M and Others, 1997).

Sleep Disruptions and Insomnia

> Dr. Danforth, Please oblige me by sending about 4 more powders. I had a miserable night last night & took the 5 you left. What is to become of this excessive wakefulness, it is impossible for me to divine.
>
> —Mary Todd Lincoln (1865) *in* Schwartz TF (1970)

With TBI, a former "day person" may suddenly become a "night owl." If a house-mate is most active at night, insists on darkness during the day, and never leaves the house without sunglasses, don't think "vampire," think "brain injury."

Sleep disruptions and insomnia after TBI are extremely common. There is far more to sleep than simply passing out. Sleep is a complex process that can be disturbed even by too little daylight. Inadequate nutrients produce levels of hormones and neurotransmitters (such as serotonin and melatonin) in quantities that are, in turn, inadequate for sleep.

Seizures

The possibility of seizures increases with severity of TBI. Seizures in an athlete are a clear signal that damage exists and further sports play is wildly inappropriate. In 1991, the NFL player Andre Waters suffered a concussion so severe that he had a seizure during the flight home. He was diagnosed with "cramps" and sent out to play the very next weekend (Carroll L and Rosner D, 2011, p. 224).

Emotional

EMOTIONAL LABILITY

During the 1981 assassination attempt on President Reagan, Press Secretary James Brady was shot in the head. Brady lost function in his left arm and left leg, had deficits in memory and thinking, and problems recognizing familiar people. He had great difficulty controlling his emotions during speech. "He would kind of cry-talk for a while," says Arthur Kobrine, his neurosurgeon (Hayden EC, 2011).

After TBI, victims can be strangely emotional, laughing one moment, profoundly depressed or angry the next. This "labile" behavior[1] may earn a psychiatric diagnosis (or victims fear that it will), but it originates in trauma. NFL star Merril Hoge suffered repeated concussions. After a hit in a Denver game, he couldn't remember plays or snap count.

He went to the sideline to sort it out and suddenly, without warning, burst into tears. He felt humiliated. Only later did he learn that this was another symptom of a concussion: If the area of the brain that controls emotions becomes damaged, people sometimes cry unexpectedly (Fainaru-Wada M and Fainaru S, 2013, p. 41).

IMPULSIVENESS AND RISKY BEHAVIOR

Prior to his accident Muybridge was a good businessman, genial and pleasant in nature; but after the accident he was irritable, eccentric, a risk-taker and subject to emotional outbursts.

—Arthur P. Shimamura (2002)

Poor impulse control and risky behavior is typical of children and teens. These are the years of drag-racing, playing "chicken" or lying down on dark roads listening for oncoming cars. Frontal lobes are still developing.

In teens or adults with TBI whose frontal lobes have been damaged, impulsiveness may extend to uninhibited speech, spending, or snap decisions involving major life issues, from quitting jobs and selling property, to divorce or suicide. Spending is a common example, but if there is plenty of money, things are a bit different. Elvis giving a car to a relative stranger or Hughes showering women with expensive jewelry is little different from other folk deciding to pop out to the store for a pizza. Their impulsivity is better thought of as ill-considered behaviors that present *unreasonable* risk to self or others. It may be financial or extend to loss of reputation, danger to personal or public health, safety and serenity.

Risky, ill-judged behavior is the setup of *The Lookout*. While speeding down a dark highway on prom night, high-school hockey star Chris Pratt turns off the headlights so his friends can better see the clouds of fireflies. For healthy brains, watching this scene is like

---

1. *Lability* comes from Latin *labilis*, meaning unstable, or likely to "slip."

watching a too-long underwater sequence; we hold our breath, knowing that this cannot end well. To Chris (who probably had previous sports injuries) turning off the lights on a flat, country road seems perfectly reasonable. He turns them on too late.

Another movie example is "Tony Stark," a.k.a. Iron Man. Cartoonist Stan Lee based the character of the wealthy industrial genius on Howard Hughes. In *Marvel's Avengers*, Stark casually zaps Bruce Banner with an electric shock just to see *if* that will cause Banner to morph into his deadly alter ego — the giant, green, super-powerful and unstoppable Hulk.

Stark is fiction. The behavior isn't. As a child, the Real Life Howard Hughes was known to lob rocks through his parents' French doors whenever he had forgotten his house key (Hack R, 2001, p. 50). As an adult, he pulled engineers off important WWII military projects to have them design a blimp advertising Jane Russell's breasts[1]. Later, he would crash and burn while testing an experimental plane with a known oil leak over a populous area.

LOSS OF A COMPLEX SENSE OF HUMOR

Quick wit and complex sense of humor requires *both* sides of the brain and fast communication between them. Story telling requires memory and sequencing; without these, the teller may become hopelessly lost in the story — then forget the punchline.

Loss of humor or age-appropriate humor is also common in TBI. A concussed brain may laugh at a pie in the face, but Gary Larson cartoons are a mystery.

After a 50-foot fall out of a window, one of Nick's many losses was his adult sense of humor. What remained (at age 30) was like that of a third-grade boy. He had the oddly happy affect and inappropriate laugh of many TBI survivors, with no awareness of his impact on others. He could play on some words and he had learned some "jokes." They rarely fit the situation, but they were all he had and his limited repertoire quickly became irritating. The return of age-appropriate humor was a welcome symptom of healing.

ANGER AND EXPLOSIVENESS

[They] have disordered thinking and electrical impulses . . . They have a minor irritation. And they just want to end it. It's like having a fly in your room and deciding to blow up your house."

—Ann McKee and Others (2009)

One of the most frightening symptoms of TBI is mood swings. A once mild-mannered person may fly into a towering rage or violent action — from assault to suicide — at the smallest provocation. Normally, the frontal lobes control our internal waves of emotion, but if they are damaged, the slightest annoyance may be blown out of all proportion.

---

1. Star of Howard Hughes' movie, *The Outlaw*.

A classic joke told at Alcoholics Anonymous meetings is that when a normal person gets a flat tire, he calls AAA. When an alcoholic gets a flat tire, he calls the suicide hotline.

Alcohol damages impulse control but so does TBI, often with tragic results. When high school football star Austin Trenum was told to do his homework before going out with friends, he stormed off to his room — then hanged himself. On autopsy, he was found to have had CTE at age 17 (Hruby P, 2012).

Not all anger is a sign of brain damage. There are different *kinds* of anger. Raging anger can be genuine loss of control. It can be a carefully calculated tool to control others. It can also be a survival strategy.

As explained by a veteran interviewed by Chris Buchanan for his documentary film[1],

[Anger] helps you get your job done as a soldier . . . . If you're on patrol and a car cuts in front of you, if you're too chilled out about it, that car will kill you. You have to be angry at the car, at the driver, and you draw on that anger, and that's what fuels you to act — to shoot the car to stop it from possibly killing you. The problem is when you come home after a year of living with that kind of adrenalin-pumped up anger. It takes time to bleed that fuel out of your system.

—Christopher Buchanan, *In Search of the Lost Platoon (2010)*

FLAT AFFECT

He left the States 31 months ago. He was wounded in his first campaign. He has had tropical diseases. He half-sleeps at night and gouges [enemies] out of holes all day. Two-thirds of his company has been killed or wounded. He will return to attack this morning. How much can a human being endure?

—*Life Magazine (1945)*

Flat affect is a lack of visible emotional reactivity, a failure to display normal emotion through words or body language. Speech may be a monotone, with little vocal inflection, few or no gestures and little facial or emotional expression.

This, like other symptoms, may range in severity, from the blunted emotions of depression to the unfocused round-eyed gaze, the "2,000-Yard Stare," seen in severe trauma, PTSD, and the battle-weary soldier.

The phrase was popularized through a painting by Tom Lea[2], the real-life portrait of an exhausted young Marine at the 73-day Battle of Peleliu in the South Pacific during World War II.

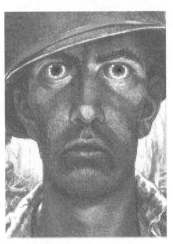

FIGURE 3-4. Flat Affect

1. See http://www.pbs.org/wgbh/pages/frontline/woundedplatoon/journey.
2. *Marines Call It That 2,000 Yard Stare*, by Tom Lea.

LOSS OF SOCIAL SKILLS

The social skills appropriate to human society are a complex dance of connections, position and flow, depending on flexibility, timing, and even sound and tone. In concussed adults these skills may be lost; in children they may fail to develop. Results may include lack of boundaries, inappropriate familiarity, talking too loudly or boisterously, or long rants on socially unacceptable topics.

Without intent to offend, people with injured brains may fail to hear others, may fail "to pass the ball" in conversation or other interactions, or may interrupt persistently while unaware that these things are happening. Or, they may be aware but unable to stop them and later embarrassed by their own behavior. They may interrupt purposely because, if they don't, then the thought, the idea, the memory will vanish. Or they may fail to see why any of these things matter. Or they may not interact at all.

POOR HYGIENE AND SELF-AWARENESS

The main thing that threw [Ava] off, and me, too, was his body odor. Howard never bathed, he never used a deodorant. And I'm sure he never cleaned his clothes. They were always dirty, and he never bothered to change. I remember standing next to him at Ciro's one night, and I smelled him before I knew who it was. . . Ava couldn't get past the body odor, and neither could I.

—Arlene Dahl *in* Gardner A (1992, p. 127)

Victims of concussion often become invisible to themselves. They may lose all interest in grooming, forget or refuse to bathe or to eat. Damaged self-awareness can result in inappropriate social behaviors (both personal and professional), including clothing, from age-inappropriate dress to the downright goofy or bizarre.

I'll never forget seeing Howard in that outfit, the pants starting six inches above his ankles and the jacket sleeve starting six inches above his wrists. It was no use telling him about it; to my knowledge he wore that same outfit night and day for at least five years.

—Ava Gardner (1992, p. 78-82)

A person may ignore an entire side of the body — or more. At his trial, serial killer Ted Bundy was astonished that other people claimed to have *seen* him. In his world view he was invisible (Von Drehle 1995, p. 288).

ANXIETY, PANIC, AND PARANOIA

Anxiety is a natural result of all the losses resulting from the injury, many of which are not believed or acknowledged by others. Anxiety and panic attacks, like depression, can come from an injured brain, from damage to the inner ear, from guilt and pain over others injured or killed. The result is often friction in families, with friends, or at work. It may be impossible to hold a job, resulting in financial disaster and an uncertain future.

As a diagnosis, *paranoia* has been argued in and out of existence (McKenna PJ, 1997). Today its features and boundaries remain controversial. Nevertheless, it is generally thought of as delusions and irrational beliefs combined with a sense of persecution. Paranoid behaviors have followed many head injuries and are associated with sleep disorders.

King Henry was terrified of plots and rebellions which his own behavior had inspired.

Lord Nelson became convinced that the Prince of Wales was sneaking into Emma's bed.

Mary Lincoln feared poverty and starvation despite a government pension of $3,000 per year (the modern-day equivalent of about $44,000). She refused to trust banks, travelling with the bulk of her estate as cash and convertible bonds (payable on demand), in her petticoats.

Howard Hughes was terrified of germs and spies. *Part* of the reason for blocking windows in his penthouse suites with plywood was to keep people in helicopters from looking in.

Football veteran Cookie Gilchrist was reclusive, estranged from friends and family, and so paranoid that he taped all conversations.

DEPRESSION

Depression (or a diagnosis of depression) is extremely common after TBI.

Part of this may be natural grief and mourning. Very often one loses one's sense of self, the skills and abilities, even the memories that make a person unique. While struggling to heal, one loses the *now*. One may also lose a future long seen, planned and worked for, and be unable to imagine any other.

Part of depression is the brain itself. Depression appears when a brain slows down, especially in the left and front. It appears in people who don't even realize they have been injured, who know no loss, who have no clue why they feel the way they do, why they are so tired, why they need to sleep so much. Anti-depressants may be so poorly effective that patients question the diagnosis. "I don't feel *depressed*," they may say, "I just feel *not there*."

There are also physical reasons for depression. Depression is a first symptom of many nutritional deficiencies, and malnutrition is a common *secondary* symptom of TBI.

Secondary Symptoms

> The post-concussion label is often a dead end with no agreement upon treatment, pathology, or prognosis . . . [P]atients tire of describing their experiences and resent the implication that they malinger or unconsciously promote their troubles. They may remain silent about odd perceptual experiences and cognitive slips, as such are not intuitively linked to their accident, or for fear of being taken for mental cases.
>
> —Grimm RJ and Others (1989)

A wide array of secondary symptoms can follow the initial injury and symptoms.

Table 3-3. Secondary Symptoms of Concussion / TBI	
Physical and Sensory	**Cognitive**
Malnutrition	Inability to multi-task
Alcohol and drug addiction	Obsessive / compulsive disorders
Apnea, both sleeping and waking	Clutter and hoarding
Hormonal changes	**Emotional**
Environmental sensitivities	Shame and humiliation
Auto-immune disorders	Social isolation, loss of relationships
	Suicidal thoughts

Symptoms remaining three months or more after a concussion earn a diagnosis of post-concussion syndrome. Symptoms may be treated individually. For example,

- Depression is addressed with anti-depressants.
- Weight gain triggers a stern lecture on diet, exercise, and self-control.
- Sexual disinterest or dysfunction may bring a prescription for Viagra® (for men) or psychiatric counseling (for women).

One of the most common and damaging secondary symptoms — which can lead to so many others — is malnutrition.

MALNUTRITION

Malnutrition does not mean "starving," it means "bad-feeding." It is damaging and deadly in its own right. It may arise from many other symptoms, ranging from impulsivity to desperate calorie restrictions due to weight gain, or simply from overwhelming fatigue.

Throughout the 17 years following his TBI, Bill was too fatigued to function. He could stay awake only for a few hours a day and it took him almost a week to do laundry (see page 49). The kitchen revealed another sign of TBI; no food and no pots in the cabinets because he could no longer cook. But cooking also requires groceries and after TBI, grocery shopping is a huge challenge. Like many others, Marie couldn't even make a grocery list.

> When I looked in the refrigerator to get ideas, I realized that it didn't help because I could only see the things that were *there*, not the things that were *missing*. I would drive to the store and walk the aisles hoping that the sight of something would remind me that I needed it. I bought paper towels because it seemed the kind of thing you only get every once in a while so there was a good chance I would need them. But because I kept thinking that, when I got home I would find that I already had *many* paper towels.

At the store, a full cart may be abandoned because check-out is too long and too loud or because of the sudden realization that money was forgotten (again) at home. Food that does make it home may spoil because it is left in the car. Food that gets into the house may spoil on the floor or counter tops before it is put in the refrigerator. In the refrigerator, it may rot long before being used. And that's just the beginning.

Cooking is an extremely complex process. It requires cognitive skills that may no longer be available. It requires prioritizing and sequencing, multi-tasking, a sense of time and memory. One of the best popular books on the realities of "mild" TBI is *I'll Carry the Fork*. Author Kara Swanson ran a successful catering business. After her TBI she found herself pouring kitty litter into the washing machine and lost in familiar places with no idea where she was or why she was there. The book title refers to her inability to remember that food was in the oven; it would burn unless she carried the fork in her hand as a reminder (Swanson K, 1999).

Cooking may also require *reading* a cookbook when reading has become difficult or impossible. Fast food menus come with *pictures*. Crackers, ramen noodles, or other heavily processed or junk foods are even easier, but can make the problem worse. They tend to be high in flavor enhancers such as MSG (monosodium glutamate) which can be actively harmful to an injured brain.

Glutamate is a neurotransmitter. Normally it is combined with and controlled by other molecules but tissue breakdown sets it free. Levels high enough to kill neurons accumulate within 24 hours of injury and may peak from 48 to 72 hours later (Baker AJ and Others, 1993).

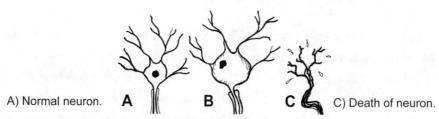

A) Normal neuron.   **A**   **B**   **C**   C) Death of neuron.

B) Swelling in presence of free glutamate.

FIGURE 3-5. Destruction of Neurons by Free Glutamates

Areas with the most glutamate receptors are most vulnerable to glutamate damage. These include the hypothalamus, control center for appetite, endocrine glands, sleep-wake cycles, immunity and emotional balance. Another area is the heart. Some speculate that high-MSG food may lurk behind many "restaurant coronaries" (Blaylock R, 1996), especially in combination with a magnesium deficiency.

ALCOHOL AND DRUG ADDICTION

It takes energy and organization to cook a decent meal and to clean up afterwards. Easier to order pizza. Even easier to drink alcohol which provides fast calories, pain relief, and requires no chewing. Unfortunately, alcohol can also destroy nutrients, cause more brain damage, and end in addiction. But when pain is too terrible to endure and sleep won't come, alcohol and drugs become increasingly attractive. One client was downing a fifth of whiskey a night in a desperate attempt to win a few hours of unconsciousness. Unfortunately, alcohol damages sleep even more, continuing the cycle of sleep disruption and its many side effects. Sleep loss can also increase pain, which may have been bad enough on its own.

In Civil War days, when medicine was heavily based on opiates and mercury, morphine addiction was known as "the Army Disease" (Personal communication, Zeih D, 2012). It could just as easily have been called "the Women's Disease." Addiction of women (and their teething children) was extremely common, if unseemly. Opium and its derivatives were the wonder drugs of the day. Paregoric was for fussy children. The stronger laudanum ("tincture of opium") and morphine were standard treatment for menstrual and labor pains[1], migraine, and every other pain including that of fever, infection, and trauma. Mary Lincoln suffered all of these. As a young woman, she was afflicted with migraines, especially in the spring, but after her 1863 TBI, migraines became her "constant companions."Unfortunately, while opiates soothed the pain, they often ensnared the user in an incurable addiction.

---

1. Heroin for labor pains was still common in England as recently as 50 years ago (Sacks O, 2012, p. 258). In the US, codeine cough syrup was freely available until 1970.

It is almost impossible that Mary did *not* become an addict. In terrible pain, both physical and emotional, she appears to have become increasingly dependent on laudanum and then stronger opiates. Eventually her behavior resulted in her infamous sanity trial. On hearing the verdict for her commitment, she immediately made a frantic attempt to buy laudanum but was thwarted by several alert pharmacists (Beidler AE, 2009). Historically, this has been seen as a suicide attempt. More likely, it was the response of a woman desperate to secure drugs before being locked away from her supply. Drug addiction in addition to TBI is a viable explanation for Mary's increasingly disturbed behavior after 1863.

It is difficult to realize how very different things were in her day. Pasteur had just begun work on germ theory in France. The first medical paper on the novel notion of disinfecting wounds and surgical instruments before surgery would not appear until 1867 in England. The first antibiotics (sulfa drugs and penicillin) were almost a century away. Even aspirin would not be isolated until 1897. But the hypodermic needle (invented around 1853) could deliver opium and mercury to the patient more efficiently than ever before.

But that was then and this is now. Things have changed. Well maybe, because when we try to treat TBI symptoms with our standard arsenal of drugs, it doesn't seem to work much better than it did in Mary Lincoln's day. Today, millions are addicted to opiates such as hydrocodone, oxycontin, and Percocet®. They may be scorned for their weakness, but very often their addictions began with brain injury.

When Howard Hughes died with five broken needles in his arms and high levels of codeine in his blood, he was assumed to have been a drug addict. Working with medical records and autopsy reports, Dr. Forest Tennant concluded that Hughes (who never smoked or drank) was *not* an addict in the usual sense. Codeine was not injected into veins for a "high" but into muscle, for pain control. Blood levels of codeine five times the lethal dose — for a *beginner* — reflect increasing tolerance for the drug over 30 years. This pattern suggests a severely damaged man trying to control pain arising from the continuing effects of TBI, broken bones, burns and scar tissue (Tennant F, 2007).

DEHYDRATION

Trauma to sensory centers can leave a person unaware of thirst or unable to translate awareness into action. Sometimes dehydration is purposeful; when it is too awkward or painful to get up to urinate, the obvious solution is to avoid fluids.But dehydration alone can produce many serious secondary symptoms: depression, constipation, headaches, even body odor due to accumulating toxins that cannot be resolved by deodorants.

APNEA

Just as it is impossible to heal without healthy sleep, it is impossible to heal without healthy breathing.

Apnea ("no breathing") can cause *anoxia* ("no oxygen," that is, low oxygen) which can damage the brain (Gainer R, 2011). It may also cause nightmares, possibly as a warning system that something is terribly wrong (Cloud J, 2012). Apnea is of at least two types: *Obstructive* (caused by a blockage) and *central* (coming from the brain itself).

Obstructive apnea is usually blamed on overweight, flabby tissue, or enlarged tonsils. Children can have obstructive apnea from enlarged tonsils, leading to brain anoxia and cognitive problems. This is not uncommon, but it is made worse by changing fashions in treatment. Through the 1950s, children's enlarged tonsils were taken out. No question. With the discovery that tonsils were an important part of the immune system, their removal became less automatic. Today treatment has gone to the other extreme. Now, we will "wait and watch," but in children's developing brains, years of untreated apnea with reduced oxygen can result in cognitive, social and physical problems[1]. It has been found to cause high blood pressure in children as young as two and is suspected to predispose children to cerebrovascular disease, pulmonary hypertension, and performance deficits (National Academy of Sciences, 2006).

It can also appear in a brain that "forgets" to breathe. This is known as *central apnea.* and is often seen in persons who have had concussions. There may also be "neuromuscular" apnea related to problems with the phrenic nerve which controls the muscle of the diaphragm but comes from the neck.

In driving tests, sleep-deprived adults did as poorly as those who were blatantly intoxicated (Fairclough SH and Graham R, 1999; Powell NB and Others, 2001). Sleepy drivers are less aware, fail to stay in their lanes, have slowed reaction times and lose steering control (Colten HR, 2006, p. 148). Compared to healthy drivers, their risk of traffic accidents doubled and the worse the apnea, the higher the risk (Terán-Santos J and Others, 1999; Young and Others, 1997). Given these effects, apnea helps to pass TBI on to others.

---

1. So can anesthesia before age three (Ing C and Others, 2012).

HORMONAL CHANGES

Symptoms of endocrine injury or failure may appear soon after, or long after the initial injury. In the luckiest patients, the problem is immediately recognized and treated. In others, onset is amazingly slow and sneaky; visible symptoms appear months or even years after the injury, long after we think the patient should be better, long after support services have ended, and long after the patience of family and employers has run out.

Damage to hypothalamus or pituitary can trigger a cascade of problems, sometimes months in the making, impacting all hormone systems. These can involve everything from growth and repair to changes in water balance, thyroid problems, abnormal sweating or low body temperature, fatigue and depression to sleep problems, weight gain, sexual dysfunction and infertility.

The pituitary, master gland of the body, nestles in the sphenoid bone at the base of the skull. (See Figure 4-4 on page 84.) If brain or bone shifts in the course of TBI, the pituitary and communicating blood vessels and nerve fibers from the hypothalamus can be damaged. The results impact body, brain, and quality of life.

Temperature Dysregulation and Dysautonomia

If you are reading this, you are a mammal. Mammal bodies work best within certain operating temperatures, of around 98–100 °F (36.5–37.5 °C). If they "freeze to death" it isn't because they turn to ice. It is because they are too cool, too "un- warm," for critical enzyme and other reactions to take place. Subnormal temperatures offer slow death by hypothermia[1]. After concussion, body temperature can fall, possibly due to malfunction of the hypothalamus, the part of the brain that regulates body temperature.

After several TBIs, Phyllis had a documented body temperature of around 95 degrees F. "Poikilothermic,"she said, and kept a hot-tub (at 98.6 F) to bring her temperature down in summer, up in winter[2]. Her body, unable to properly regulate temperature on its own, was an extreme example of *dysautonomia*, dysfunction of processes that should be automatic.

Most people with this condition feel cold, but there may also be severe sweating, often at night, a symptom mentioned by Lord Horatio Nelson[3] and many veterans returning from Iraq and Afghanistan. Often it is inability to self-regulate after TBI, but they believe they feel cold at home "because it was so hot over there." Brian ran a temperature of 96.5 F.

---

1. To die of *hypothermia* is to die of "low-temperature," defined as 95.0 °F (35.0 °C) and lower. Below 86 °F (30 °C) the system progresses towards major organ failure and death.
2. *Poikilothermic* (Greek, *poikilos*, varied) refers to organisms such as amphibians (frogs) and reptiles (snakes) whose body temperatures must vary with the temperature of their surroundings.
3. Nelson may have had lingering symptoms of malaria, but inappropriate sweating is a common symptom in other war veterans with blast injuries.

"In my ER," said a trauma nurse, "he would have been within half a degree of emergency re-warming for hypothermia." But Brian never made it to the ER because he was Fine; he thought he was cold because of "moving north" from Florida to Virginia — *in July.*

Katherine, after multiple concussions from an ex-husband, ran a temperature of 95.6 F. Extreme depression, fatigue, and all-over body pain were attributed to abuse, but symptoms did not respond to anti-depressants. Her rheumatologist diagnosed fibromyalgia but refused to do thyroid testing, insisting that fibro and hypothyroidism were entirely separate, but low body temperature alone can cause severe pain.

Phyllis had subnormal temperatures and persistent pain after a ski accident and TBI. Figure 3-6 shows the extent of her pain on beginning neurofeedback treatment. Over the course of 33 FNS sessions at Brain Wellness and Biofeedback Center of Washington (BWB), temperature normalized and pain levels fell significantly.

Low temperatures also come from poor nutrition, too few calories, and/ or the sedentary lifestyle that often follows traumatic injury. Meanwhile, AD(H)D meds reduce appetite and anti-depressants can block thyroid and B vitamins, lowering metabolism.

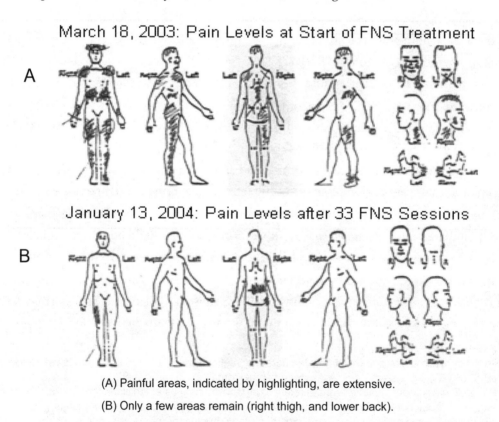

(A) Painful areas, indicated by highlighting, are extensive.

(B) Only a few areas remain (right thigh, and lower back).

FIGURE 3-6. Pain Patterns Before and After FNS Neurofeedback Only

Sexual Dysfunction

Hormone disruption after TBI can cause a wide range of sexual dysfunction: impotence in men, menstrual or fertility problems in women. In both sexes there may be low libido or complete loss of interest, which creates yet another strain on a relationship.

Changes in Appetite, Weight, and Body Composition

A common finding after TBI is growth hormone deficiency, which changes weight and body composition.

Like many modern-day football players, Henry VIII was an outstanding athlete. He grew to be 6-ft 1-in., a young giant in his day. His custom-made armor shows a gradual increase between his 20s and 30s, but by age 45, he was morbidly obese. He died with a Body Mass Index (BMI) greater than 50[1]. Modern endocrinologists suspect that Henry's symptoms reflect hormone changes following brain injuries from his jousting accidents of 1524 and 1536 (Ashrafian H, 2012).

After TBI, gains of 20, 30, 50 pounds or more are not rare. We usually mistake post-TBI weight gain as "laziness" or lack of self control, but even when the cause is understood, we rarely understand how it affects the victim or how it leads to further disability. A glimpse of this appears in judo students. The one most likely to be injured on the mat is not the complete novice; it is the returning adult who studied as a child. Neural pathways were laid down to analyze and respond to the body's position in space, *but now that body has changed*. Posture and weight and center of gravity are different.

The strain and discomfort of putting on weight can be experienced by *putting on weight*. Going about your regular day in a 20- to 50-pound backpack will get the idea across. But post-TBI weight gain is often in the waist, especially in the belly. Sudden weight gain here can be debilitating and painful in many ways — much like pregnancy. Some childbirth trainers use a weighted body suit, The Empathy Belly®, to get across the sensation of new weight.

Although it weighs a mere 33 pounds (primarily in the belly), *some* of its effects include pressure on internal organs, fatigue and shortness of breath, increased heart rate and blood pressure and restricts physical movement and abilities.

Most users (often men, seeking empathy with pregnant wives) rip it off in minutes. Those who leave it on report changes in self-image and confidence; both fall when a body can no longer do what it used to do.

These apparently simple changes can produce so many problems that the rental agreement includes a waiver warning against use by persons who weigh less than 100 or more than 300 pounds, or who have the following conditions.

---

1. Body Mass Index (BMI) is the relationship between mass and height. See Glossary.

- Chronic back pain; disorders of spine, neck or pelvis (including scoliosis or disc problems).
- Fractured, broken, or dislocated bones; strains or sprains of muscles or ligaments.
- Damage or weakness in ribs, knees or ankles.
- High blood pressure, vertigo, dizziness, fainting, asthma or other breathing difficulties.
- Heart problems (including heart attack or stroke).
- Epilepsy or history of seizures.
- Any serious abdominal skin bruises, recent wounds or scars, or organic disorders such as a hernia, enlarged liver or spleen, or infections.
- Any other condition for which your physician has advised you to avoid strenuous activity[1].

The waiver goes on to warn that use of the product with any of the above conditions — *common side-effects of injuries that can be associated with TBI* — may make them worse or cause additional injury.

Weight gain is not trivial. It places serious demands on the body. Avoiding further damage may involve avoiding many normal behaviors and many of life's joys. The company advises that you should not do the following.

- Behave frivolously.
- Twist while simultaneously bending over[2], or bend over without bending knees.
- Make any abrupt, jerky or swift movements in any direction.
- Bounce, jump or run.
- Wear high-heeled or slippery shoes.
- Go on stairs, steep inclines, or slippery surfaces.

In real life, that may translate into: No bouncing about on a horse (never mind jousting!), no dancing in the rain, no sports, and being afraid, *very* afraid, of suffering further injuries should you do anything beyond the sedate and boring.

So how does that make you feel?

---

1. See the complete waiver at www.EmpathyBelly.com.
2. The combined motion of standing while twisting strains the quadratus lumborum muscle. The resulting muscular pain is horrific and the cause of many failed back surgeries. Bend and lift properly, no matter what your weight or condition.

ENVIRONMENTAL SENSITIVITIES

The blood-brain barrier (BBB) refers to tightly bound walls of blood vessels in the brain. In general, it blocks:

- Many harmful toxins, bacteria and viruses.
- Hormones and neurotransmitters intended for the rest of the body.
- Large and low-fat molecules.

The BBB is often said to be uncrossable, but it is not. Even under normal circumstances there are areas of the brain where it is especially weak or actually lacking. These are in the *circumventricular organs* which include the hypothalamus, pituitary and the pineal gland[1]. The BBB is also weak or lacking when actually torn by trauma, eroded by imbalances of electrolytes, or strained by high intracranial pressures, all common in TBI. When it breaks down, toxins, pathogens, and environmental chemicals can easily reach the brain.

INFECTIONS AND AUTOIMMUNE FUNCTION

Skull fractures, tears in the dura, and breakdown of the BBB greatly increase risk of brain infections such as meningitis. But breaks and tears are a two-way street. Things don't just get *in* to the brain; brain materials also leak *out* into areas where they don't belong, where they are seen as alien invaders. There they trigger immune responses, then autoimmune disease, one of the issues found during autopsy of Elvis Presley (Tennant F, 2013).

This process was documented in a group of boxers, active or retired, their ages ranging from 17 to 53. Of these 61 men, 13 had antibodies to chemicals from the hypothalamus, and 14 to chemicals from the pituitary. In the normal control group, *no such antibodies were found* (Tanriverdi F, De Bellis A, and Others, 2010). That is, with repetitive brain injury, the boxers had developed antibodies to their own brains.

Boxers, as a group, have long been known for brain injury. An odd riff on that awareness was the peculiar claim (page 30) that they were the *only* group[2], that other athletes (such as NFL football players) were somehow exempt. Continuing studies of CTE by the intrepid Ann McKee and other researchers ended that notion. In 2012, a landmark study by Lee Goldstein, McKee and others showed that the source of the TBI didn't matter; the brains of young men dead with football injuries, or from soldiers who had suffered blasts all showed the same damage, the same tangled and broken neurons, and the same auto-immune responses.

---

1. And also the *area postrema*, known as the "vomit center" due to its extreme sensitivity to toxins. These organs, linking the CNS and the blood stream, are an integral part of neuro-endocrine function. Lack of a BBB allows them to test the blood for what is or isn't there, and to send out peptides and hormones that drive the brain-body system.
2. Aside from "steeplechase riders."

Cognitive

The secondary symptoms of TBI flow from deficits that have come before.

INABILITY TO MULTI-TASK

Multi-tasking requires multi-skills. It requires alert energy, executive decisions concerning what goes where and why, and in what order. It requires memory. Traditionally, women are the multi-taskers while men talk about the importance of doing One Thing at a Time. In a Scottish-American folksong, "Father Grumble" swears that he does more work in one day than his wife does in three. So one day she goes merrily off to do the plowing, leaving him to care for cow, pigs, and chickens, and to wind the yarn. Of course it ends badly for a man unaccustomed to multiple demands.

Modern life ends badly for men and women who lose lost these skills, the ability to hold things together. Bill and Carol could not remember how to cook; Marie could not remember to do laundry or how to shop for groceries. These things may seem small and trivial, but without them, lives and families and worlds collapse.

OBSESSIONS

> In all likelihood, Muybridge's brain injury included at least the orbitofrontal cortex and probably more extensive damage such as damage to the anterior temporal lobe. . . . Patients with orbitofrontal damage exhibit inappropriate risk-taking behavior, obsessive-compulsive disorder [OCD], and social disinhibition.
>
> —Arthur P. Shimamura (2002)

After TBI, compulsive behaviors may appear involving talking, writing, hoarding, gambling, or Obsessive-Compulsive Disorder (OCD).

Talking or Writing

TBI may trigger compulsive non-stop talking (*logorrhea*) or writing (*hypergraphia*, the polar opposite of writer's block). French essayist Michel de Montaigne began his massive writings after falling from a horse. The NFL's Mike Webster wrote thousands of letters and notes on any available paper even though he had to wrap his twisted fingers in duct tape in order to hold a pen (Fainaru-Wada M and Fainaru S, 2013, p. 4). Howard Hughes wrote incredibly complex instructions for the simplest acts, such as a nine-step procedure for opening a can of peaches.

> Step #7. Removing Fruit from Can. Under no circumstances does HRH want any contact between the fruit itself and the outside of the metal can. In spearing peaches or whatever fruit is being used, under no circumstances should the fork itself touch any part of the can whatsoever. In removing fruit from the can to the sterile plate, please be sure that the fruit is not pressed or pushed into the side or the bottom of the can while spearing. This part of the job should be done very slowly and gently, so as to keep the fruit from accidentally brushing

against the inside of the can. The man may use his sterile spoon to lift the fruit out of the can if this will prevent any further contact between the fruit and the inside of the can.

Obsessive / Compulsive Disorder (OCD)

This may appear after TBI especially after frontal lobe injury. Like other symptoms, there may be a family tendency to OCD, but TBI can trigger it or make it worse.

Besides his germ phobia, Howard Hughes was infamous for his obsession with peas. There had to be 12 on his plate and they had to be exactly the same size.

Henry VIII may also have suffered OCD after his concussion. Terrified of dirt and infection, his most sumptuous garments were worn for only about three days, then burned. He strictly forbade his courtiers' time-hallowed custom of pissing against the palace walls and he became a champion hoarder.

Spending and Hoarding

A typical episode of the A&E TV series *Hoarders* begins with a detailed tour through living conditions that leave healthy brains aghast ("clutter porn"). Then comes a cleaning crew (often in hazmat suits) to remove dead cats and rats, piles of trash, rotted food, and vermin. They sweep and tidy to prevent the city from condemning the property, to prevent the State from taking the children, to provide a fresh start. But all too often, as the show admits, this is not enough. If underlying problems (always assumed to be psychological) are not addressed, the hoard returns. In many of these cases, the real problem may be brain injury, unrecognized and untreated. Making a decision to keep or discard becomes overwhelming, so is postponed while the hoard grows.

Henry VIII eventually owned 60 palaces and the largest and most costly collection of tapestries in the history of the world. When he died, the Crown was essentially bankrupt.

When Mary Lincoln left Europe and returned to Illinois, she brought with her 40 trunks, stuffed with clothes both new and unworn, old and shabby. She spent hours "sorting" her trunks with such little progress that a servant quit the house for fear the floor would collapse under the weight of the hoard. Meanwhile, she wrote endless letters to Robert demanding that he return things she had given to him and his wife years before, including household goods and baby clothes long worn out or thrown away.

SHAME AND HUMILIATION

Shame can come from or lead to depression, but it can be a category all by itself.

Our brains create and shape our abilities, our past and our future, our lives. When they are damaged, it can be absolutely shattering to lose skills in which we took pride, that fed and supported our families, that identified us as *who we are*. If there are no obvious external signs of injury (and often when there *are*) it is easy to assume that a person's behavior is a matter of choice, under their control. Failure to make the right choices is, therefore, *failure*.

One may fail to manage affairs so that a home is no longer a refuge but a stress and an embarrassment. Taxes are unfiled and bills unpaid. Despite a heavy load of credit card debt, it seems perfectly reasonable to buy expensive, or needless items (like Mary Lincoln and her 300 pairs of kid gloves). It will all be paid off someday, but meanwhile, it also seems reasonable to hide problems from more functional friends or family members, who will certainly be critical and horrified. "What's *wrong* with you?" They don't know, and they can't imagine. Perhaps you can't either. All you know is that you're *wrong*.

Difficulty making good choices or carrying them out reflects poorly on the individual whose behavior may be criticized. "I often felt judged," said Marie, and if I tried to explain, my family thought I was using TBI as an excuse."

Attempting to hide shameful symptoms leads to confabulation, denial and lying, trying to re-direct attention to a fault in others, behaviors that are never good for interpersonal relationships. There's always an explanation for the most outrageous behaviors and if there isn't, it must be someone else's fault.

Sam was a promising young lawyer until injured in a motorcycle accident. Fired from job after job for various inappropriate behaviors (including failure to show up for work), his only remaining option was dog-walking. He was late or no-show for almost half of his appointments but there was always a reason. Family and friends suffered countless emergencies, grandparents died by the dozen. Thieves had broken into the car to steal his dog grooming supplies (but left the car and everything else in it).

Strangely, there is truth behind the lies. It may be truly impossible to get out of bed, to remember appointments, to find the energy or courage to get out the door, to find and organize tools and equipment — but what employer believes that? What spouse wants to? Even if they do believe, work must be done; dogs must be walked. Good will can last only so long. But for a long time, everything that is wrong may be someone else's problem, because *you* are Fine. Many people withdraw to hide their symptoms, another strain on relationships.

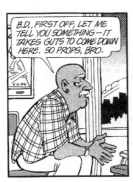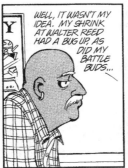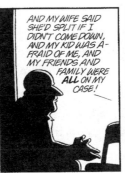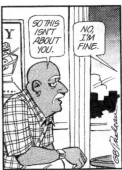

FIGURE 3-7. On Being Fine

SOCIAL ISOLATION AND LOSS OF RELATIONSHIPS

He was a 27-year-old former Marine, struggling to adjust to civilian life after two tours in Iraq. Once an A student, he now found himself unable to remember conversations, dates and routine bits of daily life. He became irritable, snapped at his children and withdrew from his family. He and his wife began divorce proceedings.

—Nicholas D. Kristof (2012)

There is much more to being alive than not dying. Life is interests, activities, and friends. TBI victims often lose these. Many isolate themselves in a room for years, the end result of extreme sensitivity to sound and light, the inability to take in words, to form coherent thoughts. Easier to just stare at the wall. After his riding accident, French essayist Michel de Montaigne mentioned poor memory and such inability to tolerate company, that he retired to the tower of his chateau where he intended to pass the rest of his life. He emerged eight years later, but only because he had kidney stones.

The mother of an injured Iraq veteran reports that her son has not left the basement in two years. A retired professional football player hasn't left his room in five. These people, and so many others, exist in a "conscious coma." Technically they are alive, but without an actual life. This withdrawal is hard for normal brains to understand. Even if crowds or noise are unbearable, surely you could have a few friends over?

Not if the energy isn't there. Think of a 100-watt light bulb — and a brownout. No matter how brightly that light *should* be able to shine, if the power isn't getting through from the power station or due to overwhelming demands, that bulb will dim and fade.

Not if you are essentially sleepwalking. Difficulty following a conversation, words, ideas can be intensely stressful. Words are too loud, too sharp, even when spoken in a normal tone of voice. More than one person speaking sounds like babble and it just makes you more tired.

Not if you're living in chaos. Even dealing with one person can be too much. A kitchen that is a pile of dirty dishes and rotting food, a room where every flat surface is covered with overdue bills and junk mail, is not the place for a quiet time with anyone. Trying to clean is overwhelming. Trying to hide it only adds to the pain and shame.

Strong men and women who lose their strength and skills, also lose their place in the world. TBI may be suspected when teams cut once-promising players, when a husband or wife is suddenly "not the person I married," when a manager can no longer manage, when you are far from the person you were and no obvious way of getting back[1].

Mary Lincoln is remembered as a shrewish madwoman, but she was far more than that. Mary left her affluent privileged life to marry a poor country lawyer whom she truly loved, to care for home and family without a flock of servants or slaves, and was an affectionate and loving wife and mother. Many historians believe the broken carriage seat (page 9) to have been an assassination attempt. If so, it missed the president, but left Mary damaged and broken in ways that impacted her family and possibly American politics for years to come (Cornelius J, Lincoln Library, personal communication, 2012).

A standard US divorce statistic is that 90 percent of marriages fail because of arguments over money and problems with debt. With TBI alone, up to 75 percent of marriages fail (Carroll L and Rosner D, 2011, p. 79). Combining lost income with the expense of treatment can be a terrible strain on a family. After her injury, said Carol,

> I was furious with my husband for not understanding what I was going through, even though I didn't understand it myself. But he had his own injuries, dating at least from our wedding day when we gave each other mountain bikes. When he rode his new bike up the steep bank in front of our house, it flipped. The back of his head hit concrete, and fluid gushed out of his ears and nose. He refused to see a doctor, swearing that he was fine. It was years before I understood that he wasn't fine, that there was a reason for his increasingly odd behavior and anger issues, and that there were *two* brains spiraling down into confusion, desperation and divorce. But I was the one who didn't understand first — and it destroyed our marriage.

---

1. *Hans Brinker* or *The Silver Skates* published in 1865 and filmed by Disney in 1962 addresses the impact of a father's TBI on his family.

LOSS OF SENSE OF SELF

Accommodation is the process of recognition, acceptance, and adjustment to a new set of limitations, in this case as a result of *minor head trauma*. It is the point at which the head injured person is able to reform his sense of self, not grasping futilely at his old self, but recognizing, accepting, being comfortable with, and building his life around a new self that incorporates a new set of capacities and limitations.

—Thomas Kay, Ph.D. (1986)

You just moved your head! Doesn't that make you happy?
— Fezzik the Giant to The Man In Black
The Princess Bride (1987)

We are our memories, the things we have done, the people we know, and the skills we have to offer. Their loss can be devastating. Suggestions that failure to accept new limits — especially before there has been sufficient time to mourn their loss — is sometimes seen as yet another personal failure by the victim. For those who have not suffered traumatic losses themselves, some imagination is necessary.

In the *Princess Bride*, The Man In Black, a superb athlete and swordsman, lies paralyzed.

Are you a musician? Imagine losing a hand, your sense of pitch or timing.

A ballerina? Imagine losing your balance, your center, your legs.

A student, researcher or instructor in an advanced and exciting field? Imagine losing your brain. And then imagine that the injury that put you in this terrifying situation is referred to as "mild." How does that make you feel?

SUICIDE

In patients who have depression after TBI, suicide is not rare.

Historically, suicide rates have been lower in the military than for the general population. However, following the Iraq / Afghanistan wars, military suicide rates are now double the rates for males in the general population (Kaplan and Others, 2009). The highest rates are in Army veterans. There is a strong relationship among TBI, PTSD, and suicide.

From 1993-2002, suicide became the leading cause of death for female veterans, and the second leading cause of death for male veterans (LeardMann CA and Others, 2013).

Concussion and Intelligence

Brain injury does not necessarily destroy intelligence, at least not to the point that we tend to associate with the concept of "Brain Damage."

While in England, after his TBI, Edweard Muybridge filed two patents: one for plate printing, another for a washing machine. Howard Hughes may have managed badly, yet made many contributions to aviation. On the other hand, intelligence can't balance out the symptoms of TBI. Table 3-4 is a log of the difficulties experienced by an intelligent and once capable college professor after injury.

Table 3-4. Professor's Log of Difficulties Upon Return to Work Life[a]

- Experiences seem often new if I haven't done them for a month or two, e.g., friends I don't recall (names and faces). Not entirely unpleasant, but distressing. Seems to be especially a problem with people I've met the past year or two, less with friends of longer standing.

- Don't know people's names when I meet them in the hall; in meetings which meet several times I can't identify people or names.

- Writing proposal, could not remember previous one . . . what we measured or found.

- Found a paper and proposal I had written just before the accident; have no recollection of having written them. They sound OK, but it's like reading someone else's work. I have to think about what's said and try to understand it.

- A few hours after I told real estate agent about a co-op, forgot that I had discussed it with him; didn't remember telling W about the notebook computer; couldn't recall I had returned call from X: he called Saturday, I returned the call Sunday, by Monday I had forgotten and called him again.

- Couldn't remember a confrontational conversation I'd had with Y a few months ago. After he mentioned it, I could only vaguely recall where it happened, nothing about what was said.

- Forgot:
  - to send attorney letter and release,
  - committee meetings,
  - appointment with the Dean,
  - teaching presentation,
  - to grade student papers and bring next essay assignment.

- Could not remember simple traffic instructions.

- Couldn't figure out how to get possessives, e.g., *earth's*: apostrophe or not? Couldn't spell *diligence*, *useful*, *repetitious*, *concentrate*, *mystic*.

- Hard to concentrate on things, e.g., review of Z's paper, kept forgetting and getting distracted. Left it for four days and forgot most of what I had thought about it.

---

a. Reproduced by permission from Table 3 in Suchoff IB, Ciuffreda KJ, and Kapoor N (2001, p. 52).

The Contagion of Concussion

TBI has long been associated with adult prisoners. The Centers for Disease Control and Prevention (CDC) found that between 25% and 87% of men and women imprisoned for violent crimes have suffered a TBI prior to incarceration. That's a big range, but even at its low end, it is about three times higher than the rate of TBI in the general population (8.5%).

—Meredith Melnick (2010)

Concussion affects life immediately but its effects may linger for years afterward, unseen and unappreciated. As we have seen, it does not affect only the person concussed. TBI can be contagious[1].

TBI brings with it inability to protect ourselves and the inability to protect others. Being unable to protect children has terrible impact on the family and the world. Raising young children is demanding at best, and even more difficult when a parent's reaction time is slowed, and memory impaired.

"It is too bad," said a young mother, "that my children are growing up brain-injured."
My memory is so bad that I've forgotten they were on the changing table, so they fell off. Once I put my infant daughter in the car seat but forgot to buckle the straps; when I had to brake hard on the Beltway she flew into the front seat, hitting the dashboard.

On the roads, people with slowed reaction times, sleep apnea or insomnia due to concussion are more dangerous to themselves and others than most of us realize. Familiar actions come to seem so innocuous that we lose all sense of risk (Diamond J, 2013). Sitting atop a missile streaking towards the city at 60 MPH would be a terrifying experience. Sitting *inside* that missile, in the form of a motor vehicle, gives us a sense of security; a false one, as we can't know about the addled guidance systems of the missiles around us whose specs are off kilter.

Adding cell phones, medications, drugs, alcohol and other distractions or impairments to an already challenged brain is a prescription for disaster.

Rear-ending the car ahead may add to your own injuries. It can also damage occupants in the car ahead, passing the injury on — and the cycle continues.

Consider concussion and violence. TBI contributes to problems with impulsiveness, anger, and judgment. Not too surprisingly, it also contributes to crime. Treating TBI and the cognitive disabilities that led to crime would be a far more effective approach than throwing the injured into prison.

---

1. Contagious: capable of being transmitted by contact; disease; tending to spread from person to person, as a disease or as contagious laughter. From Latin *contangere*, to touch.

Mild Traumatic Brain Injury Redux

> The term "mild" brain injury has shortcomings and is overly simplistic. When individuals have lost their marriage, their job, their health, and even their whole outlook on life, that doesn't define *mild* to me.
>
> —Alisa Gean, M.D. *in* Walsh N (2012)

> You keep using that word. I do not think it means what you think it means.
> —Inigo Montoya in *The Princess Bride* (by William Goldman, 1973)

A diagnosis of "mild TBI" is much like a claim of "simple surgery." It may be simple for the *surgeon*, but not necessarily simple for *you*. It should be taken seriously, but often it is not.

One problem is that diagnosis depends too heavily on whether or not the patient is *said* to have lost consciousness. Often this information comes from the victim, the same person who may have been unconscious, who wasn't really there, who was "out."

Another problem is that in standard English, *mild* means "mild," as in "minor" as in "no big deal." In TBI, it means nothing of the sort. Nevertheless, when TBI victims (especially those diagnosed with *mild* TBI) fail to recover, the patient is suspect, no matter how extreme the differences between their pre- and post-TBI behavior.

Consider an athlete who, every morning at daybreak, would leap out of bed, run to the ocean and surf for an hour before setting off to work. After a a mild concussion, he was unable to work and ended on disability, spending his days sitting numbly at his computer. He was accused of malingering — as if he would purposely have chosen to give up a joyful vibrant life in exchange for a few dollars and a life of computer Solitaire.

There are many estimates of the yearly cost of TBI. Most are based on loss of productivity due to absences from the workplace, loss of basic abilities and professional skills. At best, there is loss of income (and often health insurance) if one must take a job below one's original abilities. Health care for other family members may be delayed because all resources must go to the TBI victim There are more costs when a family member must quit work or school to be caretaker, when a person ends on disability or an entire family ends on welfare.

All of these possibilities are costly, in the now and in the future, but there is far more to it than money.

What is the cost when a parent can no longer protect or play with a child, can no longer read or help a child to learn? Imagine or remember the parent unable to be patient, unable to tolerate a child's giggles or the loud squeals of delight that every little kid should enjoy. Imagine the parent who can no longer bear the light or laugh or smile.

These are the true costs of TBI. No dollar signs can capture these losses.

What Happens in Concussion

WHERE SYMPTOMS OF TBI COME FROM AND WHY. BRAIN ORGANIZATION AND WHAT'S GOING ON (OR NOT) UNDER THE HOOD.

I n any group of humans, brain anatomy and physiology are about the same. If the group shares a common traumatic event, such as a train wreck, variations in sex, size, health, position, and direction of forces can produce injuries from trivial to catastrophic.

What happens to bodies and brains (and what will happen to them later), is different from person to person. Nevertheless, all treatment begins with classification of injuries.

Primary Injuries

In TBI, *primary* injuries refers to the "first" injury, the trauma as a direct result of the dive through the windshield, the fall from the roof or bicycle. Primary injuries are divided into "closed head" or "open head" trauma. *Closed head trauma* has no obvious break in the skull. It is generally less deadly than *open head* trauma in which the skull is cracked open, possibly with visible bone and brains. From here, injuries are further classified as *focal* and *diffuse*.

FOCAL

Focal injury is *localized* injury. It is the spot we can point to in a scan or image and say "*Here* is where you are hurt." It is the point of impact or "blow" (*coup*), it is the hematoma, it is the gunshot wound, it is local ripping and tearing of tissue.

- A *coup* injury is the site of a "blow" where an object strikes the head.
- A *coup-contracoup* injury typically occurs on the side opposite the impacted area inside the skull. The brain strikes or is struck by one side of the skull, bounces off, then hits the *opposite* side.
- *Hematoma* ("blood-swelling") is an area where blood has collected following bleeding.

Diffuse

> When brain damage is visible, as it was with . . . Phineas Gage, it's a straightforward task to correlate a specific set of symptoms with injury to a certain part of the brain. When damage to the brain can't be seen — as is the case with most concussions and even severe closed-head injuries — it's a lot harder to tie the wide-ranging, and sometimes very subtle, symptoms to the jolt to the head. Not until the 1980s would scientists begin to understand how the brain could be damaged by an injury that was, for all intents and purposes, invisible.
>
> —Carroll L and Rosner D, *The Concussion Crisis (2011)*

Focal injury may be accompanied by *diffuse* injury, which can be even more severe.

Think of a delicate flower or a spider web floating in a glass or metal bowl of Jello. When the bowl moves, the flower moves with it. If it stops suddenly because it was hurled into a brick wall at highway speeds, the Jello may slosh and shear, petals or cobweb connections may be stretched or torn. There will be far more damage than a simple dent or break in the container. Similarly, when a moving head stops suddenly, the brain keeps right on moving, possibly rotating, shifting, and compressing or horrible combinations of all of these.

Axons are the delicate spiderweb connections that link millions of individual and widely separated neurons (brain cells) into a functioning whole. When these fragile connections are stretched or torn over a widespread area, the result is known as Diffuse Axonal Injury (DAI). Symptoms worsen, seemingly out of all proportion to the injury.

Shaken Baby Syndrome is an all-too-familiar example of DAI. Adults may experience a similar result from rotational injuries in auto accidents; a common cause of DAI is the roll-over, or being spun in a car, even with no blow to the head at all.

Diffuse injuries involve damage over a large area of the brain, yet outside (and on CT and MRI images) there may be no visible damage. The explanation was long believed to be due to broken blood vessels, a break in the supply system. But then Dr. J. Hume Adams noticed dead and dying axons plugged by black tar-like balls of protein. Right next to them, clearly visible under the microscope, were *healthy* cells and blood vessels. Their presence suggested something other than a direct blow to the damaged areas. These developed hours or days after the injury. Most frightening, they appeared even in *mild* TBI (Adams JH and Others, 1982).

Forming these damaged areas did not require massive trauma.

Stretch an axon slowly and it adapts and grows. Rapid stretch is a different matter. Even minor stretching can damage *microtubules*, the delicate internal scaffolding that supports and supplies the axon and neuron.

D. H. Smith and others documented this process by placing neurons on opposite sides of a strip of thin film. When their axons had grown toward each other and connected, the researchers lightly stretched them, by bending the film with a tiny puff of air.

A stretch far too small to tear tissue was enough to leave the formerly smooth axon wrinkled and wavy, like elastic that has been overstretched, or like the contours of a parking garage after an earthquake has collapsed its supporting internal beams. Microtubules not only lost structural integrity, they dumped their loads of protein and other nutrients in a pile at the point of injury (Figure 4-1). From that point on, the rest of the axon would starve, wither and die.

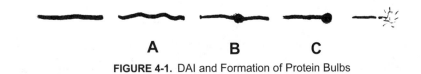

A   **B**   **C**

FIGURE 4-1. DAI and Formation of Protein Bulbs

A. Axons stretched with a tiny puff of air, enough to break the microtubule support "beams."
B. Nutrients dumped at point of injury. C. Axon from that point withers and dies.

Smith went on to prove that several very mild hits could be more damaging than a single larger impact, set the stage for Second Impact Syndrome, and explain many of the continuing symptoms of Post-Concussion Syndrome (Tang-Schomer MD and Others, 2010).

New studies of athletes playing high-school football have documented a continued decrease in brain function even without dramatic collisions. Their injuries consisted of seemingly minor, but repetitive hits. These small hits, *subconcussions*, were enough that the brain needed to adapt, to compensate in academic tasks. They were small enough that the brain learned to adapt, to accommodate — to a point. But even these seemingly minor strains, small injuries, perhaps equivalent to the damage from a tiny puff of air, were too much. The mental skills that were the birthright of these boys began to disappear, not with a bang but a whisper (Talavage TM and Others, 2013).

For serious injury, it isn't even necessary to actually *strike* the head. All that is required is a rapid acceleration or deceleration of the head (Gennarelli T and Graham DI, 1998).

That is, a simple whiplash will do the job.

WHIPLASH

A subset of the Hollywood Head Injury that does no harm is the Hollywood Whiplash Injury which also does no harm aside from triggering a lawsuit which is always fraudulent.

In the 1966 film, *The Fortune Cookie*, a football player collides with a network cameraman. The cameraman's injuries are minor, but a sleazy injury lawyer ("Whiplash Willie" Gingrich) persuades him to feign paralysis in hopes of a huge insurance settlement. This simple tale has been retold over many years in many different versions. In all of them, the supposed victim is eventually seen engaging in sports, heavy physical labor, or hauling home heavy and expensive luxury items bought in anticipation of windfall court settlements. The ending is always the same. Fraud is revealed. Truth triumphs. Whiplash is debunked.

Technically, *whiplash* is a "forced hyperextension / forced hyperflexion" injury in which the head whips too far back then too far forward. We tend to imagine this motion (and nearly all illustrations present it as) occurring in a single plane of movement (straight forward and straight back), but life is rarely that simple. A better image is the "bobble-head" moving and responding to forces from *all* directions. In either model, the forces involved can strain or tear muscles, connective tissue and other structures in head and neck. One of the internal structures of the neck is the spinal cord. Injury there is never trivial.

In the Real World of human bodies and brains, these injuries can be extremely damaging and long-lasting. They always have been. In the 1800s, *railway spine* was the term for post-trauma symptoms reported by passengers injured in railroad accidents[1]. Collisions were common and the flimsy wooden rail cars of the day offered little protection. Then as now, when there was little obvious external sign of trauma, claims of injury were rejected as fake.

At the modern ER, accident victims who have no visible bleeding or obvious impairments (that is, their CT scans show no fracture or hematoma and they can walk and talk), will be advised to "take it easy for a few days." Otherwise, they are "Fine."

Two days later the same patients may feel *terrible*. If they return to the ER, they will get "The Look" because ER docs "know" that when patients reappear after 48 hours, it is because they think there may be money in it and by now they have had time to talk to a lawyer[2].

A more likely explanation is this: *Injured neurons have begun to die.*

Another possibility is that strained and distorted structures, uncorrected, remain in strained, distorted — and painful — positions.

1. The first detailed medical study of railway spine was published in 1867 by a Dr. John Erichsen, who noticed that injuries were most common after rear-end impacts. Dr. Hermann Oppenheim, a respected German neurologist, attributed symptoms to physical damage of spine and brain. An equally respected French neurologist, Jean-Martin Charcot, dismissed them as "hysteria."
2. Personal communication from an (anonymous) ER physician.

STRUCTURES OF THE NECK

It has justly been said by one of the greatest masters of the Art of Surgery . . . Robert Liston . . . that no injury of the head is too trivial to be despised. The observation, true as it is with regard to the head, applies with even greater force to the spine.

—John E. Erichsen, *On Railway and Other Injuries of the Nervous System* (1867)

The brain does not stop at the head. It continues through the canal of the neck vertebrae in the form of the spinal cord. The neck is packed with positional sensors and nerves that convey pain and other messages to a brain that may be too traumatized to handle them.

Even minor neck dysfunction can be painful and disabling. A common example is the straight or "military neck" with loss or even reversal of the normal curve due to trauma to cervical muscles. Strangely, loss of the curve may be dismissed as "normal," despite muscle strain and nerve compression known to produce neurological problems, pain and headache.

The curve of a normal neck (Figure 4-2-A) acts as a spring. In motion, discs and vertebrae compress and rebound vertically and obliquely forward. In the straight "Military" neck (Figure 4-2-B, also slightly *reversed*), discs compress vertically with every step, leading to disc narrowing, bone spurs, and nerve compression. Figure 4-2-C is reversed at the skull. Note that even if there is minimal damage to spinal cord, brain, discs, spine and nerves, there may be significant injury to the neck muscles, producing pain and headache. X-rays do not show the subtle soft tissue damage that accompanies whiplash injuries.

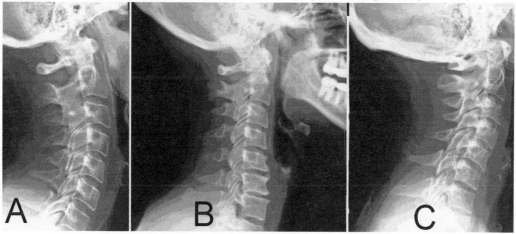

FIGURE 4-2. Cervical Curves

A Normal cervical curve, B Straight or ("Military") reverse curve, C Partially reversed.

Follow the white spots on vertebrae to see curves most clearly. In B, neck bones rise straight up from the shoulders; at the middle of the neck, the curve is slightly reversed. In C, the curve is reversed at the shoulders, normalizing somewhat towards the skull. Note the closed space between the upper vertebrae and skull compared to A and B. Courtesy Dr. Michael Karafa.

THE PHYSICS OF WHIPLASH

Today, once-invisible damage can be seen with high-tech imaging tools, but these are expensive. When victims seek reimbursement, defense lawyers often dismiss them as fakers and the medical personnel who documented their injuries as dishonest and conniving. This is especially likely if injuries are claimed from a low-speed accident, especially if the vehicle had little or no damage. Strangely, low-speed accidents can be *extremely* damaging.

Why was the plaintiff hurt so badly if the vehicle was not?

Because the vehicle was not.

We may know this instinctively. At some level, we realize that standing between a wall and an oncoming 6,000-pound SUV is a really bad idea, no matter how slowly it is moving. Yet we also believe that if the victim is sitting *inside,* the same forces are harmless. They are not.

Low-speed collisions can actually be more damaging to human tissue than high-speed crashes. At low speeds, crumple zones do not crumple. Inflatable air bags do not inflate. More rigid materials transmit more crash forces to and through the passenger; *forces on a passenger in an undamaged vehicle can be almost double those in a damaged vehicle* (Emori RI and Horiguchi J, 1990). The large mass of motor vehicles means that even slow impacts create enormous forces. And, they must be *conserved.* That is, "before" energy must equal "after" energy plus energy required to damage the vehicle. *Less* energy absorbed by the vehicle (as shown by *less* vehicle damage) means *more* energy available to damage the passengers.

In the 1970s, to save weight and gas, cars were built with light frames and plastic body parts that bent and crushed in the most trivial of accidents. This protected passengers, but prompted cries of outrage from owners and insurance companies. Now stiffer frames and bumpers protect the vehicle, leaving passengers to take the hit (Miller DB, 1996).

A woman with a long slender neck is most susceptible to whiplash injury, but men are not immune. When healthy male volunteers with healthy male necks were subjected to extremely low-speed impacts of 3.6-6.8 m.p.h., accelerometers measured forces of 10 Gs and higher (McConnell WE and Others, 1995). This was said to cause no injury, but according to another investigator (Brown C, 2000) all of the once-healthy young men later developed classic symptoms of whiplash.

Skull Bones and Fractures

We tend to think of the skull as a solid thing, like a bowling ball with a view-screen behind the eyes. In reality, it is a complex 3D jigsaw puzzle made up of 22 separate bones. Even eye sockets are not simple holes but an intricate joining of seven separate bones.

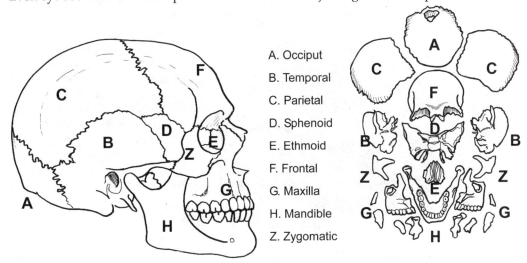

A. Occiput

B. Temporal

C. Parietal

D. Sphenoid

E. Ethmoid

F. Frontal

G. Maxilla

H. Mandible

Z. Zygomatic

The seemingly solid skull is actually made up of 22 separate bones.

FIGURE 4-3. Bones of Skull

On the inner side of the bones there are grooves and canals that hold blood vessels and nerves, and bumps and ridges that serve as attachment points for various structures.

A skull *fracture* is any break in or between the bones of the skull. Forces strong enough to break bones are certainly strong enough to damage the brain inside. Fractures can tear the meninges and blood vessels resulting in hemorrhage and hematoma, and greatly increase risk of meningitis or other infections (Dagi TF and Others, 1983). They can also damage cranial nerves. Fractures are always dangerous, but one of the most serious is *basal* skull fracture, breaks between any of the bones forming the skull base and supporting the brain. These are: the frontal, occipital, temporal, sphenoid and ethmoid.

- OCCIPITAL (FIGURE 4-4 A). Commonly injured in backward falls and able to shove other bones and structures out of position. This is one reason why a blow to the back of the head can cause black eyes and loss of sense of smell.

- TEMPORALS (FIGURE 4-4 B). The two temporal bones hold the jaw joints. It is hard to correct jaw joint dysfunctions[1] if these are misaligned. A space between temporal and occipital forms the jugular foramen.

---

1. The lower jaw (*mandible*) attaches to the temporal bone, hence shifting the temporal bone can cause temporo-mandibular joint dysfunction (TMJD), heavily involved in migraine headaches.

Chapter 4

- SPHENOID (FIGURE 4-4 D). Its name means "wedge," it looks like a bat, and it sits like a cross-beam across the skull. At its center it cradles the pituitary gland. Connects to all bones of the skull base, knocking any one of them out of position can shift the sphenoid and its connections.

- ETHMOID (FIGURE 4-4E AND FIGURE 4-6). Its name describes its texture ("sieve-like"), which in turn explains its fragile nature, the odd symptoms that come with damage, and why a broken nose may be the visible marker of an unrecognized brain injury.

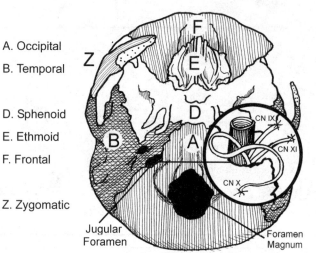

A. Occipital

B. Temporal

D. Sphenoid

E. Ethmoid

F. Frontal

Z. Zygomatic

Jugular Foramen

Foramen Magnum

A blow to the back of the head and the wedge-like occipital bone (A) can shift other bones out of place.

Jamming the occipital bone against the temporal bone (in basal skull fracture) can narrow the jugular foramen ("hole") through which the jugular vein and three cranial nerves leave the brain[1].

Inset shows jugular vein, hypoglossal nerve (CN IX), vagus nerve (CN X), and accessory nerve (CN XI).

Z, zygomatic, the cheek bone (removed at right for clarity) is not in the skull base.

The foramen magnum ("big hole") allows the spinal cord to pass from brain to neck.

FIGURE 4-4. Underside of Skull (Skull Base)

Classic signs of basal skull fracture are:

- LEAKS OF CEREBRO-SPINAL FLUID (CSF). Fluid may leak into middle ear, out through a torn eardrum, or into sinuses, or drip from nose.

- RACCOON EYES (panda eyes in the UK). Two black eyes (bruising in the orbits of the frontal bone) after a blow to the *back* of the head (Figure 4-5 A)

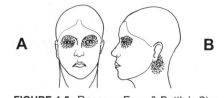

FIGURE 4-5. Raccoon Eyes & Battle's Sign

- BATTLE'S SIGN. Bruising of the rounded bump behind the ear (mastoid process), part of the temporal bone (Figure 4-5 B).

Compressing the jugular vein slows drainage of blood from the head, increasing pressure in brain and eyes (Talty P and O'Brien PD, 2005; Jonas JB, 2005). Results may range from headaches (whose victims prefer to sit up rather than lie down) to symptoms of glaucoma.

Besides loss of sense of smell, compressing or straining cranial nerves (CN) can cause a wide range of frightening effects, from severe autonomic symptoms to problems with vision, hearing, difficulty swallowing and severe headaches. The accessory nerve (CN XI) can cause spasms of muscles of neck and upper back (sternocleidomastoid and trapezius muscles), which can, in turn, trigger severe headaches.

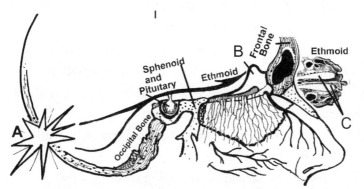

B is an exaggeration of the *crista galli* ("rooster's crest"), the bony central ridge of the ethmoid bone. Grooves on either side hold the *olfactory bulbs* (C). Holes allow odor-sensing nerve branches to pass through the bone to the nose.

A blow to the back of the head (occipital bone, A) can set off a chain of bony shifts: pressure on the sphenoid bone to ethmoid to frontal bone. Results may include shearing of olfactory nerves, damage to the pituitary, and fracture of the ethmoid with damage to its many sinuses.

FIGURE 4-6. A Blow to the Back of the Head

The following symptoms can result from fracture of the ethmoid bone (Figure 4-7).

- LOSS OF SENSE OF SMELL (ANOSMIA, "NO SMELL"*)*. The olfactory nerves (CN I) pass through the cribriform plate on the bottom of the ethmoid. A fracture or shift here can slice the nerves. Sense of taste may also suffer, in part because *taste* is so heavily based on *smell*.

- LEAKING BLOOD AND BRAIN FLUID. Breaks in the ethmoid combined with rips of the dura allow blood and/or cerebral spinal fluid to leak from ear and nose. If fluid is free to drip out, bacteria are free to come in, bypassing the blood-brain barrier and greatly increasing risk of infection, from sinusitis to meningitis.

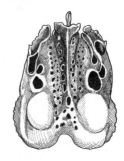

FIGURE 4-7. Ethmoid

- SQUIRTING TEAR DUCTS. If fluid squirts onto your glasses or innocent bystanders when you blow your nose, you have fractured the paper-thin portion of the ethmoid that separates the nasal passages from the tear ducts. *Avoid* blowing nose; let it drip, let it heal.

- CHRONIC SINUS PROBLEMS. The ethmoid is a bit like an English muffin; although it may appear smooth in models and surface illustrations, it is actually a complex labyrinth of holes and air spaces (sinuses). Tears and breaks can result in infections, pain and pressure.

SUTURES AND JOINTS

The major skull bones fit together along *sutures* with interlocking edges that look very much like dove-tail joints. They are joined by *fascia* (fash-uh), the tough connective tissue that links every cell of the body[1]. These fibers contribute to skull elasticity by permitting a tiny but critical amount of normal movement. Of course, *normal* does *not* describe the shifts in a head thrown through a windshield, slammed into concrete or stepped on. It does not include rippling from blast injuries, or fractures in which the skull splits open along sutures.

Movement was long dismissed on the grounds that frontal sutures ossify in childhood, and all others "by adulthood." OK, *when* in adulthood? Not until age 20-30 (for the sagittal suture), or 30-40 (coronal). The lambdoidal suture (surrounding the occipital bone) isn't expected to close until 40-50 (Schuenke M and Others, 2010, p. 7), and other ages have been reported into the 60s and 80s, when many things harden or fuse, whether they should or not.

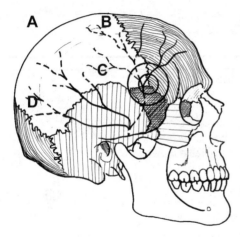

Sutures remain throughout life as zones of weakness (or movement). Skulls may fracture along these lines: (A) *Sagittal* (down center of parietal bone, (B) *coronal* (across the "crown" of the head), (C) *temporo-parietal*, and (D) *lambdoidal* suture.

The *pterion*, at the intersection of four sutures, is also known as "God's Little Joke." It is the weakest part of the skull and a major artery (the middle meningeal) runs directly underneath.

The dark "wing" is the sphenoid, the bone that articulates with every other bone of the skull base (Figure 4-4). Fracture can occur from a direct blow or by a blow to front, back, or side.

FIGURE 4-8. Pterion

Fascia is our original nervous system. It is also *piezoelectric*, meaning that it generates an electrical signal in response to pressure and strain. Throughout our lives fascia continues to send information, including pain signals, throughout body and brain. Strain on fascial fibers due to untreated distortions between skull and cervical bones can cause pain and dysfunction — especially headaches — for many years to come.

---

1. How tough? The iliofemoral ligament of the hip (which connects the thigh bone to the pelvis) has a tensile strength exceeding 772 pounds per square inch or 350 kg per square centimeter (Kahle W and Platzer W, 2004).

Secondary Injuries

Damage by a penetrating object that shatters the skull, such as a bullet or battle-axe, is not hard to understand. Others injuries are more mysterious, even to those who have them.

Damage doesn't stop with the original (primary) blow or trauma. It can continue with changes in blood flow and internal pressures.

- In *hemorrhage* there may be too much "blood-flowing" into or out of the brain.
- With reduced blood flow, the brain does not receive the oxygen it needs to function (*hypoxia, or* "low-oxygen") and toxins are not removed.
- *Cerebral edema* (swelling of the brain) can raise intra-cranial pressures to the point of *ischemia* ("strangling") of cells and blood vessels, or *herniation* (squeezing brain tissue out of a "rupture" or break in the skull). High pressures can also break the blood-brain barrier.

The most insidious damage is the cascade of chemical and hormonal disruptions that can continue for hours, days, months, or years.

PITUITARY AND ENDOCRINE PROBLEMS

Months after [he] came home from Iraq, he began having dizzy spells and radical mood swings and had lost all interest in sex. Army doctors diagnosed him with multiple brain injuries — he had endured several head-rattling bomb blasts — along with depression and post-traumatic stress disorder. But it was another symptom, the sudden gain of 50 pounds, that led to deeper investigation.

—Alan Zarembo, *L.A. Times* (2013)

Endocrine problems are relatively common after TBI, especially when there has been basal skull fracture, edema, coma, electrolyte problems, and low blood pressure, infection and inflammation. And, rather than getting *better* over time, problems may get *worse*.

The result is chronic fatigue, problems with memory and concentration, insomnia, mood disturbances, sexual dysfunction and infertility. For some people they last a lifetime and will never be resolved by anti-depressants or talk therapy.

Wilkinson CW and Others (2012) found pituitary damage in 42 percent of TBI cases they examined that were caused by blast injuries (bTBI).

HYPOTHALAMUS AND PITUITARY

The hypothalamus monitors body status and reports any necessary corrections to the pituitary gland. Together (Figure 4-9) they control the hormones behind body temperature, sexual behavior, appetites and interests.

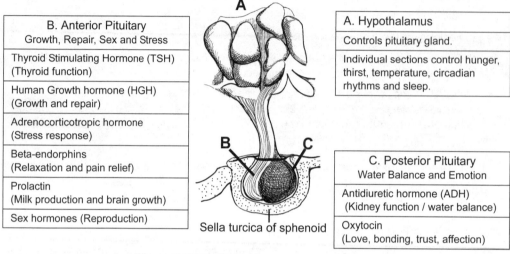

B. Anterior Pituitary Growth, Repair, Sex and Stress
Thyroid Stimulating Hormone (TSH) (Thyroid function)
Human Growth hormone (HGH) (Growth and repair)
Adrenocorticotropic hormone (Stress response)
Beta-endorphins (Relaxation and pain relief)
Prolactin (Milk production and brain growth)
Sex hormones (Reproduction)

A. Hypothalamus
Controls pituitary gland.
Individual sections control hunger, thirst, temperature, circadian rhythms and sleep.

C. Posterior Pituitary Water Balance and Emotion
Antidiuretic hormone (ADH) (Kidney function / water balance)
Oxytocin (Love, bonding, trust, affection)

Sella turcica of sphenoid

FIGURE 4-9. Hypothalamus and Pituitary

The pituitary isn't actually in the brain; it hangs below the hypothalamus like a tiny grape at the end of a slender stalk that passes *through* the dura on its way to a pit in the center of the sphenoid bone (Figure 4-6 on page 85). If brain or bone shifts in response to injury, strain on the dura can squeeze and strangle the stalk like a tourniquet, blocking blood supply and nerve signals between hypothalamus and pituitary, or pituitary, thyroid, and adrenals. The pituitary can also be squashed by high cranial pressures or even yanked out of its little "seat" (*sella*), a condition known as "Empty Sella Syndrome" (Figure 4-10).

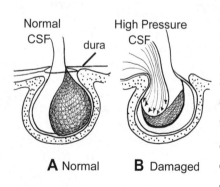

Normal CSF   dura   High Pressure CSF

A Normal   **B** Damaged

FIGURE 4-10. Empty Sella Syndrome

Endocrine disruptions after TBI have long been lumped as Post-Concussion Syndrome while ignoring the very real hormonal imbalances behind the symptoms. Papers on the problems have been largely limited to endocrinology journals. Now, growing attention to the issue has produced startling findings that help explain the brain fog, personality changes, and weight gain. After TBI, *some* chronic hormone deficiency has been found in 30 to 40 percent of selected patients. In these, *multiple* deficiencies have been found in 10-15 percent.

Brain Organization: A Peek Under the Hood

You will never ever hear anyone say "Hey! It's only a brain injury!" and yet patients, friends and families are often surprised that a concussion, an injury to the brain, could actually cause such a wide range of frightening and seemingly bizarre symptoms. Can you point to the spot on your body that is not affected by your brain?

OK, trick question. There isn't one.

Like computer software, specific program modules handle specific skills and abilities. Specific symptoms of concussion depend on the area of injury. These areas are not as localized as once thought (the brain can "rewire" itself).

For example, one advantage of learning a foreign language as an adult is that it is processed differently than language learned in childhood. A native right-handed English-speaker with damage to the left brain's language areas loses all speech. If he learned French at 30, he may still be able to speak — in French. With several languages (and depending on the severity of injury), some patients retain the language learned most recently, with other languages and skills returning as healing of connections progresses (Aglioti S and Others, 1996; García-Caballero A and Others, 2007; and Martinell-Gispert-Saúch M and Others, 1997). Temporal

THE PARTS

Like the skull, the brain is not just one thing; it is a jigsaw puzzle of parts, add-ons, apps, and the critical connections between all these pieces.

Pre-frontal: Emotional control.

Frontal: Reasoning, planning, and language.

Sensory-Motor strip: Controls muscles and sensory inputs.

Parietal: Integration of spatial and sensory information.

Occipital: Visual processing.

Temporal: Auditory cortex.

Cerebellum: Motor learning and coordination.

Brain stem: Basic life support. Breathing, blood pressure.

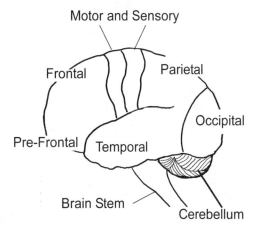

FIGURE 4-11. Lobes of the Brain

BRAIN STEM AND CEREBELLUM

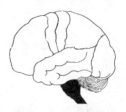

The most advanced software of our brains is built up from earlier versions just as the most advanced versions of Microsoft Windows still contain commands from DOS 1.0[1]. The brain stem is the oldest part of our human brain[2]. It contains triggers and controls for the most basic functions of life: breathing and heart rate, appetite and digestion, circulation, sexual attraction and territorial drive. A dozen cranial nerves (CN) branch off from the brain stem; these handle the basic senses of sight, hearing, taste, and emotion.

The brain stem is also involved in consciousness; un-consciousness can imply shock or injury. There is an old medical belief that with no loss of consciousness, no harm was done. Not so. One can suffer severe brain injury but remain fully conscious[3].

The *cerebellum* ("little brain" at the back of the big brain) provides balance, coordination and fine motor control. New research suggests that it may also have some cognitive functions such as attention and fear and pleasure responses. Damage to the cerebellum may cause inability to balance (even with eyes open), and impact posture and motor learning.

LIMBIC SYSTEM

Structures of the *limbic system* provide the advanced capabilities of mammals: temperature control (from the hypothalamus), memories (from the hippocampus) and emotion (from the amygdala, involved in fast, protective responses but also PTSD). Sense of smell (from the first cranial nerve (CN I) is part of the limbic system and strongly linked to memory and any of its accompanying emotions. The limbic system is often injured in abused children (Teicher MH, 2002).

CORTEX

The cortex (the "bark" of the brain), is a thin outer layer of cells, is the most human part of the brain, the last to develop, the first to be injured. Its main function is to moderate the storm of impulses bubbling up from the limbic system.

---

1. The original Microsoft Disc Operating System.
2. Commonly known as the reptile brain, a sort of Brain Version 1.
3. Part of the NFL's claim that football players suffer few or no concussions was because they counted only those resulting in *unconsciousness* (Fainaru-Wada M and Fainaru S, 2013). Players were routinely revived with smelling salts and sent back to the field; presumably those "dings" didn't count either.

Our Two Brains

> The right hemisphere functions like a parallel processor, while our left hemisphere functions like a serial processor. They think about different things, they care about different things . . . they have very different personalities.
>
> —Jill Bolte Taylor, TED presentation (2008)[1]

The two hemispheres of the brain have different functions, different specialties. They communicate via the *corpus callosum*. Without this bridge, brain and body split into two separate worlds, each reflecting the capabilities and limitations of the controlling hemisphere.

In general, the right hand (controlled by the left brain) will be unable to write a coherent sentence. The left (controlled by the right brain) will be unable to draw a simple 3-D figure. The left brain is cheerful and positive (often inappropriately so) while the right is more wary and tends towards depression.

Right hemisphere abilities are older, the right brain deals with space and interprets and creates facial expressions. With its more complex connections to the limbic system, the right brain handles emotion. The left hemisphere provides the words that describe that emotion. It is responsible for language, for splitting the hairs of time and color and sequencing, for creating an overall sense of self.

These two worlds are joined by a bridge of white matter, the *corpus callosum*.

CORPUS CALLOSUM

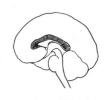

The *corpus callosum* ("hard body"), the largest white-matter structure in the brain. Its 300 million connecting fibers form the major communication cable, the "phone cord" between the two halves of the brain. The connection can be damaged in TBI. It may also fail to develop properly or be purposely cut (a desperate remedy for severe cases of epilepsy).

The resulting slowed or impaired processing can produce dramatic symptoms, many involving anger and rage. Putting words (left brain) to emotion (right brain) helps make sense of feelings and emotions. But if the message can't get through, the right brain keeps upping the signal to no avail. "Like UPS," says neuropsychologist Angelo Bolea, "it keeps on trying to deliver"[2].

A split brain is not a normal brain, but neither is a traumatized one. Distinct brain changes are visible in children who have been abused, and later, in the adults they become (Teicher MH, 2002). Changes include:

---

1. See Jill Bolte Taylor's book *Stroke of Insight*, or her presentation at www.ted.com.
2. Personal communication, November 2013.

- LIMBIC IRRITABILITY. Changes in the emotional brain, and an abnormal EEG associated with self-destructive behavior and aggression.
- LEFT HEMISPHERE DEFICITS. Smaller, less functional, leaving the right hemisphere more active than in normal brains, with problems with depression and memory problems.
- POOR FUNCTION IN THE CORPUS CALLOSUM. The connection is smaller in abused brains. This allows shift in activity between hemispheres more extreme than in normals, resulting in dramatic shifts in mood and personality.

In animals, neglect and trauma increase cortisol and decrease thyroid production. Hormone changes impact development of neurochemical and neurotransmitter receptors in the hippocampus, amygdala and other areas that control fear and anxiety. These same changes in humans may lie behind depression, anxiety, PTSD, AD(H)D, and suicidal thoughts.

Damage to the corpus callosum (due to emotional abuse and/or TBI) may also lurk behind borderline personality disorder, a mysterious condition characterized by a tendency to see things in black and white (Teicher MH, 2002). "Borderlines" typically put people on a pedestal, then see them as completely bad after some perceived slight. There may also be a hair-trigger temper and paranoia. Some suspect that the condition occurs when the two hemispheres are left to act relatively independently with the outside world, rather than interacting, moderating, and supporting each other as they were designed to do.

LOBES OF THE BRAIN

These have the same names as the bones that they lie beneath.

OCCIPITAL

Eyes may be front, but visual information is processed at the back of the brain. The occipital cortex has point-to-point mappings with the retina of the eye. Damage here can produce blindness, in spots or fields, unrelated to the eye itself.

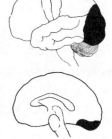

Injury in this area is typical of falls on slippery surfaces, such as skateboard and snowboard accidents, followed by loss of dreams and impaired reading ability; victims may buy reading glasses that never seem to work, even after repeated returns to the eye doctor. There may also be "face blindness." The *lingual gyrus*[1] (an area of the occipital cortex) is involved with facial recognition. Sally (page 35), hit in the head as a child, can't recognize her husband in old pictures because he no longer has that face.

---

1. It is named not for "language," but for its shape (from Latin, *lingua*, tongue).

PARIETAL

The parietal lobes handle spatial sense, providing a cognitive map of what's going on. It can tell your right from your left, is aware of body parts, touch and other sensory information. It also handles math, and in right-handed English speakers, some language skills.

The left notices differences in size and colors. Although math skills are usually attributed to the "logical" left brain only, left-sided math skills are those of arithmetic: addition, subtraction, division, multiplication. The right side handles *spatial* math such as geometry and even estimating. Both sides are involved to the extent that mathematical concepts such as calculus and ranges of numbers have spatial, as well as numerical, components.

TEMPORAL

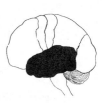

The temporal lobes are responsible for audio-visual perception and memory. The right handles visual and short-term memory (such as the fleeting memory of dreams). The left specializes in verbal and long-term memory. Together they carry the brain's "dictionary" of language as it relates to understanding words, speaking, and the emotional inflection (*prosody*[1]) of those words. They are heavily involved in temporal skills (awareness and management of time) and in *temperament*.

Violent rages are often linked to temporal lobe damage in combination with damaged or undeveloped frontal lobes. They can also be caused by tumors or cysts. Although many are asymptomatic, others are not so benign.

Louise had no sense of humor or time, and was notorious for her explosive temper. She beat her children daily, and made her husband's life (as she said at his funeral) "a living hell." Yet after her most violent rages, she would collapse weeping in remorse, unable to understand why she did these things. "I don't *want* to be like this," she would cry. "It isn't *me*." A brain scan done after a fall revealed cysts in the left temporal and frontal lobes.

Temporal lobe epilepsy can cause illusions in any of the five senses (Teicher MH, 2002). The right can also produce hallucinations of faces, such as those often seen at night before falling asleep. These images can be frightening but are not "psychotic"; they are *neurological* (Sacks O, 2012, p. 168). The right side also contains an area known as "The God Spot." It can produce feelings of spiritual connection. Activity here may produce a saint or philanthropist. It may also produce an all-knowing Jim Jones and a Jonestown.

---

1. From Greek, *prosoidía*, a "song sung to music." *Prosody* is the rhythm, stress, and intonation of speech that carries information far beyond the meaning of the word itself. In popular media, a common contrast is presented in the flat speech of robots or Coneheads versus normal humans.

FRONTAL LOBES

What we think of as "personality" is largely the creation of this most human part of the brain. Different areas handle different tasks.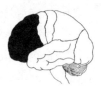

- The most frontal portion (the dorsal *pre*-frontal cortex) is the "executive" brain. It organizes, sequences, establishes priorities, makes lists.
- The area behind the eyes (the orbito-frontal cortex) handles emotional decisions.
- The area towards (but in front of) the motor strip sets the motor cortex into action.

The frontal lobes are last to develop and commonly damaged. Many believe that any trauma serious enough to produce symptoms of concussion will also damage the fragile frontal lobes. Skull bones are especially rough behind the eyes; movement of the brain across bony points and ridges can tear tissue in the orbitofrontal cortex, often with damage to the front (anterior) of the adjacent temporal lobe. These injuries result in problems with "executive function," that is, problems with organization, inability to make lists, bad or snap decisions, poor life choices, impulsiveness, and other behaviors seen as "immature." A pleasant and highly functional person may change into someone described by family and friends as "a complete stranger," fitful and aggressive, with wild emotional swings from rage to weeping, subject to inappropriate or obsessive behaviors.

After age 24, auto insurance rates for male drivers drop precipitously; frontal lobes are still developing through the teens and early twenties. This is the age of gangs, martial arts, young terrorists, and high death rates. It is also the age of military enlistees whose brains are more vulnerable to damage than adults and whose injuries may damage further development.

Damage after TBI, stroke or brain disease has been linked to OCD and hoarding. In a study of 87 patients, only 13 of them began hoarding after injury, but all 13 had damage to the orbito-frontal area (Anderson SW and Others, 2005; Brown WA, 2007). Brain imaging in patients who hoard and display OCD tendencies reveals an abnormally strong response to emotional triggers, such as the thrill of a high gamble or a big purchase on overloaded credit cards.

Researchers track this behavior with a gambling game (Shimamura AP, 2002). Players can choose a deck with cards that give rare high gains ("Win $100!" with steady losses) or a deck offering frequent small wins ("Win $5!" with fewer losses and potential of a modest win). Patients with orbito-frontal injury choose decks that offer the thrilling but rare big win, failing to notice or care that in the long run they are losing money. They choose (or can't control their craving for) risky situations. Even if they function well during the day they may lose control when fatigue sets in, one reason why late-night surfing on E-Bay can be a terrible idea.

Frontal damage may also increase artistic expression, not by increasing skill or innate ability, but by failing to suppress or edit emotions and creative ideas (Miller BL and Others, 1998).

Part 2

The Road Back

CHAPTER 5   # Evaluating the Damage

ADVANTAGES AND LIMITS OF TESTING AND WHY "NORMAL" RESULTS DON'T
NECESSARILY MEAN THAT YOU ARE FINE. WHAT SHOULD BE DONE WHEN
SYMPTOMS PERSIST AND WHO YOU NEED ON YOUR TEAM.

Better trauma care after TBI has decreased death rates but increased the numbers of survivors living with disabilities. For many, problems are just beginning. Part of this is the hurdle of tests and evaluations.

In the ER, basic tests are done, but for some, it is too soon. For example, diffuse axonal injury is not readily visible on CT or MRI and not immediately after trauma. Eventually it appears as spots (tiny hemorrhages) in the white matter. It takes time for edema or atrophy to develop. It takes time for neurons to die, which is why the person who seems fine at the ER may be in terrible shape 48 hours later. Tests done later show a bigger picture, but they must also be the right tests: X-ray, CT, and MRI show *structure*. None of these show *function*.

After the ER, symptoms that continue for more than a few months deserve a full hands-on exam: medical, dental, neurological and endocrine. Otherwise, too much weight is given to the easy but often superficial diagnosis of post-concussion syndrome.

In 1909, 10-year-old Hope was riding home from her one-room schoolhouse when her horse bolted. Hope clung on until they reached the barn. The lower barn doors were open, the upper ones closed. The horse galloped through the opening, but Hope's head and upper body slammed into the upper doors. She was torn off the horse and hurled to the ground. She was never again the merry little girl she had been before the injury. She lost her energy and zest for life. As a young woman, she suffered weight problems, depression, multiple miscarriages and endless fatigue. "I was just born tired," she would say, a history strongly suggesting endocrine disruptions. In her 60s she was diagnosed with gallbladder problems, but there was something in there besides stones — a *rib*, broken in her fall some 50 years before.

That was then, this is now. Medical care has vastly improved, except, it seems for TBI.

Over a century later, Robert was skiing when he caught a tip and flew headfirst into a tree trunk. At the ER, because he did not *remember* losing consciousness, he was declared to be "Fine," and released with a warning that he might be sore for a few days due to the severe bruising of his collarbone and chest. Ten days later he began a nightmarish two years of weekly and sometimes twice-weekly late-night trips to the ER. A history of asthma inspired treatment with ever stronger asthma medications. When those didn't work, he was assumed to be suffering seizures. Anti-seizure drugs were added with no result except their side effects of fatigue and confusion. Eventually depression and low oxygen levels were attributed to apnea, and he was fitted with a mask for a CPAP (Continuous Positive Airway Pressure) machine. This once-athletic young man could not climb a single flight of stairs without gasping for air. A physical therapist found the truth: the blow to the collarbone and inflammation of bruised upper ribs had drastically impaired breathing. Normally, collarbones rise during inhalation to allow lungs to expand. Robert's jammed collarbone, unable to rise, essentially left him breathing with one lung. The result was anoxia, with all the symptoms that brings.

On an especially wild Saturday night, Wayne was smashed in the head with a bar stool. Years of nausea, headaches, and mysterious infections were finally found to be coming from his teeth; the blow had cracked roots below the gum line, invisible to casual inspection.

After their concussions, all of these people had continuing symptoms, but only *some* symptoms deserved to be lumped into the mysterious post-concussion category. None of these people were healed purely by *time*. Proper testing and treatment of brain *and* body, could have prevented years of pain and disability.

Testing

The past few years have seen huge advances in imaging. X-ray, CT, and MRI remain as basics. Other systems are currently enjoying rapid development and new applications that reveal function help to paint a far larger and more accurate picture than ever before.

IMAGING

X-RAY AND COMPUTERIZED TOMOGRAPHY

X-ray and Computerized Tomography (CT, a computer-driven X-ray) are the two most common imaging tools used in the ER. They clearly reveal bone fractures and also show bleeds, hematomas, and fluid in facial sinuses. CT shows hemorrhage best.

Neither one shows subtle soft tissue injuries or diffuse axonal injury. Because these are invisible to X-ray, an X-ray declared to be "clear" does not eliminate their possibility.

MAGNETIC RESONANCE IMAGING

Magnetic Resonance Imaging (MRI) has long been seen as the ultimate test. But an MRI is not just an MRI; there are many *kinds* of MRI. The best for TBI is Gradient-echo MRI. What it "sees," better than others, is the iron (from hemoglobin) left in brain tissue by small hemorrhages, including those from diffuse axonal injuries.

However, if symptoms continue or new ones appear, investigation should not end with a report of "normal" MRI. There are many examples of "normal" MRIs from brains that aren't normal at all and are suffering a long list of devastating symptoms. Before Nathan Stiles (page 30) died of second-impact syndrome, an MRI indicated that everything was fine, yet autopsy revealed that he had CTE at age 17.

When symptoms don't match what appears on images, one should trust the symptoms rather than the images or test results alone.

DIFFUSE TENSOR IMAGING

Diffuse Tensor Imaging (DTI) is based on MRI technology. It tracks water as it moves through brain tissues showing damaged or broken connections in the "wiring" of the brain. Although still experimental and rarely available outside research laboratories, it holds enormous potential for showing what is really going on — or not — in an injured brain.

SPECT

Like PET and fMRI, SPECT (Single-Photon Emission Computed Tomography) provides an image of active brain function and ongoing metabolism. The system uses radioactive technetium, which emits gamma rays. It measures the rate at which different areas of the brain absorb the technetium. Specific areas that are over, or under-active can appear as dark and "cold" (or even missing) or bright and "hot."

QUANTITATIVE EEG

Quantitative EEG (QEEG, often referred to simply as "Q") uses standard EEG to record the brain's electrical patterns. The difference between traditional EEG and QEEG is that data from the client's brain is compared to a "normalized database," that is, a database of normal brains — uninjured and drug-free — of the same age[1].

---

1. Such as the database developed by Robert Thatcher, PhD. See www.appliedneuroscience.com

QEEG data is collected via a flexible cap with sensors and attached to a laptop computer. It is non-invasive, involving no contrast materials and it can be used even with infants and children. As in EEG, analysis of QEEG results assumes that distinct mental functions produce distinct electrical patterns which reappear whenever that mental function or state re-occurs (Kaiser DA, 2006, p. 40)[1]. The Q provides detailed information on what is happening then *quantifies,* shows "how much," the current state differs from the norm.

Although sometimes resisted as "experimental," QEEG research is extensive and data meets current requirements for admissibility to court[2]. Admissibility was long based on a the 1923 "Frye" ruling using the vague concept of general acceptance by the scientific community. In 1993, the U. S. Supreme Court replaced "Frye" with a new ruling ("Daubert") specifically requiring evidence based on the Scientific Method[3].

Few of us understand a raw EEG; we must trust the expert to explain its meaning. In vivid contrast, the QEEG translates data into colorful charts and graphs, such as the TBI Probability Index (Figure 5-2), a graph that allows anyone to see deviations from normal[4].

The real concern with QEEG may be that it shows too much too clearly. Defense attorneys for insurance companies, satisfied with more standard tests showing that the plaintiff is Fine, have tried to throw QEEG data out of court. A possible reason why appeared at a seminar on sports injuries.

When an attendee asked why QEEG was not being used to evaluate concussions, the question produced a definite deer-in-the-headlights response. The stammered response was essentially that QEEG is a *problem* because it shows continuing deficits. It shows that injured players do not heal as quickly as teams might wish, even after passing standard sideline tests that all too often, are intended to get the injured player back in the game.

1. The same assumptions underlie fMRI and other scans. Marked variations are seen as abnormal.
2. This applies to *Federal* courts. State courts decide admissibility individually, hence there are now "Frye" states and "Daubert" states. For a list, see: www.atlanticlegal.org/daubertreport.pdf.
3. That is, not just vague "general acceptance," but a history of hypothesis testing, estimates of error rates, and peer reviewed publications that lead to and support "general acceptance."
4. *Quantitative* comes from Latin, *quantus,* how much, how large? For a sample QEEG report, see www.AppliedNeuroscience.com. Under the Service & Workshops tab, see "Our Services."

NEUROLOGY TESTING

> One running joke on the team involved three words — Red Brick Broadway — that Pellman had players recite to determine if they were able to play after a concussion. According to Kevin Mawae, who played center for the Jets for eight seasons, "The three words were always the same. He would leave you and come back before the next series, and you'd go, "Red Brick Broadway. I'm ready to go."
>
> —Mark Fainaru-Wada and Steve Fainaru (2013)

After a TBI, victims should have at least a basic neurological exam. "How many fingers am I holding up," is not an exam. It is a joke. Very often the joke is that the coach always holds up the same three fingers. An even worse joke is the idea of having an injured player repeat a few words. Former players on the New York Jets football team report that team physician, Dr. Elliot Pellman, often allowed concussed athletes back on the field based on a standard phrase.

A more realistic field test is to have the person follow (track) a moving finger with his eyes. This is a good basic exam for head injury because eye movements require many cranial nerves. The problem is that this test is also highly subjective; problems may be missed or ignored by untrained, biased or busy examiners.

Best is a full neurological exam by a neurologist. Even then, more may be needed.

Damage to the frontal lobes is evaluated by Luria tests of focus and adaptation. These are named for Alexander Luria, a Russian neuropsychologist who correlated clinical observations with surgical and pathological findings in persons with known brain injuries. He found that those with frontal lobe lesions could not adapt to changes in programmed motor tasks. For example, a subject asked to raise his right hand in response to one tap by the examiner and left hand in response to two taps could remember the rules and respond without difficulty. But when the order was changed after several repetitions, the subject continued to raise right and left hands in the original pattern.

The following tests for frontal lobe function (Table 5-1 on page 102) are adapted from *Base Instincts* (2002), by neurologist Jonathan Pincus. Because of the importance of the frontal lobes in planning and inhibiting motor responses, abnormal results on two or three tests suggests frontal damage.

Table 5-1. Tests for Frontal Lobe Function[a]	
TAPPING	Tapping the bridge of the nose will cause blinking which should stop after 2 or 3 blinks. If it does not, subject is considered unable to adapt to new situations.
WORD FINDING	How many words can subject think of within 60 seconds? Normal is 14 (plus or minus 5). Fewer than 9 is abnormal and indicates frontal dysfunction.
TOUCH PERCEPTION	Examiner touches subject's hand and foot simultaneously. Normal subjects will notice both; abnormal clients will notice only one site being touched.
TURNING	With subject seated on a swivel chair and eyes closed, examiner places hands on subject and turns subject quickly to L and R. If head does not move, subject is considered unable to adapt.
MOVING FINGERS	Subject, while holding hands at sides, is asked to move R and L index fingers alternately and to look at each movement. After a series of movements, the subject is asked to look at the finger that is *not* moving. Difficulty suggests problems with impulsivity and inattention.
MOTOR SEQUENCING	Subject is asked to strike thigh with R palm, R fist, then side of R hand. Repeat for L palm, L fist, then side of L hand.
THIGH STRIKES	Subject is asked to strike thighs simultaneously with R palm and L fist, alternating fist and palm with each strike.
VISION TRACKING	HORIZONTAL: Subject asked to track finger movement out to 45 degrees. Abnormal if subject cannot maintain gaze or movements are jerky. PERIPHERAL: As subject looks upward, examiner moves an object side to side. —1. Subject watches object with peripheral vision (without moving eyes). —2. Subject closes eyes, sticks out tongue and holds for 30 seconds.
RELAXATION	Examiner supports client's arm or leg then lets go. In severely abnormal clients, the limb will remain suspended (*paratonia*).

a. R=Right and L=Left.

NEUROPSYCHOLOGY TESTING

> The issue of cerebral lesion location based solely on neuropsychological assessment techniques has largely been supplanted by neuroimaging methods . . . . However, neuropsychological assessment techniques remain the best descriptors of behavior and are essential to the mission of improved understanding of brain-behavior relationships. The task now at hand is to integrate the behavioral neuropsychological assessment with the various forms of neuroimaging analysis to provide a more refined understanding of human brain—behavior relationships.
>
> —Bigler ED, Porter SS, and Lowry CM *in* Maruish ME and Moses JA (1996),

> Specifically, measures often fail to capture the complexity of a real-world environment that places multiple simultaneous demands on cognitive processing.
>
> —Schoenberger N (2001, p. 272)

When patients continue to insist that they are *not* Fine (and especially when a lawsuit is involved), a neuropsychological exam may be ordered. Neuropsych tests have long been seen as the gold standard for objective evaluation of brain function, but results often depend on who ordered the test and the results they want to see. Using the tests alone is limiting, like customs agents trying to guess the contents of a closed black box with a game of 20 questions. Now, as in new airport security systems, the box can be scanned, revealing the actual contents. Imaging can add more information on the underlying biological reasons for symptoms than can traditional neuropsych (NPsy) exams alone because,

- NPsy: Processes are measured in seconds or minutes.
  Imaging: Processes are measured in *thousandths* of a second.

- NPsy: Many patients are dismissed as malingering based on "lack of effort," but there is no consensus definition of what "effort" is (Bigler E, 2009). It is a judgment call by the examiner.
  Imaging: An fMRI can't be faked. Connections communicate, brain areas light up or they don't.

- NPsy: Evaluations of "effort" cannot evaluate how hard a brain is working in order to muster additional resources, in order to cope.
  Imaging: Can show *functional* activity.

Working with TBI victims and forensic data, neuropsychologist Erin Bigler (2012) found poor correspondence between their test results and fMRI images, concluding that patients with very real neurological injuries fail tests of *effort* for neurological reasons. Patients who react slowly are suspected of *trying* to do poorly, but concussion itself causes slowed reaction time and apathy. Patients with damage to the frontal, temporal or limbic areas can become apathetic, and lose their motivation, drive, and goal-directed behaviors (Lezak MD, Howieson DB, and Loring DW, 2004). Strangely, tests of "effort" are assumed to be relatively insensitive to such injuries and to place *minor* demands on cognition; poor test results imply poor effort (Willis PF, Farrer TJ, Bigler ED, 2011, p. 1426). That is, actually *finding* certain symptoms of concussion in a patient with a documented concussion is sometimes taken as proof that the patient doesn't really *have* these symptoms; it is that he just isn't *trying* hard enough.

This is an odd assumption, especially when a big part of the problem is the testing experience itself. A professional in the field of brain injury rehabilitation with more than 30 years of clinical experience notes that some clients have appreciated the tests because they "showed me where I am." For many others, the tests provoked anxiety or were downright frightening.

1. EXCESSIVE DURATION. Tests may continue for as long as 8 hours. Is this the way to test clients with mental endurance issues? Validity of results must suffer with increasing time.
2. ARTIFICIAL FORMAT. One variable is tested at a time, through short sub-tests with a single focus. Qualitative observations of clients are not used to modify results, thus the results do not reflect function in the real-life settings where clients fail. They are not even reported from the history.
3. REDUNDANCY IN SOME TESTS, LACK OF OTHERS. Concentration and short-term memory are tested repeatedly. Others (such as delayed recall of more than 30 minutes, divided attention, writing, and social skills) are often ignored.
4. MEASURES OF EFFORT AND VALIDITY ARE NOTORIOUSLY WRONG AND INVALID. Reading over 100 questions and filling in the little boxes is hard on the subject's eyes, comprehension, and endurance. Yet if they do not or cannot finish, they are accused of lack of effort.
5. PRIOR FUNCTIONING IS RARELY CONSIDERED. Tests results are compared to an approved population of matching educational background, not to what the subject could do prior to injury. Yet even persons with the same apparent educational background vary tremendously in skills and abilities. Dismissing loss of advanced skills because the subject is now "average" ignores potential loss of income and can also lead to a devastating loss of sense of self.
6. VOCABULARY AS A MEASURE OF PRIOR ABILITY. Vocabulary is not necessarily preserved in TBI.

Neuropsych testers are also constrained by guidelines in presenting a realistic picture of post-concussion changes. This is especially true of "effort."

How much can the examiner miss? A lot.

Neuropsychological assessment of brain injury is sometimes challenging, especially when identifying cognitive deficits in people who were high functioning and with superior intelligence prior to injury. Most contemporary neuropsychologists focus on tests of language function such as Verbal Memory and Executive Function. If a person has superior before-injury function in this area, their after-injury scores may show in the "Average" range. They may be assessed as "normal," completely missing the prior superior function — and its loss. Additional tests[1] can provide a more complete picture of brain injury. One such test is the Tactual Performance Test.

—Angelo Bolea, Ph.D.

---

1. Including Muriel Lezak's Neuropsychological Assessment, the Luria and the Halstead-Reitan tests.

Morgan, a brilliant scientist, won a hotly contested position out of 3,000 candidates — then she tripped and fell down a flight of stairs.

The first neuropsych exam declared her to be average, although she had never been that before; exceptional, superior, outstanding, and awesome, yes, but never *average*.

Dr. Bolea added the Tactual Performance Test. The seated client is blindfolded, then asked to fit a series of shapes into the corresponding

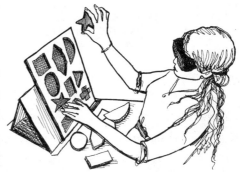

FIGURE 5-1. Tactual Performance Test

holes in a wooden board (Figure 5-1). This is essentially identical to children's toys that teach shape matching.

The entire test should take 15 minutes, but 30 minutes later, Morgan had been unable to fit any of the shapes into their holes. She couldn't even find the board directly in front of her. At times her hand was up in the air beyond the board or even behind her head. Dr. Bolea's diagnosis: Subcortical Brain Dysfunction and Bilateral Posterior Dysfunction, completely missed by the neuropsych examiner and the MRI.

Morgan was also given a QEEG (see page 99) comparing her brain function against a database of normal, uninjured brains. Results showed a 99.5 percent probability of TBI.

A. Bell-shaped curve showing normal brain function. The solid line shows where most uninjured human brains function.

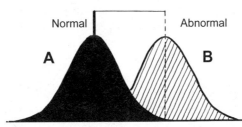

Normal   Abnormal

A   B

B. Morgan's brain function (dashed line) is offset from "normal" by a large amoun' Probability of TBI is 99.5%

FIGURE 5-2. Morgan's QEEG Showing Probability of Brain Trauma

Neuroimaging and QEEG are a shift towards examining actual neurobiological processes. But, neuropsych testing should not be abandoned. Ideally, all these tools should work together, with compassion and understanding of TBI, awareness of previous abilities, and with consideration of the aftermath of difficult and frustrating symptoms.

BLOOD TESTS

Is there actually a blood test for TBI and its symptoms? There may be.

MARKER PROTEINS IN TBI

On comparing 787 TBI patients with normal controls, researchers found a strong link between mild TBI and two proteins appearing in their blood: S100B and apoA-1[1]. The study was done *pro-actively*, that is, testing whether a blood test could *predict* what would show up on CT scans. Measuring the two proteins proved to be a highly accurate, highly predictive test for TBI (Bazarian JJ and Others, 2013). They present the possibility of an objective diagnosis that may even be able to predict future healing. ApoA1 is not specifically a brain protein; it does housekeeping and repair. The higher the pile-up of damaged neurons, the higher the levels of ApoA1 that converge to help with clean-up operations.

The idea of biomarkers has come up before. Because serum S100B rises with damage to the nervous system, it has been used in Europe and Asia to screen patients *before* doing CT scans. The US, however, has long relied on the notoriously untrustworthy reports of concussed patients and witnesses (who may have arrived after the injury), which is why "most of the time," says Jeffrey Bazarian, an ER doc, "I'm guessing" (Walsh N, June 21, 2013). In contrast, this research may add an important tool to the diagnostic toolbox and reduce the need for many CT scans, a source of radiation to the brain, and a major ER bottleneck.

ENDOCRINE DYSFUNCTION

Tests revealed damage to [the soldier's] pituitary gland. It was a rare finding in the military, but that may be because few doctors have been looking for it.

—Alan Zarembo, L.A. Times (2013)

Even "mild" TBI can damage endocrine function. Growth and sex hormone imbalances are most likely; thyroid and adrenal deficiencies are less so but equally devastating. There is little relationship with severity of the TBI, but problems are most likely in patients who developed diabetes insipidus and electrolyte abnormalities (Tanriverdi F and Others, 2011). Signs of endocrine dysfunction (including low body temperature and weight gain) may earn no more than a basic TSH test. If it appears "normal," blatant physical symptoms may be ignored.

Endocrine damage can heal on its own. Only 3-6 percent of TBI patients with known endocrine problems continue to show deficits for more than a few months. Some policy makers

---

1. S100B (a calcium-binding protein) is found in glia and astrocytes, components of the white matter of the brain. It rises after damage and breakdown of these structures. ApoA-1 (apolipoprotein A1) transports high-density lipoproteins (HDL, "good" cholesterol, the primary component of neurons).

have argued against standard screening because these percentages are low. However, for the person who has them, the rate is one hundred percent and life can be hell.

Hormones are the very stuff of life. Their dysfunction results in an increasingly poor quality of life that has long been attributed to post-concussion syndrome but investigated no further[1].

In adults, symptoms can linger for a lifetime that ends before it should. In children and adolescents, *all* hormones can be affected, disrupting puberty with poor growth and sexual development that may persist five years after injury (Rose SR and Auble BA, 2012). These lives are damaged before they really begin.

The US military can no longer ignore endocrine issues. Blast injuries are especially likely to produce endocrine problems because of the raised intracranial pressures involved in explosions. Table 5-2 shows current DCoE recommendations for endocrine testing (DCoE, 2012). Testing is not done immediately after injury, but should be scheduled if symptoms remain for more than 3 months and if new ones appear up to 36 months after injury. Referral to an endocrinologist is advised if lab results suggest endocrine dysfunction or *even if they do not but symptoms remain* after other possible causes have been excluded.

Table 5-2. Endocrine Testing Recommendations by DCoE		
Hormone	**Symptoms**	**Test**
Growth Hormone	Loss of lean muscle mass and strength, weight gain with increased body fat around waist, reduced heart rate, low blood pressure, poor memory and concentration, fatigue, depression, anxiety, constipation, and decreased sex drive.	IGF-1 (Insulin–like Growth Factor)

Gonadotropin Deficiencies:
  Testosterone, Estradiol
  Luteinizing Hormone (LH)
  Follicle Stimulating Hormone (FSH)
	Infertility, anemia, hair loss, decreased muscle mass and strength, amenorrhea and mood disorders, loss of libido.	Males: Testosterone
		
		Females: Estradiol, LH, FSH.

Adrenocorticotropic Deficiency	Low blood pressure, weight loss, malaise and fatigue.	Morning Cortisol levels (<12 mcg/dl)
TSH Deficiency	Weight gain, cold intolerance, poor short-term memory, constipation, and dry skin.	TSH and Free T4

1. Perhaps another example of the need to rethink classifications of TBI severity.

Roadblocks

Webster was often laced with a varying, numbing cocktail of medications: Ritalin or Dexedrine to keep him calm. Paxil to ease anxiety. Prozac to ward off depression. Klonopin to prevent seizures. Vicodin or Ultram or Darvocet or Lorcet . . . to subdue the general ache. And Eldepryl, commonly prescribed to patients who suffer from Parkinson's disease.

—Greg Garber (2005)

There are no currently FDA-approved medications for the long term treatment of psychiatric symptoms due to brain injury.

—Taber KH and Hurley RA (2009)
Defense and Veterans Brain Injury Center (DVBIC)

TBI patients are told that their status one year after the injury "is as good as you're going to get." This is partly because time and drugs (on which our medical system relies so heavily) have thus far failed to show good results in healing cognitive symptoms. By necessity, therapy has long focused on helping clients to accept the injury and the loss of sense of self, and to deal more gracefully with enduring pain and disability.

This is a reasonable approach if nothing more can be done, but, for many injuries, the idea that nothing more can be done is no longer true. Healing from TBI can be a long and difficult road, but is often worse than it should be. Problems often begin with failure to recognize that an injury has occurred at all — even in the ER.

POOR ASSESSMENTS

Although mild TBI is one of the most common neurologic disorders, its evaluation and management are not formally taught in medical school or residency programs. . . [it] is considered an unpleasant clinical exercise that is neither intellectually compelling nor associated with academic rewards, while too often associated with litigation. Thus, TBI patients are cared for by neurologists, internists, or family physicians who received no instruction in their care during residency programs or by neurosurgeons who are "too busy" to care for them in their private practices. Consequently, old myths persist and patients return to work, school, or competition earlier than advisable. The neuro-forensic implications of this situation can be devastating for patients.

—Roberto Masferrer, Neurologist (2000)

When dealing with a brain-injured person it is extremely important to remember that one is dealing with *a person whose brain is injured*. Memory and perceptions can be wildly unreliable. Nevertheless, this information, deeply flawed though it may be, drives the diagnosis, future treatment, legal and insurance issues.

Most TBI victims rescue themselves rather than being retrieved by others. If they know they were unconscious, they probably have no idea how long. No matter how long they were "out" they may not remember ever having been unconscious at all. In essence, patients are required to self-diagnose, to describe what happened when their brains were switched OFF. When they try to answer, the actual event may be unavailable to memory and mis-reported; the jostled brain is an unreliable reporter yet most concussed persons are asked about their symptoms while they are in that incompetent state. Symptoms may also be dismissed or misinterpreted.

At the ER, Carol was diagnosed with a basal skull fracture. The young physician who did follow-up had never heard of "raccoon eyes," the classic sign of basal skull fracture. He did ask about problems with sense of smell; she said she had *not noticed* any. On that basis he dismissed the ER diagnosis and insisted that she "admit" that her husband had beaten her, blackening both eyes (but failing to injure nose or face in any way). The implication was that she would not be treated until she told the truth and only the one he wanted to hear. Several days later, she was sitting at the kitchen table trying to read the newspaper when her husband burst into the kitchen screaming, demanding to know what was going on. With her back to the stove, she hadn't noticed the smoke and stench of dinner burning just three feet away. He smelled it from the other end of the house.

Neurologically, sudden loss of sense of smell is as significant as sudden loss of vision. Because the physician did not test her sense of smell, that symptom, unnoticed by the patient, went unrecognized.

There are other ways to test an impaired sense of smell short of burning down the house. Commercial test kits are available, but a quick home check can provide valuable screening. After a TBI, a sudden inability to tell the difference between a whiff of lemon or lime, coffee or chocolate (or to smell them at all) is far more meaningful than a claim that everything is "Fine" — especially when that claim is untested, and especially when made (cognitively speaking) by a person who *wasn't even there*.

LIMITS OF UNDERSTANDING AND TECHNOLOGY

A physician fell off a roof, but despite the memory problems, confusion, depression and job difficulties that followed, he denied any concussion. Why?

"Because I never lost consciousness," he said.

"You most certainly did!" said his wife, "that's why I called 911. And when you woke up you thought you were in Hawaii!"

"Nice place to wake up," said the therapist.

"Oh," he said, now remembering for the first time. "Oh! That's what the EMT said."

For far too long, TBI has simply been misunderstood — by nearly *everyone*. A striking feature of Chris Nowinski's book on TBI, *Head Games*, is how long it took him to find good information about his symptoms because even his physicians were at a loss. Many TBI patients receive little or no exam beyond "Can you touch your nose? Can you follow my finger with your eyes?" Important information, but more is needed.

An EEG may be done but limited to a brief check for seizures. If there are no seizures *during* an EEG (never mind *after*), you're Fine.

"Nothing seen on the MRI" is often confused with "Nothing is wrong." But standard MRIs show *structure*. They do not show *function*, nor does it follow that continued problems are imaginary. Actual damage may be revealed only at autopsy, too late to help the patient.

Inner ear damage too tiny to be seen on MRI or CT scan can cause disabling vertigo and vision problems. Even when an underlying TBI is recognized, traditional treatments have had limited success in restoring function. Many baffled therapists blame the patient.

- To a patient with reversed cervical curve after whiplash: "Maybe you were just born that way."
- To an 11-year-old boy kicked in the head resulting in hearing loss: *"Malingering."*
- About a child who suddenly developed explosive temper and problems with impulse control after falling from a tree: "It can't be brain injury because he didn't have amnesia afterwards."
- To a soldier thrown 30-40 feet resulting in crushed vertebrae, a two-inch loss of height, non-stop headaches and inability to read: "Your problems are all psychological."
- To a formerly high-level executive with extreme post-TBI sensitivity to light, sound, and motion, who could no longer drive, read, or do math: "You lack motivation."
- Per a 10-year-old girl whose fall from playground equipment resulted in concussion and constant headaches: Insurance would not cover physician's fees "because," explained the nurse serving as medical contact, "a concussion is not a medical condition."
- To a woman suffering from post-concussion depression after a fall: "You just need to get more exercise." At the time of her injury, she was training for the Marine Marathon.

People with any or all of these symptoms and living in terrible pain and confusion have been told: "You need to get out, exercise, get a job, get a grip. You're Fine!"

On Being Fine

> "Fine!" said Troy Aikman[1].
> "Fine!" said Steve Young.
> "Fine!" said Wayne Chrebet.

Even among physicians, it is commonly (but wrongly) believed that if there was no loss of consciousness, then no serious harm was done.

Some doctors have told patients after a fifth concussion or a two-week coma, "It's OK to go back, you're Fine." Dr. Pellman, the infamous "Dr. Yes" (the *rheumatologist* put in charge of the neurological health of NFL players), became notorious for his claims that it was perfectly safe for a concussed player to return to the same game. In 2003, Wayne Chrebet was knocked out by a knee to the head. "I'm fine," said Chrebet and, with Pellman's blessing, staggered back onto the field. After that game, Chrebet never played again.

Many believe they are Fine despite obvious injury. Others *say* they are Fine, but more as a social convention than anything approaching medical accuracy. A victim of a head-on car crash had tumbled out of the wreck and was sitting dazed on the curb when a harried EMT asked her how she was. "Fine," she said politely. After loading up other victims who were actually bleeding, the ambulance crew drove off without her. She now sits alone in her basement apartment, unable to work, on disability, chronically depressed and morbidly overweight. She was not fine and she hasn't been fine since the accident.

"The first rule," notes neurologist Peter Dunne, "is this: *Do not allow a TBI patient to decide he/she is Fine*. This is true for all trauma and illness. Some people exaggerate symptoms, but others minimize them, something a lot of people apparently don't understand."

> The number of patients I have seen over the years having a [heart attack] (especially men) who say: "Oh, it's nothing, just a bit of indigestion," is frightening. Especially with TBI, the culture (football, hockey, paratrooper, and certain national cultures) may promote minimizing. I know of cases, back to when I was in Vietnam, who died because they said they were Fine. They were believed and allowed to wait or were turned away from care that might have saved their lives.
>
> —Peter B. Dunne, M.D.[2]

A fascinating example of Fine-ness based on superficial appearance appeared on a blog about a newly discovered image of Phineas Gage. As one reader observed, it is a Rorschach test for perceptions of the individual viewers.

---

1. All three careers were ended by head injuries (Carroll L and Rosner D, 2012, pp. 29, 75). For the Wayne Chrebet story, see Keating P (2006).
2. Personal communication, 2013.

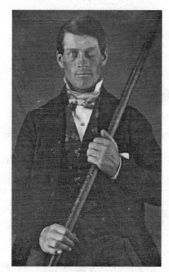

FIGURE 5-3. Phineas Gage

Many questioned whether this man could actually be brain damaged when he was *so handsome and so nicely dressed.* Many handsome corpses go to their graves nicely dressed, but that does not mean they can hold jobs or be sociable. Some saw reports of Gage's poor post-injury behavior as a symptom of the eternal class struggle between the working man and management. But Gage's contemporaries were observing distinct post-injury personality changes in a man well known and once highly regarded by all. They were not addressing social hierarchy, economics, or freedom of speech. When a doctor reports cleaning a wound so severe that "half a tea-cup of brains" falls out, his concern is neither philosophy nor economic theory.

Afterwards, the brain injury may still be very real, but it may not be visible. Invisibility brings its own difficulties. Many therapists refuse to believe or to treat a patient who may profit from a lawsuit based on dysfunction. No matter how poor the trade-off, the patient is suspect. This is especially true if symptoms can't be seen by others.

And then, even if the symptoms you *claim* to have are actually *real*, well what did you expect at your age anyway?

Whatever you expect, maybe now you can expect much *much* more.

Today, new treatments and new technologies can help a brain to heal in ways that time alone cannot.

CHAPTER 6 # Helping a Brain to Heal Itself

BIOFEEDBACK AND NEUROFEEDBACK IN TREATING SYMPTOMS OF
CONCUSSION AND OTHER CONDITIONS. THE HISTORY AND RESEARCH
BEHIND THEM, HOW THEY WORK, AND WHAT HAPPENS IN A SESSION.

Biofeedback is a process that enables an individual to learn how to change physiological activity for the purposes of improving health and performance. Sensors track brainwaves, heart function, breathing, muscle activity, and skin temperature. These instruments rapidly and accurately "feed back" information to the user. The presentation of this information — often in conjunction with changes in thinking, emotions, and behavior — supports desired physiological changes.

—Joint Statement on Biofeedback by AAPB, BCIA, ISNR (2008)

iofeedback is an umbrella term for techniques that help improve relationships between brain and body in order to promote health and well being. A simple biofeedback device is a *mirror;* it allows us to change hair or clothing to a more desirable state.

Traditionally, biofeedback techniques in which sensors are applied to the head have been known as *EEG biofeedback* or, more recently, as *neurofeedback.*

A mounting body of clinical evidence documents their powerful positive effects, showing that *they can modify the activity of the brain and ease the symptoms of TBI.*

Interesting claim. But is it true?

It is.

The Electric Brain

One of the problems with the current drug paradigm is the attempt to fix *everything* wrong with your earth vehicle by pouring yet another chemical additive into the gas tank. Sometimes this works, but sometimes the problem is not the gas; sometimes it is the fuel line that provides the gas. Sometimes it is the tires or their alignment.

Sometimes it is the electrical system. Like other computers (and the rest of the body), the brain gives off tiny electrical impulses. Brainwaves are the products of neurons turning on and off. These are detected by an EEG (Electro-Encephalo-Gram)[1]. A raw EEG can be filtered and split into different frequencies. The four most commonly recorded by clinicians are known as *alpha, beta, delta* and *theta*[2]. Different brainwaves have different characteristics ranging from the fast high frequency beta waves needed for quick thinking, to the long slow delta waves typical of deep, restorative sleep.

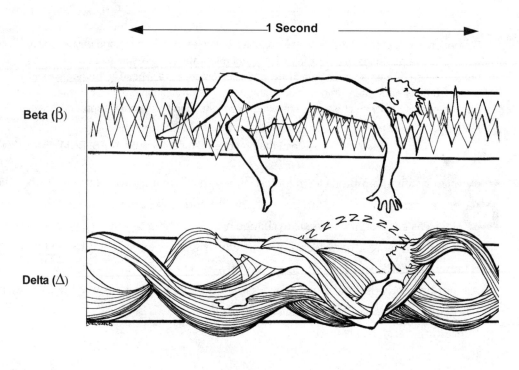

FIGURE 6-1. Brainwaves and Sleep

1. Literally "writing by the electricity in the head." Comparable to the ECG (Electro-Cardio-Gram, formerly EKG or Electro-Kardio-Gram) which displays "writing done by the electricity of the heart."
2. The Greek letters *alpha (α)*, *beta (β)*, *delta (Δ)*, and *theta (θ)* were assigned to the different wave patterns, roughly in order of their discovery (not speed).

No brainwave is *good* or *bad*. What matters in the brain and in any successful team — whether business, ball games or band — is balance, timing, and appropriate interactions. Imagine a concert in which the violins are constantly overwhelmed by the trumpets, or the delicate notes of the harpsichord are drowned out by the bagpipes.

Per function, you might think of brainwaves and frequencies in terms of how many balls you can (or need) to keep in the air while juggling the demands of daily life. Restful sleep requires strong slow waves; fast ones lead to insomnia (Figure 6-1). During waking hours, fast response and multi-tasking require strong fast waves (Figure 6-2); excessively slow ones bring fatigue and "brain-fog."

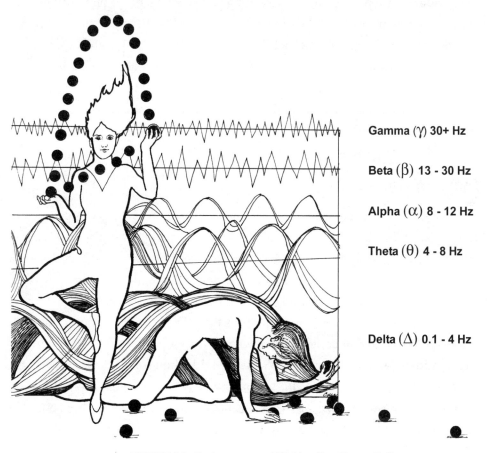

Gamma (γ) 30+ Hz

Beta (β) 13 - 30 Hz

Alpha (α) 8 - 12 Hz

Theta (θ) 4 - 8 Hz

Delta (Δ) 0.1 - 4 Hz

FIGURE 6-2. Brainwaves and Waking Function or Fatigue

Brainwave Changes

> An adult should not have theta or delta patterns in the waking record and if they appear, they are called *slow wave abnormalities*. The slower the frequency and the more often it appears, the greater is the degree of abnormality. Abnormal slow waves appear when the brain cells are damaged regardless of the cause of the damage.
>
> — Hughes JR (1994, p. 15), *EEG in Clinical Practice*

Brainwaves change in response to changing requirements. For example, rats respond to errors with a burst of low-frequency (below 12 Hz) brainwaves to the medial frontal cortex. Destroying these areas destroys ability to adjust after errors (Narayanan NS and Others, 2013).

When brains are injured, when there is bleeding and swelling, blood and nutrients are decreased leading to a hibernation-like state referred to as *EEG slowing*. While the brain is stuck, behavior cannot change. Dr. Michael Tansy likens this to having a great car but, the windows are mostly blacked out, it has only one gear, and can make only *right* turns.

Like the car that cannot self-heal, a damaged and hibernating brain can't necessarily wake up without help. Neurofeedback is like AAA for the brain; it can wake it up, get it "unstuck," back on track and on its way.

100 Years of Research

Research on the electrical behavior of the brain began as soon as there was equipment available to record it. One of the earliest research tools in psychology was the *galvanometer*, used to measure change in electrical resistance of skin in response to stress. This is known as the Galvanic Skin Response (GSR) or Skin Conductance Reaction (SCR), first described by Russian physiologist Ivan T. Tarchanoff in 1890. It was used by Freud and Jung who read lists of words to their patients. Words and questions that triggered GSR responses pointed to areas to be addressed in that patient's treatment.

In 1915, graduate psychology student William M. Marston found that GSR changes when people lie[1]. This was the origin of the *polygraph*, named for the "many" physiological changes it tracks and "graphs" in subjects, including heart-rate, breathing, and GSR, that is, the basis of modern biofeedback systems for health and healing.

In 1924, Hans Berger recorded a human brainwave, *alpha*, also known as the *Berger rhythm* (Figure 6-3).

---

1. In some venues this became the lie detector. Marston later created the comic book character Wonder Woman whose magic lasso forces villains to tell the truth.

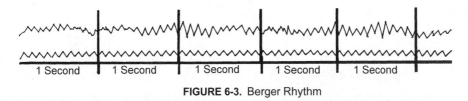

FIGURE 6-3. Berger Rhythm

The top line is a burst of alpha and beta. The lower line is a 10 hz reference. After Berger H (1929).

In the 1960s, at the University of Chicago, researcher Joe Kamiya found that subjects could learn to recognize when their brains had entered an alpha state, and, to produce alpha on demand. His research brought the phrase "alpha state" into common use.

In the 1970s, at the Menninger Voluntary Controls Laboratory, Elmer and Alyce Green researched biofeedback and neurofeedback effects for treating stress-related conditions including those from cancer treatments. Working with an Indian yogi, Swami Rama, they documented his ability to produce atrial flutter at will and to change temperature by 11 degrees F between two spots on opposite sides of the same hand. He had learned to do this by visualizing one spot getting red (for increased blood flow and heat) and the other blue (reduced flow and cold). A first rule of all forms of biofeedback is: The faster and more accurate the feedback of information, the faster the learning. Using biofeedback monitors, an intern learned to do in two weeks what had taken Swami Rama 10 years to master[1].

Meanwhile, Dr. Barry Sterman studied brainwaves in cats while they were still and alert, waiting to pounce on food presented at random. Their *alert stillness* (calm in brain and body) produced a rhythm of 12-15 Hz (cycles per second) over the sensory motor cortex. This rhythm is known as Sensory Motor Rhythm (SMR). The next step was to teach the cats to enhance SMR. When they did, they were immediately rewarded with a squirt of chicken broth and milk; the cats learned to produce that specific rhythm in abundance. Results were published in the highly respected journal, *Brain Research* (Sterman MB and Wyrwicka W, 1967).

---

1. The Menninger Voluntary Controls Laboratory (in Topeka, Kansas) was associated with the Menninger Clinic but closed in 1994 when the clinic closed. The current-day Menninger Clinic is a standard psychiatric facility in Houston, Texas. It has no relationship to the former research facility.

Epilepsy

Shortly after, NASA asked Sterman to study hallucinations and seizures in workers exposed to rocket fuel. When exposed to rocket fuel, *most* of the cats suffered severe seizures, *but not those remaining from the SMR study.* Learning to change their brainwaves had raised their resistance to seizures. That is, SMR biofeedback had very real physiological effects. Would this work in humans? In 1971 Sterman began training a young woman afflicted with gran mal seizures[1] since falling off a horse as a child. A year later she was declared seizure-free and had a driver's license. Epileptics will know how very unusual this is, but these results were repeated in other subjects and published in *Epilepsia*, the leading peer-reviewed medical journal for epilepsy (Sterman MB and Macdonald LR, 1978). In the study, 6 of 8 patients reported significant and long-lasting reductions in seizures.

Attention Deficit and Hyperactivity Disorder

> Sterman's paper said there is a brain wave frequency known as SMR that may be dysfunctional in epileptics, and when that rhythm is partially restored, a resistance to seizures occurs. As soon as I read that, I said, "My God, I think this will work for controlling hyperactivity in children because the circuitry is very similar." If you could quiet the motor responses for epileptics, then quieting the motor responses in hyperactive children should be a piece of cake.
>
> —Dr. Joel Lubar quoted *in* Robbins J (2008, p. 136)

On reading Sterman's reports on epilepsy, Dr. Joel Lubar suspected that Sterman's findings might apply to his work with hyperactive children. They did. As Lubar's hyperactive children trained with biofeedback, their symptoms disappeared. And, as had happened with Sterman's epileptics, when subjects were given random feedback or trained in the opposite way, problems returned.

Benefits have been repeatedly documented over the years and yet "no research" is still a common claim. *No research* is a far cry from *not reading the research that exists.* In reality, there is enough solid neurofeedback research that in 2012, the American Academy of Pediatrics included biofeedback as a "Level 1 Best Support Intervention"[2]. That is, *not only has biofeedback [neurofeedback] been found effective for AD(H)D, it is recommended as a primary option* (AAP, 2010).

In July 2013, the Food and Drug Administration (FDA) approved a system that helps diagnose AD(H)D in children and adolescents by comparing the ratio of theta and beta

---

1. "Big Bad" in French, now known as "Generalized Tonic Clonic Seizures (GTC)."
2. For the category of "Attention and Hyperactivity Behaviors," Level 1 AAP recommendations begin with Behavior Therapy and Medication and *Biofeedback*," however, the studies cited by APA are actually *neurofeedback* studies.

waves. Children with AD(H)D tend to have stronger theta waves than normal children. Approval was based on a study of 275 children (ages 6-17) with attention or behavioral issues. Patients were evaluated with the Neuropsychiatric EEG-Based Assessment Aid (NEBA) to calculate the ratio of theta to beta brainwaves, plus a battery of standard tests including DSM-IV criteria, behavioral questionnaires, IQ tests and physical exams. Independent experts then reviewed the data to reach a consensus diagnosis of AD(H)D or another, separate condition. Compared to traditional clinical assessments alone, diagnosis was more accurate when theta to beta ratios were also considered.

The test takes 15 to 20 minutes, and is intended to supplement information from the medical and psychological exams to confirm an AD(H)D diagnosis or guide further testing (US Food and Drug Administration, 2013). This may sound very new and cutting edge, but FDA approval is actually for the device, *not the technique*. Dr. Mary Jo Sabo was evaluating AD(H)D by measuring theta to beta ratios and effectively treating AD(H)D nearly 20 years ago.

In 1990, a mother was at her wit's end in dealing with a severely ADHD child. When she heard of neurofeedback, she brought her son to Dr. Mary Jo Sabo. Nothing else had worked, but soon his mother began to notice changes at home and school. The improvements fueled a growing conviction that this treatment should be available in schools. Linda Vergara, an assistant principal at the Enrico Fermi School in Yonkers, New York, asked Dr. Sabo to start a pilot program. And so began the famous Yonkers Project on neurofeedback in school kids.

THE YONKERS PROJECT

Dr. Dennis Carmody, Psychology Professor at St. Peter's College, volunteered his services in setting up the research design using an educational model to evaluate children through parent, teacher, and student input. Dr. Mary Jo Sabo, school psychologist Jim Giorgi, and Dr. Sabo's staff of Biofeedback Consultants Inc., did pre-treatment testing[1]. Each child received a neurofeedback evaluation with a mini-brainmap documenting the ratios of beta to slower brainwaves (theta and delta). They purchased two computers with printers; treatment space was found in a small book storage room. Children were recommended by their teachers, then staff met with their parents who were overwhelmingly enthusiastic.

The program began with 16 children. Eight would receive 40 treatment sessions. Another eight, who served as controls, were wait-listed. They would have their chance the following

1. Tests included McCarney teacher and parent forms, TOVA, and Piers-Harrison Self Esteem questionnaire. Tests were given pre-, mid- and post-neurofeedback training. Systems used were Neurocybernetics, CapScan, and Peak Achievement Trainer. "We didn't have Heart Math in those days," notes Dr. Sabo, "so we played baroque music."

year, but Vergara was so pleased with results that she placed 20 more children in the program that first year. Technicians worked from early morning until the school closed at 6:00 pm.

In most cases, the positive results began to show up after 20 sessions. Behavior improved. Impulsive and oppositional children became less of a challenge in the classroom. Grades went up. Parents began reporting that children were doing better at home.

All of this happened in an inner-city school under the most unlikely conditions. Despite its lofty name, Enrico Fermi School for the Performing Arts and Computer Science had a population of children from hard working families that were struggling to keep their children off the streets of tough, drug-filled and extremely dangerous neighborhoods. "One morning when we came to work," reports Jim Giorgi, "we had to step over the chalk outline of the body of a man who had been murdered in front of the school building."

The first eight were the children who, out of a school of 1,000, were the most disruptive, the ones who made life most difficult for themselves and others[1]. Kids like "Joe." At age 10, Joe tried to drown a cousin in the bathtub. At recess, he wasn't allowed out to play with other children; he spent most class time in the principal's office. Eric, a child of alcoholic parents, being raised by a 17-year-old sister, would hide in the closet. But with training, violent children become calmer, classrooms became quieter, gang leaders calmed down. "Teachers would ask us to train them earlier in the morning," recalls Dr. Sabo, "so they could have a more peaceful day."

Eric and Joe both began to return to the classroom. Eventually, the worst that Joe could be accused of was being involved in a cafeteria food fight in fourth grade. He was not drained of life as can happen with AD(H)D drugs; his personality remained, but he was no longer the surly, hostile child he had been before. He was able to pay attention, able to learn and grow. Five years later, in junior high school, he spoke on local Public Television presenting his own testimonial to the value of the treatment. "It saved my life," said Joe.

Eventually the program expanded to School #9 and School #13. Both reported the same inspiring results as those seen at Enrico Fermi. But the upshot of this pioneering program for school children was *cancellation*. Despite the pleas of parents and teachers to School Boards, the small amount of public funding was seen as too much; it was needed elsewhere. After the program ended, Dr. Sabo was contacted by many private schools, but treatment was lost to the very children who needed it most and who were most unlikely to get it privately.

Too often, the dollars for 21st century, non-medicated, non-invasive help for children with issues just don't fit the budget.

---

1. These were fourth graders (ages 9 to 10). By 1995 we were admitting children as young as preschool because we found they responded so quickly. — Dr. Mary Jo Sabo

Biofeedback and Neurofeedback

In my opinion, if any medication had demonstrated such a wide spectrum of efficacy it would be universally accepted and widely used . . . [Neurofeedback] is a field to be taken seriously by all.

—Frank H. Duffy, MD (2000)

Neurofeedback is a kind of biofeedback. Information coming from a sensor placed on the back of the neck is known as *biofeedback*. Information from a sensor placed an inch or two higher, on the back of the head, is called *neurofeedback* and focuses on brain activity, or more specifically, on signals coming from the brain.

There are now two basic approaches to neurofeedback: "traditional" and "passive."

TRADITIONAL NEUROFEEDBACK

Traditional neurofeedback is an active learning process. It teaches your brain (typically below the level of consciousness) to recognize, control and work with your own brainwaves, to restore and repair vital brain activity. Using only their brainwaves, patients have been taught to play games ranging from PAC-Man to rocket ship races (keeping the purple ship out in front of the red one). Traditionally, the reward was a light or tone or game points. Newer systems offer a video or movie; as long as a brain remains focused, on task, the movie plays. When the brain loses focus, the video fades.

What is common to all these systems is that the brain gradually learns to function with more appropriate and productive cognitive and emotional responses. This occurs unconsciously and automatically so we engage appropriately in real life situations.

PASSIVE NEUROFEEDBACK

Different forms of noninvasive brain stimulation techniques harbor the promise of diagnostic and therapeutic utility, particularly to guide processes of cortical reorganization and enable functional restoration in TBI.

—Demirtas-Tatlided A and Others (2012)

Newer neurofeedback systems change EEG patterns in a different way. Rather than actively focusing on rocket ships or space aliens, subjects sit quietly with eyes closed while being treated with brief pulses of extremely tiny electromagnetic signals. It is like tickling the injured brain awake with a feather or a gentle whisper compared to the baseball bat of drugs or surgery. Their tiny signals are barely above the background noise of our surrounding electronic soup, smaller than those put out by cell phones, small enough to be in the range found to be involved in healing and regeneration of tissue (Becker RO, 1998). They are so very tiny that a common skepticism is that any positive results must be due to placebo effect. There is ample evidence that something else is going on.

- The literal meaning of *placebo* is "I please." Medically it refers to an improvement or cure due not to chemistry or physiology of intervention (such as a pill or surgery) but to *expectations*. The pill can be bitter, unpleasant, and still have a placebo effect. Clients with TBI may experience headache or fatigue during or after the *first* treatment, possibly with startling (but small) somatic recall of the original trauma (see page 129). Long term outcomes are the documenting evidence that symptom improvements are not due to *expectation*. Hence, while treatments aren't necessarily "pleasing," neither are the results imaginary.

- Teenagers (often resistant), small children (unaware they are being treated), and disabled persons (lacking the impulse control and focus that would enable them to train with traditional neurofeedback techniques), nevertheless have significant changes in symptoms and behavior.

- Explosive behaviors have normalized.

- Treatment requires no effort or attention from the client, but often is completed more quickly than Traditional Neurofeedback. Positive results can appear within 3 - 6 sessions, with more appearing over the following sessions.

There are advantages to both traditional and passive approaches. Both work miracles for some, but not for *all*, simply because biofeedback can't do *all* that may be needed.

Neurofeedback does not replace appropriate medical care or psychotherapy.

It can't provide the nutrients missing from a terrible diet.

It won't work well if there is an active chronic infection or parasites.

It can reduce spasticity and relax muscles caught in flight-or-fight loops of stress and tension, but it does not repair scar tissue or remove adhesions. It won't correct bad posture that inhibits breathing and reduces blood and oxygen to muscles and brain.

You can move a person very effectively by tickling him with a feather, but not through a locked and barred steel door. That is, the feather won't work if bones are misaligned or jammed too tightly to allow proper neurovascular function.

Clients who fail to recover fully with neurofeedback (especially those who were hit in the head with a windshield or a planet) may need direct, hands-on bodywork to correct structural problems that can block improvements.

Nevertheless, neurofeedback alone has restored cognitive function, and relieved pain and depression after TBI.

A Brief history of the Flexyx Neurotherapy System (FNS)

In ancient Greece, depressed patients were treated with light flickering on their closed eyes through slits in a rotating wheel, a treatment revived in the 1900s (Sievers D, 2007). In 1993, researchers Carter and Russell found that learning-disabled boys treated with two (alternating) speeds of sound and light enjoyed improved function on intelligence tests, achievement tests, and behavior as rated by parents and teachers (Carter JL and Russell HL, 1993). Carter and Russell's work led Dr. Len Ochs to modify J&J Engineering equipment to link brainwaves to feedback frequency. That is, the client's own brain (rather than the therapist) controls the feedback. The complete system was known as Flexyx Neurotherapy System (FNS).

In 1994, Dr. Esty, intrigued by Dr. Ochs' reports of clinical results, purchased the J&J device for personal testing and later for clinical application. In 1995, she told Adriane Fugh-Berman, MD (at the new NIH Office of Alternative Medicine, now NCCAM) about the unusually positive effects of FNS on TBI symptoms. Fugh-Berman sent Dr. John Spencer to observe Dr. Esty's clients with TBI symptoms. "We are funding many treatments, but this is the first *new thing* I have seen," he said.

Because of Dr. Spencer's visit, Dr. Esty was asked to accept an NIH grant with Kessler Rehabilitation Hospital to treat TBI using FNS. One study participant, with post-TBI fibromyalgia, was able to return to full-time work after 10 years of disability. She persuaded a friend in Chicago (also with post-TBI fibro) to visit Dr. Esty and give neurofeedback a try. This woman had been disabled for 30 years, but after FNS treatment, she recovered so rapidly that her family, thrilled to have her active again, awarded a $1,000,000 grant to Chicago's Rush-Presbyterian-St. Luke's Medical Center to do a study with Dr. Esty. Wanting to do more, the family also funded, at Dr. Esty's suggestion, a systems test of J&J Engineering's I-330-C-2 device at the Lawrence Livermore National Laboratory[1]. To the best of our knowledge, FNS is still the only such system that has received outside clinical research funding.

Many readers have asked why Dr. Esty continues using FNS, now an older system no longer available commercially. It is because the research presented here continues and because good researchers don't change equipment during the course of a study, and because its effects have been carefully documented. In treating symptoms of TBI, PTSD, learning and mood disorders, FNS was — and still is — reliable and effective.

---

1. Lawrence Livermore engineers measured the tiny electrical signal carried through the cables to the scalp. It was less than what is present in other devices now in use. Some biomedical people feel that smaller signals are more effective. Greater result from lower power correlates well with Dr. O. Becker's pioneering research on tissue regeneration and "the current of healing" (Becker O, 1998).

How Does It Work?

The answer is that we don't know. Sorry, but this is what research is about: if we knew the answer, we would be *historians* rather than scientists. What we do know is that everything you have ever seen, heard, felt or thought was experienced by neurons in your brain, which is a natural miracle in and of itself.

—Susana Martinez-Conde and Stephen L. Macknik (2013, p. 4),
Barrow Neurological Institute, Phoenix, Arizona

One lingering criticism of neurofeedback is that we don't know the mechanism. But that is a work in progress as are so many other issues in brain research. For example, it was long believed that, unlike every other cell in the body, adult human neurons did not divide. The cells you were born with died off with age. Adding stress, illness, or too much beer would speed the aging process; it was all downhill from there.

In the 1960s, Dr. Joseph Altman, of the Massachusetts Institute of Technology (MIT), showed that adult mammals — rats, cats, and guinea pigs — form new neurons (Altman J, Das GD, 1965). His results were dismissed. In the 1970s, Michael Kaplan found neurons giving birth to new neurons in the visual cortex, the olfactory bulb, and hippocampus, not only in rats but in primates. His evidence was scorned and attacked.

In 1989, Elizabeth Gould, investigating the effects of stress on rat brains, found neuron degeneration and death in the hippocampus. She also found healing. "At first I assumed I must be counting [the neurons] incorrectly," Gould said, because, as everyone knew, neurons don't divide" (Lehrer J, 2006). On reviewing earlier studies, Gould realized that this was no mistake: it was real, a fact long resisted in favor of established dogma (Gould E and Others, 1989; Gould E, 2007). It changed the paradigm. It also laid the groundwork for understanding depression, and how anti-depressants work or don't work.

In 1998, Peter Eriksson and Fred Gage demonstrated the ability of the hippocampus to make new neurons throughout adulthood (Eriksson and Others, 1998). Thanks to these and other investigators, we now know that at least some brain areas can regain function on their own. This supports the concept of regeneration and of *neuroplasticity,* the ability of the brain to alter its pathways and synapses following changes in behavior and environment or after injury.

Feedback therapies seem to help neuroplasticity. How they do this is not yet known. Even if we don't perceive it, the brain responds in some way to every input, whether chemical or electrical, whether from Prozac or from light, "even," noted Dr. Ommaya[1], "a single photon."

---

1. AK Ommaya, personal communication, 1996.

Concussion and Neurofeedback

The Dalai Lama said that meditating for four hours every morning is hard work; if electrodes would give the same outcome, he would be an enthusiastic volunteer.

—Reiner PB (2009)

Neurofeedback has been highly effective in treating symptoms of mild to moderate TBI and PTSD in civilians and veterans. A 2001 study, funded by the National Institutes of Health, looked at participants injured 3 to 21 years earlier. All had completed rehab; no further improvements were expected. Dr. Esty provided passive neurofeedback treatment (FNS) in collaboration with the Kessler Rehabilitation Hospital.

Protocol included 25 treatments, pre- and post-neuropsych evaluations done by a Kessler neuropsychologist who was blinded to the subject's condition — either active or wait-listed. After treatment, and despite their bleak prospects, 7 of the 12 participants returned to their previous levels of employment or study. In the 2012 study, more positive results were again reported in Iraq/Afghanistan veterans with debilitating TBI and/or PTSD[1].

But biofeedback and neurofeedback are still considered (if considered at all) to be "alternative" or "experimental." The sticking point seems to be astonishment at the notion that brains or behavior can be altered without drugs, although it is well known that light, sound, music, and even thoughts and activities (in cognitive behavioral therapy) can change neural pathways. Neurofeedback of all kinds often produces positive results more efficiently than other therapies, but it is often the last resort, tried only after other treatments have failed. Ignoring current research and clinical successes (including the AAP pronouncements on AD(H)D), at least one "quack buster" website keeps biofeedback and neurofeedback on its list of Questionable Treatments. Grudging admission that they do actually work is followed by speculation that equally good results could be had without the electronic equipment.

The same can be said of flight simulators. It is possible to learn to fly without them, but they provide fast, safe and effective results, without the troublesome crashing and burning. When Swami Rama (page 117) returned home to India, he brought with him thousands of dollars of biofeedback equipment. Obviously the traditional yogic training techniques work quite well (eventually!) but by using the electronic equipment, "I can teach my students quickly what it took me many years to do."

---

1. Results of both studies (Schoenberger NE and Others, 2001 and Nelson DV and Esty ML, 2012), were published in peer-reviewed journals. Such successful outcomes led to Dr. Esty's ongoing treatment study with the Department of Defense Traumatic Injury Research Program of the Uniformed Services University of the Health Sciences (USUHS), the US military medical school.

Getting Started With Neurofeedback

At Brain Wellness and Biofeedback Center of Washington (BWB), medical specialties referring clients for neurofeedback include neurologists, psychiatrists, internists, rheumatologists, neurosurgeons, psychologists, nurse practitioners, chiropractors, osteopaths, speech pathologists, vision therapists, neuropsychologists, social workers and counselors.

Two Institutional Review Boards (IRB) oversee BWB's two ongoing military studies: Chesapeake Research Review, Inc. and the IRB of Sam Houston State University.

Intake and Treatment

FNS neurofeedback evaluation begins with a detailed history and a functional map of the client's brainwave activity.

INTERVIEW

Clients are asked to rate their main symptoms on a scale of 1-10. They are also asked to recall injuries and stressors that may contribute to the presenting symptoms. When asked about concussion or traumatic events, most are dismissive of what happened to them. Many will protest that they weren't unconscious "for very long" or that, if they were, they were in the hospital "only for a few days."

Often, with discussion, they begin to remember other injuries. They begin to realize that falling from a second-story window or a hit hard enough to make them miss school or work almost certainly involved a concussion, and that a concussion is a brain injury.

> **Note: Dr. Esty and the staff at Brain Wellness and Biofeedback (BWB) do not recommend any medication decreases, and urge clients to consult their physicians about changes in any medication. Medical supervision of medication levels is always recommended; all medication decreases must be medically supervised.**
>
> **However, physicians have often referred patients to us *because* they need to reduce medications.**

FNS Brain Mapping

Mapping involves recording brainwaves at standard sites; these are based on the International 10-20 System, a reference grid for the brain (Figure 6-4). Sites are scrubbed to remove oils and dead skin; a conductive paste is applied to improve the signal. Two of three sensors stay in place. While the client sits quietly in a comfortable chair, the therapist moves the single active sensor, recording for a few seconds at each site. The resulting map (Figure 6-5) shows current brainwave behavior, reveals imbalances and helps guide treatment.

Sites for mapping are guided by the International 10-20 System.

(A) shows the 10-20 sites seen from the top of the head.

(B) shows some of the same sites on a head.

Sites left of the Z-line are odd numbered. Those to the right of the Z-line have even numbers.

F = Frontal lobes
C = Center line (ear to ear)
Z = Zero line (front to back)
P = Parietal lobes
T = Temporal lobes
O = Occipital lobes
A = Aural (ear)

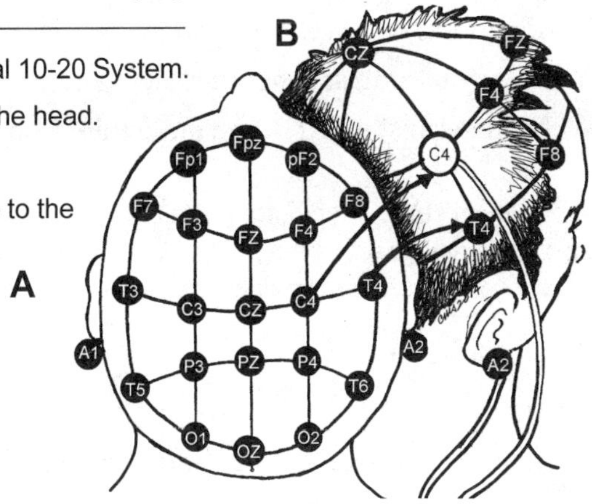

FIGURE 6-4. Brain Mapping

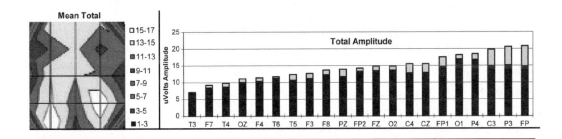

Brainwaves are graphed as if the head were a square with nose at top (as in Figure 6-4A).

Brighter colors indicate stronger power and amplitude.

Bars represent power (in microvolts) and should be about even. The light cap on top of the black bar shows variability (or "wildness") of neuronal firing.

This excerpt, showing extremely high amplitudes, suggests a problem. See Color Section for samples of complete maps before and after treatment.

FIGURE 6-5. Map Excerpt

Maps can also provide valuable clues for further diagnostic workup. When a young boy's teachers insisted that he be put on Ritalin®, his mother brought him to Dr. Karen Schultheis, hoping that neurofeedback could help the apparent AD(H)D and perhaps his episodes of "blanking out." But the boy's map was highly unusual, with extreme activity in all bands, *not typical* of AD(H)D and suggesting a serious problem. Dr. Schultheis referred him to a neurologist who immediately scheduled a scan and found a tumor.

Mapping alone has halted family meltdowns. Because she had been so fatigued, scattered and disorganized since her accident, Marie and her husband were on the verge of divorce. When her husband saw her map he was amazed.

"You mean she isn't doing these things on purpose?" She was not.

> For the first two years after my injury, my husband was in so much denial (even as he complained about all the things I was having trouble with). He was stunned when my EEG results showed abnormalities; he began checking my gas tank and filling it for me.
>
> —Marie

TREATMENT

Treatment is non-invasive and painless. The patient sits comfortably, eyes closed, and physically quiet. FNS treatment requires no attention, no effort by the patient. Guided by symptoms and the client's map, the therapist applies sensors to different sites. These detect electrical signals coming from the brain and feed back a tiny signal. The patient notices nothing from the sensor — but the brain does.

The computer (via the sensors) analyzes the speed of the strongest brainwave, and then feeds back a new signal at a different speed. Brains respond to rhythmic patterns, a phenomenon called entrainment. As analogy, think of a brainwave slow-dancing in time to slow, soulful music.

The system identifies the strongest peak brainwave in the last second, and responds with a pulsed electromagnetic wave at a higher or lower speed, as appropriate. The new signal is also rhythmic, but different than before. It is like moving from a slow waltz to a samba, or from a mad run to a quiet stroll.

In either case, the brain controls the response. It continues to respond and change with its dance partner, the computer, without conscious effort.

Results

The late Dr. Ayub Ommaya[1], neurosurgeon and TBI researcher, believed that FNS triggered a change in dysfunctional neurotransmitter function. "It is the only way," he said, "that I can explain the rapid changes I have seen in my TBI patients."

—Ommaya A, personal communication (1996)

Results of FNS treatment can be immediate, with more improvements appearing over time. As in physical therapy and massage, neurofeedback may also trigger somatic recall, a small version of the physical sensations associated with a past traumatic event.

SIDE EFFECTS AND SOMATIC RECALL

Most people have no uncomfortable side effects. The ones that do appear are brief and usually occur only after the first and second treatments. Some concussed clients may have a headache or feel sleepy after a first treatment perhaps because those are the two most common symptoms after a concussion. Any discomfort is always less than that of the original trauma and fades quickly. This can happen whether treatment is months or even decades after the trauma. Sensations are specific to the traumatic event. For example,

A 50-year-old man fell 20 feet onto concrete fracturing tibia and fibula, crushing his ankle, and resulting in concussion with loss of consciousness. At his first treatment he felt ankle and leg pain from the breaks 11 months earlier. Immediately after the second treatment, the insides of his arms began to burn, apparently a flashback to a car crash 5 years earlier when his air bag had deployed stripping the skin off the insides of both arms. The sensation lasted 5 minutes and then was gone.

A plane crash survivor, during his first session, smelled smoke and felt pain in his ribs where his briefcase hit him during impact. He then began to shiver with the sensation of the extreme cold he had felt while lying on the ground after jumping out of the plane. After treatment, he reported each of these sensations in the order they had occurred 20 years before. Within 20 minutes the sensations faded away leaving him calm and relaxed.

A two-year old girl fractured her occipital bone in three places when she fell backward onto a steam radiator. As a 70-year-old woman, she reported having always had an extremely poor memory for people she should have known well. She also spoke in a high-pitched child-like voice. Her first FNS treatment triggered a headache (unusual for her) and an astonishing change: her voice was suddenly that of an adult. The childhood voice never returned.

---

1. In 1985, Dr. Ommaya, as Chief Medical Advisor for the Department of Transportation, commissioned a report on brain injury from the Institute of Medicine (IOM). This report, *Injury in America*, led to the creation of the National Center for Injury Prevention and Control within the Center for Disease Control and Prevention (CDC).

SIGNS OF HEALING

As healing progresses the symptoms of brain injury begin to fade. Common changes (depending on the specific injury) include:

- Increased energy.
- Regained or improved pre-injury ability to do things easily and effortlessly.
- Awareness of clutter and improved organization (the "Cleaning Symptom").
- Improved sleep.
- Return of ability to remember dreams.
- Return of a complex sense of humor.
- Awareness of personal hygiene.

Positive effects remain unless or until there is a new trauma.

In the next chapter we present many brain injury experiences. Best of all, we will talk about actual healing and recovery with one form of neurofeedback: FNS.

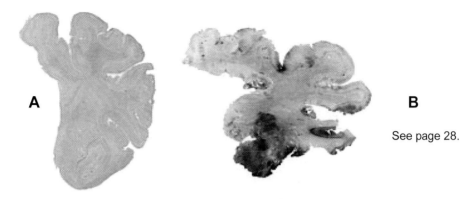

A   B

See page 28.

FIGURE C-1. Tau Staining and CTE.

A. Tissue from a normal brain (65). B. Tissue from brain of John Grimsley (45) retired NFL linebacker. Photo courtesy of Ann McKee, M.D., VA Boston / Boston University School of Medicine.

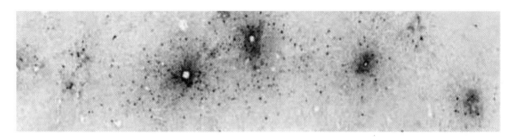

Peri-vascular tau (deposited "around the vessels") in a soldier (45), with blast injuries. White matter is also peppered with auto-immune bodies.

Photo courtesy of Lee Goldstein, M.D., Boston University School of Medicine. See page 28.

FIGURE C-2. Tau Proteins and Immune Response Staining.

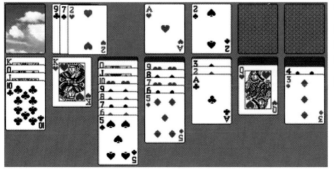

This "simple" game requires focus, sequencing, color recognition, matching, memory, and hand-eye coordination (page 39).

Players must finish in:

135 seconds for 5000 points,

120 seconds for 6000 points,

110 seconds for 7000 points.

High scores are impossible for a player who can't remember numbers or colors, doesn't see cards at the sides, must check stacks individually for a match, or is slow in dragging cards from stack to stack.

FIGURE C-3. Computer Solitaire as Memory Test.

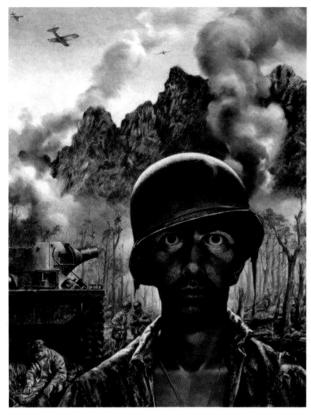

FIGURE C-4. Flat Affect.

Marines Call It That 2,000 Yard Stare, by Tom Lea (1944), *Life* Collection of World War II Art.

Lea's real-life portrait of an exhausted young Marine at the 73-day Battle of Peleliu popularized the military term for "flat affect."

See page 55.

Courtesy of the Army Art Collection, US Army Center of Military History.

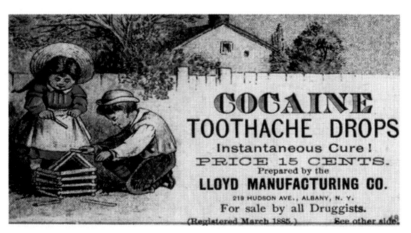

Addictive cocaine and opiates (laudanum and morphine) were standard treatment for pain in Mary Lincoln's day. This ad ran in 1885, several years after her death. See page 60.

FIGURE C-5. Cocaine for Kids.

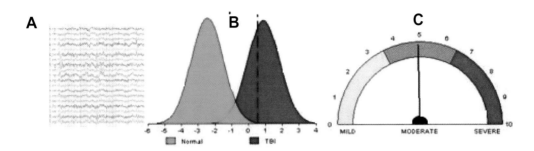

FIGURE C-6. Standard EEG Compared to QEEG.

A. An EEG shows the electrical signals of the brain. B. QEEG / computer-generated evaluation of the same information. Normal brain function is at left (green). Red (at right) shows deviation from normal, with a 99% probability of TBI. C rates the probable TBI by severity, in this case, "moderate." See "Quantitative EEG" on page 99.

Imbalances in specific brainwaves are associated with specific symptoms. High-powered levels of theta as compared to beta (the "theta to beta ratio") have long been associated with AD(H)D, a symptom which overlaps with TBI. QEEG shows many other relationships. Theta:beta ratios are just the beginning.

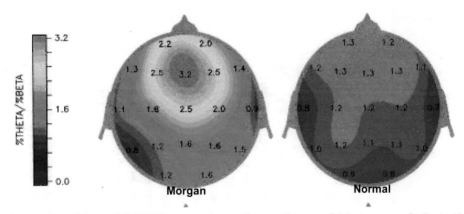

This image, from "Morgan's" QEEG report, shows abnormally powerful theta waves (indicated by warm colors) compared to low-power theta waves (indicated by cool blues) in the normal brain at right. Numbers indicate microvolts. Morgan's MRI was "normal" and her symptoms dismissed because her distinctly abnormal brainwaves were *invisible* to standard MRI imaging which does not show *function*. See page 105.

FIGURE C-7. QEEG: Theta To Beta Ratios.

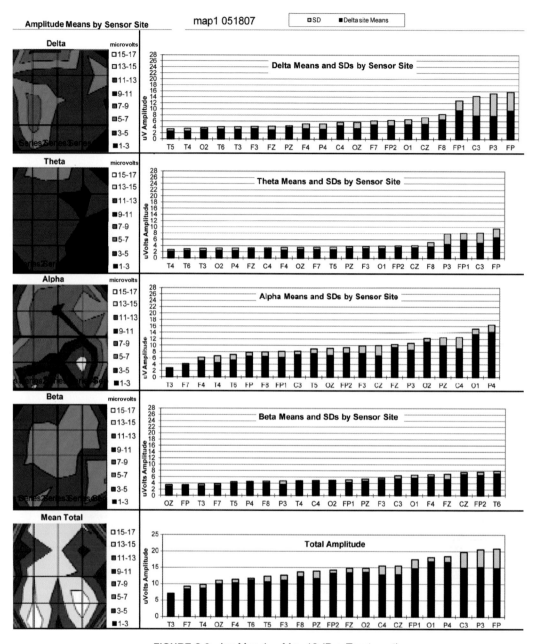

FIGURE C-8. Jay Map 1— May 18 (Pre-Treatment).

See page 127. Brighter colors indicate stronger power and amplitude. Significant imbalance in power among the bands correlates with a wide range of symptoms. Bars should be roughly equal. This map was made on intake on May 18. Notice the high amplitude slow waves especially in the alpha and delta bands. Some amplitudes shown at bottom are "white hot." Compare this map with Jay's symptoms (page 151).

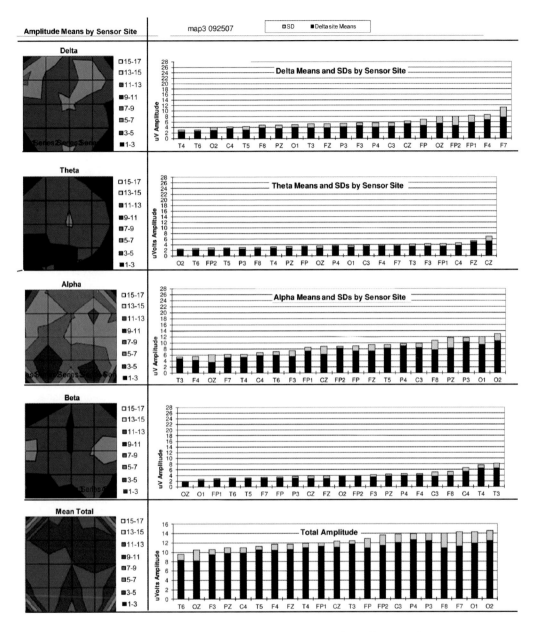

FIGURE C-9. Jay Map 2 — September 25 (Post-Treatment).

See page 127. This map was made at the end of the standard 25 FNS treatment sessions — and after additional injuries including a skull fracture. Yet despite another TBI, surgery, and severe sleep apnea (untreated until later), Jay's symptoms did not worsen, they continued to improve, a testament to the resilience that often appears with neurofeedback treatment.

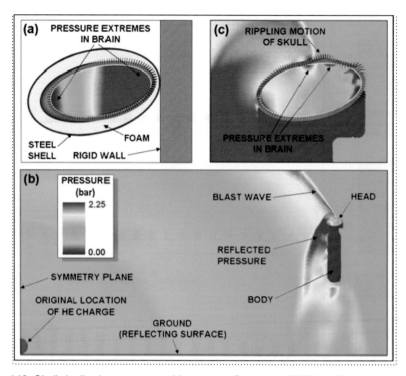

See page 148. Skull *rippling* in response to blast wave. Courtesy of William C. Moss and Michael J. King (Lawrence Livermore National Laboratory), and Eric G. Blackman (University of Rochester).

FIGURE C-10. Blast Injuries and Pressure Gradients.

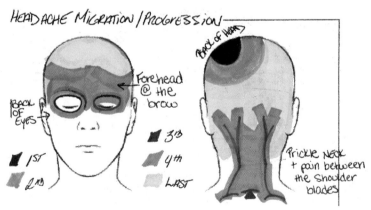

Where a headache *starts* is a clue to its *origin*. This progressive pain pattern, drawn by a chronic headache patient, suggests the splenius muscle or the nerve that supplies it. See page 191.

FIGURE C-11. Headache Progression.

Personal Choice of Most Problematic Symptoms
Average Ratings
(0-no problem; 10=severe problem)

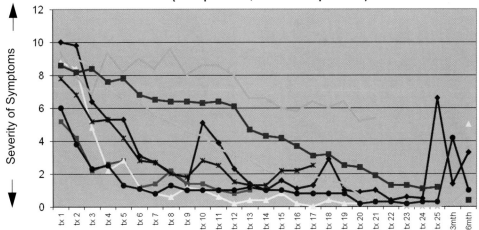

FIGURE C-12. Changes in Major Symptoms Reported by Study Participants.

Sessions 1 through 25 with 3- and 6-month follow-ups for 8 veterans. Several suffered new trauma at study end or during follow-up, but even then, symptoms did not return to pre-treatment levels. See page 150. See also Figures C-8 and C-9.

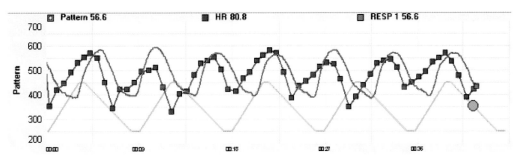

FIGURE C-13. Heart-Rate Variability (HRV) and Breath Training.

The blue line shows breathing rate which should correlate with heart rate (shown by red line).

Before breath training there was no relationship between the two lines. As the client learned to breathe at his "resonant breathing rate" (about six breaths per minute) breathing and heart rate synchronized. This promotes ANS balance and flexibility which helps body and brain adapt to demands. It triggers cellular repair, regrowth, and healing. HRV biofeedback "works to strengthen the autonomic reflexes that may be broken down with long-term stress or worry" (Lehrer PM and Others, 2008). See page 202.

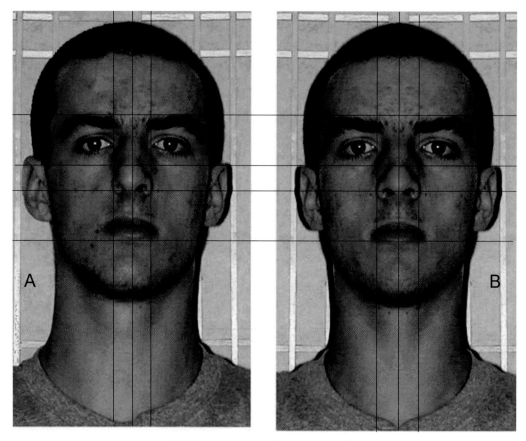

FIGURE C-14. Cranial Distortions and Repair.

See page 198. This young man was knocked down during a basketball game, then ran over by an opposing player who stepped on his head. Result: Continuous migraines with extreme sensitivity to pressure changes.

FIGURE C-15. "Wear a Helmet!"

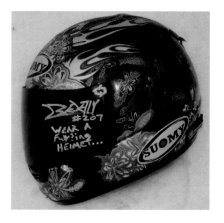

See page 226. This helmet belongs to a motorcycle racer who survived a spectacular 130 mph crash.

Besides tears and abrasions, a foot peg punched through the forehead area; there is another hole at the back. After the crash, the racer returned to a demanding executive job. That is, the helmet was disabled, but he was not.

It now hangs over the bar of the Sewickley Hotel with a message to other riders from its appreciative owner.

Courtesy of Michael Seate.

CHAPTER 7   # Children and Adults

TRUE STORIES OF MEN, WOMEN, CHILDREN WHO WERE TREATED WITH NEUROFEEDBACK AFTER NOTHING ELSE WORKED. WHAT HAPPENED TO THEM AND HOW THEY GOT THEIR LIVES BACK.

> In cases of TBI, neurofeedback is probably better than any medication or supplement.
> —Richard Brown, MD; Associate Clinical Professor of Psychiatry, Columbia College of Physicians and Surgeons, New York, NY

Neurofeedback and biofeedback have been used with great success to treat symptoms of TBI in children and adults, including military personnel. The following stories are from actual case notes.

These are just a few of many gathered over 20 years of using neurofeedback. Most of these illustrate successful outcomes. Some show the limitations of neurofeedback; these tend to involve structural and hormonal imbalances, infections, and/or degeneration.

Notice the wide variability in number of treatments. Some clients saw changes in a few sessions. Others required additional biofeedback training and other therapies for physical and structural problems.

Whatever the approach, biofeedback and neurofeedback are easily integrated into more traditional rehabilitation programs. Brain Wellness and Biofeedback coordinates treatment plans with hospital-based rehabilitation programs, physicians, and many other private providers.

Bridgett, Bruce, Archie, and Jake

The children here suffered injuries that could have lasted a lifetime.

Bridgett: The Soccer Player

HEADACHE, BODY PAIN, NOISE SENSITIVITY, NAUSEA AND DIZZINESS, ANXIETY, EXTREME LEG WEAKNESS, FATIGUE, POOR CONCENTRATION

The following story was given to us by Bridgett's mother[1].

Bridgett was a happy, sweet and driven 10-year-old. A straight-A student, she loved Irish dance, swimming and basketball, but her true love was soccer. She was an aggressive player who never sat out, even when injured to the point of tears.

By early October 2008, Bridgett had taken two significant blows to the head, but played on, reluctantly admitting to dizziness only after the soccer game was over. On October 11th, she slipped and fell on wet grass near the goal. A defender, trying to kick the ball away, missed the ball and kicked Bridgett in the back of the head. Bridgett tried to play on as usual, but when she complained of a headache, she was put on the bench and ordered to rest. That seemed to be the worst of it. Then, 36 hours later, her world fell apart.

"Suddenly," reported her mother, "concussion symptoms all started coming out at once. We rushed her to the ER. When the CT came out clean, the doctor told her just to take it easy."

But the next day, Bridgett woke up feeling terrible. Then the day after that and every day for two weeks, she woke with worse pain than the day before. She had double vision, severe fatigue, and headache. Every sound caused waves of pain. She could not bear the ticking of a clock. She was nauseated, food tasted strange, and muscle spasms rippled through her body. Stomach pain and nighttime anxiety attacks blocked sleep. The simplest tasks, such as setting the table, were overwhelming. "I can't!" she would cry, then collapse in tears.

She began to withdraw, avoid people, and show signs of depression. One of the worst symptoms was anxiety. Said her mother,

> My friendly, outgoing girl was hiding from friends and neighbors. She would cry and have anxiety attacks at least once a day, especially at night. Many nights I would sleep near her so she would know she was loved.

Her head hurt so badly that she spent most of her time in bed curled into a fetal position. She could get up if necessary — until the day that her legs were suddenly so weak that she

---

1. See her mother's full story on the BWB website at:
http://brainwellnessandbiofeedback.com/stories/belinda2.htm

was unable to crawl out of bed without help. When she finally struggled out of bed, her legs collapsed. Now, to get around at all, Bridgett needed a walker. No one knew why.

Constant headaches, mobility issues, and cognitive confusion continued for six months. The pain never lessened. Reading and writing, listening to radio, TV, or music, increased the terrible headaches. Even light schoolwork was impossible. Despite constant fatigue, it was hard for her to fall asleep at night or to wake up the next morning.

Neurologists and neuropsychologists were at a loss to explain or ease the symptoms. All said there was nothing to do but wait. Instead, the family tried chiropractic, acupuncture, physical therapy and cranial-sacral therapy. These had limited success in easing muscle spasms, but when symptoms continued, they resolved to waste no more money or emotional hope on *any* treatment without at least two first-hand accounts of success.

"In February 2009, I heard four success stories about EEG neurofeedback and Dr. Mary Lee Esty. I scheduled an appointment." Bridgett didn't want to go, certain this was just another waste of time and money. She was thrilled, however, to see her map, consistent with a contra-coup injury and post-concussion symptoms, and to hold a picture of her concussion in her hands. Bridgett wanted to make it into a T-shirt to show that her pain was real.

SESSION 1. Better sleep and less night-time anxiety, but because Bridgett felt nothing during treatment, she was sure it wasn't working.
Sessions 2-8. More anxiety issues disappeared. Could set the table, do some schoolwork, and walk with a cane. [By Session 3] Dropped the cane and could walk normally, even broke into a little Irish jig. After six FNS sessions pain level began to fall.
SESSION 9. She walked out whispering that she was "healed."

Was she joking? She was not. "This time" (as she wrote afterwards), "while I was sitting in the chair with the computer running and eyes closed, everything went instantly clear." When Bridgett opened her eyes, her six-month headache had vanished. She jumped out of the chair. "I feel great!" she said, and kept talking excitedly about how *clear* everything was. Now she could read pages and pages of text, listen to music, watch TV pain-free, and all anxiety was gone. The family celebrated by going to a noisy Kid's Night at a nearby restaurant. The girl who had been unable to tolerate the sound of a ticking clock had no headache.

Although Bridgett had been unable to write even a few sentences for six months, she finished all her schoolwork for the last eight months of fifth grade in just eight weeks. She also learned eight months of Irish dance steps in two nights and learned them well enough to place at the top of her division at an Irish Dance competition in June. There was no more anxiety, no more panic attacks, no visible effects of the concussion.

Neurofeedback produced a rapid change from an injury that could otherwise have led to a lifetime of pain and disability.

Bruce: Post-concussion Syndrome and Infection

EXTREME FATIGUE, POOR CONCENTRATION, ADD, EXCESSIVE SLEEP

During the winter of 2008 Bruce (15) was hit hard with a severe case of strep and mono. For six weeks he slept 23 hours a day. Between May of 2008 and February 2009 he needed "only" 12 -15 hours of sleep[1]. So in March he returned to lacrosse.

Within a few weeks he suffered three hits to the head, the last leaving him with no memory of the accident. He was diagnosed in the emergency room with "mild concussion." He was also confused, glassy-eyed, sensitive to noise, with sudden mood swings and impulsivity. But most prominent and troublesome were extreme physical and mental fatigue, with persistent severe headache. Because of these he could tolerate little time in school. Some days he could endure no more than an hour or two of class because "Thinking hurt."

The morning after his first FNS neurofeedback session, Bruce felt rested and went strong all day, working on geometry without needing a nap.

By the third session, he was once again making 100s on his class work and attending school full time. "We've got our Bruce back!" said his parents. By a six month follow-up, Bruce was still making excellent grades and had full energy.

Archie: The Boy Who Heard Voices

HEADACHES, AUDITORY HALLUCINATIONS, SLEEP PROBLEMS, FATIGUE, DIZZINESS, MOOD CHANGES, AND AD(H)D

Archie was an intelligent, likable and friendly boy who, in three years of elementary school, had suffered at least three Grade 3 concussions[2].

- At 10 years old, in 4th Grade, he was knocked out on the playground. On regaining consciousness, he was simply sent back to class.
- The following June, while trying to kick a ball during a soccer game, he flipped upward, landed on his head, and was again unconscious for several minutes.
- In December he was hit in the head with a ball, again knocked out. He suffered headache, dizziness and nausea when he awoke.
- The following Fall, during a soccer game, he was kicked in the head so hard that it raised a large lump. Three months later, a doctor dismissed his continuing symptoms (including hearing loss in one ear) as "malingering."

---

1. Normal sleep for that age is around 9.5 hours.
2. Grades of concussion are defined by the length of unconsciousness. With *all three concussions*, Archie was unconscious for up to 10 minutes.

This last injury triggered voices (auditory hallucinations) that urged him to harm others. The climax of his struggle was near-tasing by the police as he struggled to resist the terrifying commands of the "voices" but was unable to respond to requests to "drop the knife." Fortunately the taser wires caught in his T-shirt. Archie spent a week in a psychiatric unit with a provisional diagnosis of schizophrenia. He was put on multiple medications including lithium, Ritalin®, Tegretol®, Effexor® and Klonopin®. After his release from the psych unit, the family consulted a new psychiatrist who referred Archie to Dr. Esty.

Session 1. After the first session, he had a headache that lasted two days (not unusual with multiple concussions). On Day 3, he felt much better, sleep was better and he was calmer.
Sessions 2-6. Improvements were reported by his mother, therapist, and guidance counselor. Between Sessions 2 and 3 Archie heard "voices" twice but they were less powerful. He was still explosive, but irritability reduced, even at school. His teacher, who knew nothing of his treatments, reported that he was now learning his school lessons and sitting quietly. Energy improved, but fatigue still a problem[a].
Session 7. When asked how many times he had heard the voices, Archie had to stop and think. "Once," he hesitated. What had he actually heard? "Raid the fridge!" he replied, probably a typical adolescent boy voice speaking from the stomach. Never heard voices again.

a. Lamictal®, Effexor®, and Klonopin®, were probably contributors. Lamictal®, best known as an anti-seizure medication, is also used to calm behavior but may be too calming. By Session 6, Archie's psychiatrist had stopped Effexor® completely.

Archie's history of AD(H)D had always made schoolwork a struggle, even before his concussions. Once the TBI symptoms were resolved with FNS, Archie went on to train in traditional neurofeedback for AD(H)D with Dr. Michael Sitar.

Treatment covered two years with summer breaks. Before these sessions ended, Archie's psychiatrist had discontinued all medications.

Results support the growing body of clinical evidence and research that neurofeedback should be considered even for serious psychiatric diagnoses with a history of trauma.

Archie has graduated and is planning on going to medical school. He is also a good athlete in a competitive sport. If not for a psychiatrist who understood the connection between concussion and auditory hallucinations, this story could have had a very different—and tragic—ending.

Jake: The Diver

SEVERE TBI FOLLOWED BY INABILITY TO SPEAK, LOSS OF FINE AND GROSS MOTOR CONTROL, PROBLEMS WITH SWALLOWING, SENSORY INTEGRATION, MUSCLE WEAKNESS, AND AD(H)D

In June of 1999, 11-year-old Jake fell from a 12-foot high diving board onto the concrete deck. His skull was fractured from ear to ear and in the ambulance he suffered two seizures. At the ER, doctors induced a coma to protect against the effects of a subdural hematoma and rising intra-cranial pressures. Continued bleeding into the brain required surgery, including removal of part of the left temporal lobe. He was in a coma for 12 days.

After four months in the hospital, Jake entered a day-patient program at a children's rehab facility. He had two months of post-trauma amnesia and severe headaches. Speech was unintelligible. He could not close his lips and had difficulty swallowing. There was excessive tension in his left hand and arm, weakness with poor motor skills in both hands. All food had to be chopped to avoid choking; eating a meal took 45 minutes.

FNS neurofeedback treatment at BWB began on February 1, 2000.

SESSION 1-2. Jake's face, neck, and ears flushed, arm and hand were more open and relaxed, mouth more symmetrical. For the first time since his accident, he was able to say his dog's name with loud voice. Could only whisper before. Had trouble going to sleep, but remembered a dream for first time since injury.
SESSION 3-6. Hand even more relaxed. Could close his mouth and drink through a straw, no longer needing to hold his lips together with his hand. No more choking incidents and able to whistle and blow bubbles.
SESSION 16. Hand now so relaxed no longer needs to wear a night brace. Can control his lower lip so no longer needs the assisted communication device; he can be understood without it. Gross and fine muscle control have returned (he can manipulate small Lego blocks). On a school field trip in heat, able to walk long distance with a backpack.

By March, his mother reported that Jake was "like old Jake, more crabby and negative, but more complex." Academics, physical strength and abilities continued to improve. He never had to use the assisted communication device again. He was no longer doomed to a life of profound disability. There was no significant regression during breaks in treatment. He had 44 treatments to reach this level of functioning. Over the next six years he came for occasional "tune ups" (about 5 per year).

Pre-injury, Jake had been diagnosed with AD(H)D and sensory integration disorder. His first map in 2000 and the last in 2006 show striking differences. Seven years after beginning treatment Jake graduated from high school.

Carol, Brian, Bill, Steve and Robin

Carol: The Programmer

HEADACHES AND MEMORY PROBLEMS. LOSS OF EXECUTIVE FUNCTION, SENSE OF SMELL, READING AND SPATIAL SKILLS, ABILITY TO STAY AWAKE AND TO REMEMBER DREAMS.

In 1996, Carol stepped off an icy sidewalk and went airborne. The result was basal skull fracture, two black eyes, a concussion, and, she says, "the end of my life as I knew it."

At that time, Carol provided computer support and programming for office automation, ways of making offices run more efficiently. After her fall, she couldn't even remember how to start her computer programs, much less run them. All organizational skills were gone. She could not stay awake more than three hours at a time. Because she could no longer work in an office, it seemed reasonable to manage the house instead. Her husband declared her responsible for all housework, bills, paperwork and taxes, shopping and meals. But this was not possible. One day she found herself standing in the kitchen turning in circles with a potato in her left hand, trying to remember the next step to making dinner — by which she meant microwaving a potato; anything else was too hopelessly complex.

For three years, any changes in blood pressure (as when simply standing up from a chair) were brutally painful. Even while she was seated and calm, pain came in constant waves every three to five seconds. The (new) doctor was mystified and ordered X-rays to see if the sinuses were clear. They were, but her request for an MRI or referral to a neurologist was declared "premature because there are many drugs that we haven't tried yet." On finally obtaining a referral to a neurologist, the same drugs were offered. They did not help.

Three years later and still in pain, she persuaded another doctor to order an MRI. When it came back "normal," the insurance company ruled that it had been "unnecessary" and refused payment. She is convinced that the $800 MRI bill and a boiled chicken were the end of her marriage. Boiled chicken?

It was the most complicated meal I could manage. Severe pain and memory problems made it impossible to work or to cook a meal of any complexity. My husband called me "scatterbrained," faulted me for "failing to exercise" and for weight gain due to "laziness." I wasn't any fun any more and worst of all, I was starting to cost money. Or maybe it was simply that I could not remember how to cook. He ran off with a caterer.

FNS neurofeedback began in May 2003.

Mapping revealed abundant frontal alpha and a hot-spot of slow-wave delta activity in the right rear (occipital) lobe. "Aha!" said Mary Lee. "There's where you hit your head. It left its calling card."

Neurofeedback triggered remarkable changes. Dreams (gone for seven years), suddenly returned in vivid living color. For a few days she had trouble telling the difference between dreams and reality, but soon after, sleep stabilized, the terrible fatigue began to lift. Even more astonishing, lifelong chronic migraines began to disappear.

Session 1-4. After first session sensations of pinpricks in the injured area. Over the weekend, suddenly wrapped and mailed all of her family's Christmas presents. They were 5 months late, but sent. Greatly increased energy by Session 4: Spread mulch, spaded driveway, mucked out pond, things impossible weeks earlier. Mood irritable, but she considered irritability for good reason to be better — after losing seven years of her life — 'than cow-like complacency due to lack of energy." After years of being unable to stay awake more than 3 hours at a time, need for naps disappeared.
Session 5-12. Able to start new projects without waiting for a last-minute adrenalin rush. Made website changes she had meant to do for 5 years. Migraines greatly reduced, coming only with barometric pressure changes and rain. Cleaned house in way that had been impossible for years. Enjoyed the Smithsonian folk festival despite intense heat, crowds and noise.
Session 13-20. Two migraine attacks before storms & ragweed season. Attacks passed quickly, far less severe than before treatment. Still was able to finish a complex project. No longer turning in circles not knowing what to do. Good energy and 8-mile hikes. No headaches despite the stress helping friends move, a hurricane, & decided she needed to move. Before this, couldn't do packing/cleaning for a move. Did it in one month. No headaches for 10 days, and then only a very small one. Session 20, realized that sense of smell was returning.

Return of a sense of smell after basal skull fracture is considered extremely rare. Not only did it return fully but there are other reports of its sudden reappearance in other concussed patients treated with neurofeedback (Hammond DC, 2007).

Brian: The Martial Artist
LOSS OF EXECUTIVE FUNCTION, POOR MEMORY, LOW BODY TEMPERATURE, SEVERE AD(H)D, FIBROMYALGIA SYMPTOMS, PHOTOPHOBIA, FATIGUE, EXCESSIVE SLEEP, FLAT AFFECT AND PTSD

Brian had been a brilliant student and superb athlete, a long-time Judo player who trained and coached others in Mixed Martial Arts.

Now there were constant memory lapses, confusion, extreme difficulty reading, and symptoms of fibromyalgia and PTSD. He was extremely sensitive to light, never venturing outside without a brimmed hat and the darkest possible wrap-around sunglasses.

Looking for a career change, Brian moved from Florida to Northern Virginia. He was eager to explore the nearby Washington D.C. museums and monuments, but more than an hour of new sights and sounds resulted in sensory overload and exhaustion. He would go to bed to sleep it off and wouldn't be seen again for days. When he did reappear he would gulp down an entire 10-cup pot of coffee followed by a long, hot shower trying to warm up *before* going to the gym. Why not warm up *at* the gym? "I don't warm up," he said.

He wore a hat and heavy clothing, indoors and out, but was always cold. Muscles were tight and knotted despite constant stretching. Within an hour (often mere minutes) of getting up or working out he would disappear again for another nap. Such poor function in an intelligent and athletic man was attributed by him and others to "laziness" and "lack of motivation." But driving off and forgetting to close all four doors isn't laziness. Losing wallet and keys several times a minute is not lack of motivation.

The reaction he inspired in people meeting him for the first time was often sheer panic. He had the masklike expression ("flat affect") and Thousand-Yard Stare (page 55). He was seen as "crazy." A trauma nurse described his expression as "feral." Job interviews did not go well.

Brian attributed his feelings of cold to having moved north, from Florida to Virginia — in July when temperature and humidity was in the 90s. Another possibility came to light on checking his temperature. It ran around 95.6 degrees F, never rising above 97 degrees F, even with physical exercise. A body temperature that runs one degree low is enough to cause chronic muscle problems, fogginess and confusion (Simons DG and Others, 1999). On starting thyroid supplementation, his temperature rose and coffee intake dropped dramatically. Muscle knots melted like snow in the warm sunshine. He was far more alert, yet problems with memory and sequencing continued.

Brian denied ever having had an actual concussion. But there was a history of an extremely difficult birth, a mother four days in labor before a Caesarean. As a child he nearly died from asthma and pneumonia, and was treated with such powerful drugs that for two years he failed to grow. In college he suffered the "bends" after scuba-diving.

There was also a 30-year history of Karate, Judo, and Aikido. For Judo players and schools that emphasize breakfalls, for football players and fans of thrill rides, symptoms may not be a matter of a single serious concussion. It may, instead, be years of repetitive microtrauma. Brian reported repetitive breakfalls — "up to 300 a night for eight years." Many students simply see this as *serious* training but "I have seen stars," he admitted, "more times than I can count." Brain and body continued to deteriorate until a chance encounter with neurofeedback. A quick test to the frontal area showed severe frontal slowing.

Brian initially experimented with traditional neurofeedback, learning to inhibit theta waves. Although unable to read comfortably for years, he was suddenly able to read again, three books in three weeks starting with *Dune*, 700 pages of small print and complex plot.

He began FNS neurofeedback at BWB in May 2003.

After Session 1, Brian saw remarkable changes. For years he had never left the house without his hat and sunglasses. Then, on a brilliantly sunny and glaring August day, he went out in his usual hat and sunglasses to mow the grass. He walked right back in and put the glasses on the table. "Too dark," he said. He hasn't had to wear them since.

As executive function returned, Brian was shocked and surprised that it had previously taken so long to do simple paperwork. What had required many hours and entire pots of coffee now took minutes.

After Session 6, changes in muscular strength were just as startling (Table 7-1). The extreme changes in the amount of weight he could lift were easy; they did not involve working to exhaustion. *Easy,* perhaps because suddenly the nerve signals were getting through, when they had not before.

Session 1- 4. Problems: loss of organizational skills, inability to multi-task or focus, to filter noise, social withdrawal, problems with memory and math, flat affect "that even I notice." Now remembering dreams, able to fill orders without mixing up packages. Can work up to two hours at a stretch; before, no more than 45 minutes. No longer needs sunglasses.

Session 5-6. Light sensitivity almost gone, but, "My head feels full of light." Now easier to wake up and to go to sleep. Can remember what day it is. Less sensitive to noise. Stood for hours in the Motor Vehicles office but didn't need to stay in bed for days afterwards.

Came up with an idea for improving a web page and read a book on it. Tight muscles loosening up, can stretch, huge increase in flexibility and strength (Table 7-1). Feels as though knowledge is still there but in a locked box. "If I could open it, I could use it, but it is like a blank spot in a field of vision." Re: old diagnosis of PTSD, "Over the last two weeks a hard tight knot of fear has disappeared. It had always been there. Now it is gone."

Table 7-1. Brian's Strength Improvements	
Monday 06/24/03	Session 6 treatment followed by tingling and odd neurological sensations down back, arms, and legs.
Tuesday 06/25/03	Went to gym for regular workout of calves and legs: a set of 10-12 repetitions at 350 pounds. Was able to raise weight to 450 pounds (a 100-pound increase) for the same number of reps and sets compared to previous workout. (Increases are usually made in 5-10 pound increments. Changes of 100 pounds are unheard of.)
Wednesday 06/26/03	For the same number of reps and sets with free weights: work-out of arms and chest went from 30 to 50 pounds, a 60% increase.
Thursday 06/27	Workout of back and abdominals: estimated[a] 20 percent increase.

a. Because workout was done on cam machines rather than with free weights, the actual increase is hard to calculate directly. However, it suggests that strength testing might be a valuable part of an intake evaluation if possible. Brian notes that weight-lifting web sites are now discussing neurotropic drugs to improve physical strength.

SESSION 7-9. Calories up but losing body fat. Mood good, and now able to shift attention. Able to sequence and getting much more done in much less time. Function is so much better that he has decided not to apply for disability.
SESSION 10-14. Drove several hundred miles home to help parents move. Organized garage and kitchen. Mailing out resumes and applying for jobs. Maintaining strength despite dieting. Continues job hunt. Gets bored now because he actually has energy and options. Wants to take a break from treatments to see what happens.
SESSION 15-17. Back after a break of nearly a month of experimenting with a "nutritional supplement." This approach apparently did not work; arrived 40 minutes late for his appointment and has been getting lost again. Next session late b/c got on wrong train. Over last 2 days had migraines with scotomas.
SESSION 19-21. Vivid dreams, reading more and inspired to write again.

"When I came to Virginia," said Brian, "I believe I was dying." Brian's presenting symptoms were severe and incapacitating. The sudden improvements in cognitive and physical abilities after Session 6 helped him to realize just how poor his physical function had been after moving to Virginia and before starting neurofeedback treatments at BWB. He has now returned to teaching and a professional career.

Bill: The Biker

LOSS OF EXECUTIVE FUNCTION, SEVERE FATIGUE, COULD NOT REMEMBER FACES AND
PEOPLE. HALTING SPEECH, DYSAUTONOMIA AND MISSING 1/4 FIELD OF VISION.

Bill was a handsome young man in a highly technical field, but his bright future ended in a horrific wreck when he sailed off a slick mountain road. He was wearing no helmet and head injuries were severe. He needed multiple surgeries, including those needed to rebuild his face, after which he suffered daily facial pain. He lost a quarter of his field of vision.

Body temperature was documented at 96.5° F, and because of terrible fatigue, he was awake only three times a day for a couple of hours at a time. Sleep was haunted by flashbacks and terrible nightmares of the wreck. Cognitive function was so slowed and speech so halting that there were 10-second delays between phrases. Memory was so impaired that he had to carry a Polaroid camera at all times. Photos went into a scrap book with their identifying information. Studying the pictures was the only way he could remember people and places, and his relationship to them.

Eventually Bill tried to live on his own again, but between the crushing fatigue and loss of organizational skills, it was extremely difficult to shop for groceries and impossible to prepare a real meal. Because he could no longer cook, there was no food in his kitchen. Kitchen cabinets held books and technical papers that he could no longer read. It took him nearly a week to do a load of laundry.

In June 1998, 17 years after the car crash, Bill began FNS treatment at BWB.

SESSION 1-4. After 3 treatments, doing laundry was much easier. He could do in one morning what usually took 4-5 days. (See "Severe Fatigue and Apathy" on page 49).
SESSIONS 5-9. Suddenly able to understand a TBI report he had been struggling with for 2 years. More energy. 12 days after starting treatment, he worked from 6:30 am - 10:30 pm without "hard fatigue" and no nap. The horrific nightmares are gone. Now replaced with pleasant dreams.
SESSION 10. Reported waking with 15-20 seconds of sharp pain behind the affected eye. During a 3-week break, there were a few more episodes of pain in the right jaw and behind the eye, extending from behind eye to occiput. It felt "like a pipe-cleaner being jiggled back and forth," lasted about 30 seconds[a]. Shortly after, full vision returned.
SESSIONS 16-18. Physician verified that body temperature (documented at 96.5° F for the last 17 years), is now normal. Is excited to be reading again and remembering what he reads. A nap is now one hour rather than four.

a. Neurosurgeon Ayub Ommaya, speculated that the problem must have been a vascular event and that some sort of blockage was eliminated (Ommaya AK, personal communication, 1998). Note the similarity of Mary Lincoln's reports of "wires behind her eyes" (see page 10).

SESSION 19-22. "I feel very *present*, which is both pleasant and disturbing; it takes getting used to." On depression: "I'm afraid to be too hopeful — feels so good." Now has a full field of vision, with "no cutout, complete panoramic view from left to right. Almost makes me feel *light*."

No Tylenol and no muscle relaxant for one week. Worked at computer for 4 hours on a paper that he had started in February but had been unable to finish. Speech much more fluent. The terrible fatigue has evaporated. Describes it as "a difference in the weight around my head.

Used to sleep 10-noon, 2-4 or 6 pm, then back to bed at 8 or 9. Now up early in the morning and back to bed at 10 or 11 pm.

Session 23-25. Reading and body temperature OK with no cold spells. Vision still OK.

"Trying to not get too excited about life because I won't want to go to bed." He is enjoying the anticipation of reading something, making Making clearer decisions about scheduling events. Feeling well.

Bill's vision and body temperature remained normal. He could work through an entire day without needing a nap. Most significantly, he was able to participate in meetings, listen to conversations and track them. The daily facial pain is long gone.

———————

Bill now enjoys the challenges of day to day frustrations. He has greater choice about how to spend his energy. No longer limited to merely surviving one day at a time, he could plan months in advance and was able to handle a part-time volunteer job. He feels cautious, but no longer broken. —MLE

Steve: The Tri-Athlete
MEMORY LOSS, FATIGUE, INSOMNIA, FLASHBACKS, AND IMPULSIVITY

Steve was an extreme athlete—bicycling, hockey, kayaking, swimming, sailing, running and triathalons—with a long history of sports injuries. As a child of 5 or 6, he slid head-first into the boards at the hockey rink and was knocked unconscious for several minutes. While sailing as an adult, he was hit by the boom and knocked overboard. "I was clumsy for awhile after that," he recalls.

The final blow was during a bicycle race when he was hit by a passing car and thrown head-first from his bike. For several weeks he suffered a "mini-coma," sleeping 16-18 hours a day. Afterwards he could not stay asleep. What sleep he got was disturbed by nightmares with flashbacks of the accident. There were emotional outbursts and sudden impulsive purchases of expensive bikes and equipment.

Frightening memory problems appeared: increasing difficulty remembering client names and matching them with their files. He did not notice people speaking to him or, when he did, could not recall the conversations. He tried hypnosis, Eye Movement Desensitization and Reprocessing (EMDR), various drugs (including plenty of caffeine) with limited success. Because he avoided sharing symptoms and his fears with his wife, she thought he was purposely ignoring her. Their marriage began to suffer.

FNS neurofeedback treatment began in January 2011.

Session 1. Felt tingling in both feet and calves, a feeling as though feet were rising over his head, a flashback to the accident. Ended feeling clearer and calmer. Next day mild euphoria and improved night vision. Woke clear-headed after a long hard day— usually needs two days to recover.
Session 2. Memory better; remembered things needed for work. At work could remember client names and files. Noticed sense of smell unusually acute. Memory greatly improved. Noise sensitivity way down and is using less coffee. Feeling as if "...a new personality was dropped in my lap. Now, the frustrating negative, distracting thoughts are not entering my head. "
Sessions 3-4. Felt good enough after treatment to run in the park and go kayaking (triggering a neck spasm). During Session 4, he relived the sensation of attempting to lay down his bike and slide. During treatment felt the slide, like bubbles going up his arm.
Sessions 8-11. Good week at work. Began extreme training for a race, something he couldn't even think about a year ago. Can exercise hard without taking electrolytes. Brain feels good. There are setbacks: racing at high intensity with lots of vibration & heart rate at 190 led to headaches. Advised re not overdoing his training.
Sessions 12-16. Made dietary changes and after Session 14, best he has felt since treatment began 11 months prior.

Robin: The Hiker

HEADACHE, BODY PAIN, READING DIFFICULTY, ANXIETY, NOISE SENSITIVITY, DEPRESSION, AND LOSS OF SHORT-TERM MEMORY.

> Q. How will you know you are better?
> A. Relief from pain, able to read again and to remember what I read.

As a child, Robin was severely shocked and burned when she grasped an electrical cord with wet hands. Growing up in Canada, there were slips on ice and snow, and a fall that sent her bumping down an entire flight of stairs on her tailbone. She suffered her *first* whiplash injury at age 19. At age 30,while stopped at a light, she was rear-ended so violently that she woke up in the back seat of her car. Pain from the whiplash was so severe that she could not be touched or treated for two years.

Robin suffered all-over body pain (especially in chest, ribs and groin) and any stress triggered debilitating fatigue and anxiety. Traction, heat, cold, and laser therapy had little or no effect and she was diagnosed with fibromyalgia syndrome. Robin's Canadian clinical team which included a physiatrist and specialists in trigger point and myofascial work.But from her history and symptoms, Dr. Esty suspected a reverse curve in her neck; the diagnosis was confirmed and treated with advanced chiropractic techniques by Tony Robichaud before she came to BWB.

At BWB, sEMG evaluation, done by biofeedback therapist Emily Perlman, revealed imbalances in 16 pairs of muscles. These recovered so slowly from a movement that they never came fully to rest; they were always "on," producing chronic, escalating, pain.

At her first session, groin (psoas) muscles were so painful they could barely be touched. With sensors over these muscles, Ms. Perlman had Robin do the hip exercises prescribed by her physiotherapist. sEMG revealed that the exercises were actually *aggravating* pain by forcing other muscles to fire unnecessarily. Gluteal muscles were unbalanced and quad muscles so suppressed that they were unable to support walking. Other muscles had to pick up the slack, causing strain and pain. Release of the suppressed quads gave immediate relief. To her amazement, Robin was suddenly able to walk long distances pain free. With exercise, energy improved, allowing even more activity.

But other factors were involved. Robin's breathing was shallow and rapid and limited to the upper chest. This style of breathing changes the body's acid-base balance, excites the autonomic nervous system, and triggers panic attacks. It also strains muscles in the neck and shoulders. Some of these refer pain to the chest and Robin suffered chest pain so frequently she was even checked out by a cardiologist.

Ms. Perlman trained Robin to breathe from the diaphragm, which helped re-balance and quiet her system, reduce arousal, slow her heart rate, increased peripheral blood flow, and reduce skin conductance, all leading to a calmer state. Her chest pain vanished.

With these long-time issues resolved, Robin began FNS neurofeedback.

Session 1-4. Headache lasted for 24 hours after treatment. She was suddenly more aware of smells, could recall phone numbers, and read more easily. Pain diminished dramatically with less fatigue. As clients often do, she immediately went out and walked too far.
Session 5-8. More walking thanks to pain relief, resulting in sore muscles from the exercise. Robin considers sEMG "the most bang for the buck". She had never before been aware of muscles. On intake, Robin rated pain in her hip joints as 8.5 out of 10. After years of pain and 8 sessions, all pain and fatigue was gone, even after walking from the Capitol to the White House. Went home to Canada feeling great.

Robin returned to BWB on January 4 after another fall on ice.

Sessions 9-11. Ribs sore but no return of chest or hip pain. Cognitive recall still holding. Climbed Bethesda Metro escalator loaded with shopping bags[a], then to movie and dinner. 12 hour day!
Session 14-15. Walked 1 hour each way for cranio-sacral treatment with Eduardo Cortina. Was referred to a behavioral optometrist for evaluation of vision problems. Found near vision was extremely jerky and one eye turned "off." Planned further treatment.
Session 16-21. Planning to start Feldenkreis and Pilates. Energy good until at least 10 pm. "I get tired, but bounce back after rest." Good posture, memory, and energy. No pain, no headaches.

a. The 475-ft Bethesda escalator was once the longest in the Western Hemisphere. One can simply ride, of course. Climbing it with shopping bags is a challenge.

Response to treatment was fast and dramatic. After 17 neurofeedback sessions, 8 sEMG, and 7 HRV, symptom ratings for noise sensitivity, depression, fogginess/clarity, and short-term memory had all dropped to minimal levels. Once crippled by pain, Robin now walks easily and extensively, pain-free, something she had been unable to do for years. Extensive clinical experience treating people diagnosed with fibromyalgia points to the need for multiple interventions to get lasting relief from this painful syndrome.

Evidence of the power of these biofeedback therapies is that despite years of pain and many attempts to treat her symptoms with many different therapies, just *one week* of combined HRV, sEMG, and neurofeedback dramatically reduced the pain in her chest and ribs, and improved cognitive functioning. Cranio-sacral therapy provided additional improvements and she was referred for vision therapy as she completed FNS.

In summary, Robin wrote:

I am speechless at the turnaround you've precipitated. I feel excited about my life now.

The Wounds of War

CASE HISTORIES OF COMBAT VETERANS WITH TERRIBLE INJURIES,
DISABLING MEMORY LOSS, INSOMNIA AND PTSD, WHO HAVE COME BACK TO
THEIR LIVES AND FAMILIES.

> They put on civilian clothes again and looked to their mothers and wives very much like the young men who had gone to business in the peaceful days before August 1914. But they had not come back the same men. Something had altered in them. They were subject to sudden moods and queer tempers, fits of profound depression alternating with a restless desire for pleasure. Many were easily moved to passion where they lost control of themselves, many were bitter in their speech, violent in opinion, frightening.
>
> —Ben Shephard (2000)

These are the stories of men whose injuries were not accidental, where the intent was purposeful death and destruction. Their injuries were far more severe than most civilian injuries.

In the course of war they had been hit with bullets, grenades, shrapnel, and impacted by Improvised Explosive Devices (IEDs). They had rolled in vehicles; fallen from trucks and guard towers; been exposed to toxins including immunizations, depleted uranium (used in ammunition and IEDs), fumes from vehicles, burning oil fields, refineries, and trash pits[1]. They had done all this in searing heat, often in body armor and with packs that sometimes exceeded their own body weights.

Many are surprised that veterans, after the most ghastly experiences, are damaged. Veterans are surprised at their own symptoms, as are their families and employers. Medical workers are surprised that problems remain, for years or forever, no matter how hard they have tried to help.

---

1. When units move, they don't necessarily move their supplies. They burn them: toxic volatiles, medical equipment and supplies, plastic wrappers, heavy metals and all.

Part of the problem is that injuries are so *varied*, involving not only bullets and blunt trauma, but explosions. Explosions create many injuries such as:

- BLUNT TRAUMA. Victims are hit by flying debris. Vehicles may roll and the bodies inside may bounce off interior walls or roofs. Outside, the blast wave may pick them up and throw them through the air. They themselves become projectiles.
- BURNS OR PENETRATING INJURIES. This includes bullets, shrapnel and broken glass.
- PRESSURE CHANGES AND OVERPRESSURE WAVES, causing internal injuries. With no obvious blunt trauma, there may seem to be no damage at all but, in fact:

Invisible injuries from pressure waves may be worse than visible ones from blunt trauma.

PHYSICAL DAMAGE

Blunt trauma may create greater accelerations in the brain than a blast, yet terrible symptoms appear even from small explosions. When researchers at Lawrence Livermore National Laboratory looked at blast effects, they found a startling result: rippling of the skull. The ripples were tiny (about 50 micrometers, the width of a hair) but may effect the vascular hydraulics of blood and other fluids of the circulatory system. Alternating waves *increase* then *decrease* pressures. This might cause tissues, such as the blood-brain barrier, neurons and delicate spider-web connections, to rip and tear. Damage to lungs, liver, kidneys and *their* connections reduces oxygen supply to the brain (anoxia)[1] and the removal or isolation of toxins. This in turn changes electrical activity and metabolism, especially with injury to the HPA axis[2] (Lawrence Livermore National Laboratory, 2010). Ear damage may include tinnitus or vestibular fistula. Eye damage may include damage to the optic nerve or a detached retina. Recall Lord Nelson, blinded after a nearby explosion, with *no visible external* injury.

The researchers then discovered that, rather than protecting against these effects, helmets with webbed suspensions actually made them *worse*. Without padding to fill the air space and block pressure waves, pressures *under* the helmet can intensify, *exceeding those on the outside of the helmet* (Moss WC, King MJ, Blackman EG, 2009).

A KEY TO PTSD

We need a better way to classify TBI than the old approach based on consciousness. Too often, *no* loss of consciousness has been mistaken for *no* problem, but very often, loss of consciousness can predict future difficulties, including a greatly increased risk of PTSD.

---

1. This alone can be catastrophic; the brain requires as much as 25 percent of total body oxygen.
2. Some investigators feel that some symptoms labeled as "psychiatric disorders" are actually the *physical* result of damage to neurons and blood vessels caused by surging blood in the brain (Chen Y and Others, 2013, p. 105). During WWI these symptoms were called *shell shock*.

In 2004, researchers at Walter Reed Army Institute found changes in post-TBI mental function with or without loss of consciousness. But PTSD later appeared in 44 percent of those who had lost consciousness compared to 27 percent of those who had not (Table 8-1). In injuries that did not involve the *head*, PTSD symptoms fell to 16 percent (Hoge CW and Others (2004).

| Table 8-1. TBI with Incidence of Post-Injury PTSD ||
TBI	PTSD
With Loss of Consciousness	44%
With NO loss of Consciousness	27%
NO known TBI	16%

Blast injuries may show no outward damage at all, no hint to the chaos within, but researchers can now see injury at the cellular and molecular levels[1], damage that impairs neural plasticity, the ability of the brain to heal and change, to learn and to remember what has been learned. Swelling of the neurons resembles that seen in diffuse axonal injury. Autopsy supports that picture.

In 2011, Dr. Bennet Omalu turned his attention to deceased military veterans who had faced blasts from mortars and IEDs and been diagnosed with PTSD. One was a Marine who, after his second deployment, developed progressively worsening problems with memory, behavior and mood, insomnia and alcohol. At 27, eight months after his honorable discharge, he committed suicide. On autopsy, his brain looked Fine. No atrophy, no wounds. But a closer exam revealed broken and tangled nerve cells and lesions, the same changes Omalu had seen in dead NFL football players (Omalu B, Hammers JL, and Others, 2011).

Healing the Damage

How to help and treat soldiers with brain injuries has become a burgeoning problem. After standard medical care, most service members presented here had been through the "Wounded Warrior" program[2]. They had received individual and group therapy, yoga, massage, nutritional counseling, art therapy, music therapy, pool therapy, occupational therapy, and speech therapy. Exposure Group Therapy was done with the goal of revisiting and addressing the incidents that triggered PTSD.

1. Experimental imaging with fMRI and DTI have recently shown promise of revealing micro-hemorrhages and changes in brain function in *live* patients. Research continues.
2. Walter Reed Army Medical Center (WRAMC) Specialized Care Program Track II, a three-week program to assist the wounded OEF/OIF service members from Iraq and Afghanistan.

Despite intense treatment, these veterans still suffered difficulties with memory, anger, sleep and hypervigilance. For most, attempting to read triggered headache and fatigue after just a few lines. Before the study, three had actually attempted suicide, one was quietly planning suicide, and another attempt had been thwarted.

Most of the following accounts present the personal details of veterans who entered a treatment study to evaluate effects of neurofeedback on concussion and PTSD (Nelson DV and Esty ML, 2012). Their rapid and sometimes astonishing improvements in the face of severe injuries show why clinicians are so adamant that neurofeedback is effective, and why they are so very passionate about their work.

All veterans were treated in a FNS research study so there are extensive session notes. Excerpts from these notes appear in the boxes in each veteran's story.

The Numbers Behind the Words

These stories are compelling, but the numbers are compelling as well. The results of this exploratory study were published in the *Journal of Neuropsychiatry and Clinical Neuroscience* (Nelson DV and Esty ML, 2012). In summary: All seven service members involved had debilitating symptoms of PTSD and TBI. Symptoms were tracked throughout the study including,

- Neurobehavioral problems such as depression and memory loss[1].
- PTSD symptoms, like hypervigilance and flashbacks[2].
- A current symptom questionnaire, filled out at the start of each session, rated *current* severity of eight symptoms: Cognitive clarity, overall body pain, quality of sleep, fatigue, anxiety, depression, irritability or anger, and overall activity.

For each of these forms, participants gave a score ranging from 10 (the worst possible problem) to 0 (not a problem at all).

Treatment occurred over 25 sessions[3]; analysis showed statistically significant improvements over the course of treatment. Of the symptoms measured by the two questionnaires, most were significantly reduced, and the downward trends in the current symptoms ratings were all highly significant.

For two cases, a rise in symptoms appeared at follow-up but only after additional injury, and even then, they never returned to pre-treatment levels. One of these, Jay, had suffered some of the most terrible injuries, but also experienced a most amazing recovery.

---

1. Neurobehavioral Functioning Inventory (NRI) by Kreutzer JS, Seel RT, and Marwitz JH.
2. PTSD Symptoms Scale: Self-Report Version (Foa EB and Others, 2012).
3. Two participants dropped out early (after sessions 13 and 17) saying that they had improved so much they saw no point in continuing.

Jay and Paul, Kyle, Kevin, David and Mike

Men who went to war, what happened to them, and how they got their lives back.

Jay: The Driver
HEADACHES, MEMORY LOSS, FALSE MEMORIES, FATIGUE, SUICIDAL, PTSD AND
HYPERVIGILANCE, PAIN, DEPRESSION, EXPLOSIVENESS, SLEEP APNEA, NIGHT SWEATS

Q. How will you know you are better?
A. My memory would be better.

Jay was career military with 14 years in the Army. He was trained to drive anything except a tank. But in Iraq, from the time of the first wave in 2003, he was never used as a driver. Instead, he was placed as a gunner with ground troops, exposed to constant explosions, fire fights and night fighting.

In the course of two tours (5 and 18 months) he survived nine IED explosions, three with loss of consciousness for 20 to 30 minutes. In another incident, his vehicle and passengers were blown into the air. He crash-landed on the truck in full body armor and gear, a total body weight of nearly 260 pounds. Another explosion blew metal fragments into his leg.

Jay was left with a leg full of shrapnel, multiple concussions, PTSD, and severe loss of both long- and short-term memory. While at Walter Reed Army Medical Center (WRAMC) for PTSD, he was found to have broken bones and went through multiple corrective surgeries. He could not remember the day for more than a few seconds or remember his children's ages. He could not read more than a few lines; trying to do so made his constant headaches worse, and he had no memory of what he had just read. False memories were as true to him as real ones; he "remembered" being posted in places he had never been. His broken bones and leg wounds required a wheelchair if extensive walking was involved. Autonomic nervous system dysfunction (*dysautonomia*) left him unable to regulate his body temperature; he was always hot and sweaty, especially at night.

Impact on the family was enormous in all areas of daily living. He could not recall even the simplest steps of daily family schedules. He disliked foods that had been his favorites before Iraq. All family responsibility fell on his wife, who said she no longer knew him.

Constant headaches (with pain consistently rated at "10") were treated with Tramadol® and Percocet®, but not even these powerful medications could control the pain. He was also on lithium and Zoloft® for depression and had sleep apnea (untreated).

He was unable to drive because of his injured right leg, mobility, vision and memory problems. He had also lost his navigational skills, once so excellent that his unit, on foot, in the dark and in strange territory, always relied on him to get them home again. And he always did. Now these skills were gone. For someone who has had such abilities, losing them is like going blind. He was especially distressed by extreme fatigue, anxiety, and hair-trigger temper, knowing he had never been like that before.

Before entering the study, Jay had completed the Specialized Care Program, but he still suffered full-blown PTSD symptoms with nightmares. Seeing small piles of dirt or debris beside the road caused severe panic attacks[1]. Physically and emotionally, Jay was a wreck, but his response to neurofeedback was fast and positive.

FNS neurofeedback treatment began in May 2007.

Sessions 1-2. First session triggered a "big headache" that diminished greatly. Slept well, feeling unusually rested when he awoke. Energy and mood good, memory better. Was *happy* for about 2 hours the next morning, but while showering began to feel as had before a mission: "Physically up and nauseated, with an adrenaline rush." Lasted about 3 hours followed by calm. Reduced hypervigilance lasted through 2 days, "Even the dirt piles beside the road didn't bother me."

Session 3. Energy and mood excellent, extremely animated about changes after second treatment. Slept "like a rock. "Surprised when asked about body temperature. Since his return from Iraq, he had been sweating constantly, day and night. Hadn't noticed that sweating had stopped.

Session 3 produced the most dramatic response of all: immediate return of long-term memory. As the sensors were being removed, Jay gasped and said he was remembering things. He knew the current day and date, birthdays and anniversaries, past postings, family occasions and family memories that had been lost to him for years. His young son, wide-eyed, asked his father if he remembered going to the amusement park years before. Jay *did* remember and as they talked about that day, the little boy glowed with excitement. His joy at being able to laugh with his dad about their past experiences was thrilling to see. For the first time they had a shared history, common ground that, until that moment, had been lost to that boy and the entire family. Now he had his father back.

His wife checked him with questions such as when they were stationed in North Carolina. "We were never there," said Jay, who had long had false memories of North Carolina. He now remembers his prior tours in Korea, bases and buddies.

Throughout the session Jay was flooded with memories of family, his old car, and sports in high school. Later in this discussion he mentioned craving peas with onions. This shocked his wife who had noticed that since the injuries his taste in food had completely

---

1. Seeing roadside clutter caused intense flashbacks because dirt and trash were used to hide IEDs. The difference between PTSD and memory is that flashbacks are incredibly detailed. Unlike ordinary memory, you remember *too much*. *Every* detail is there and you cannot forget it.

changed and he would no longer eat things he had previously favored. Peas with onions had been a favorite dish.

From this point on, after just 3 sessions (his first week of treatment) Jay never again wrote down an appointment, and he never forgot one. Short-term memory also improved; he knew date and time without looking at his watch. He could also read again. On intake, he was unable to read because it caused headache and mental fatigue, but during the week following Session 3, he completed one book and started another.

By Week 2, PTSD reactions and sweating were greatly reduced and he had *no headaches all week*. Sometimes his right leg felt like jelly, possibly because he was doing more without the wheelchair, and the leg was tired from unaccustomed use. Anxiety was also down; he might notice something and feel some anxiety, but nothing like his previous reactions of wanting to stop the car and get away despite knowing there was no real danger. He is still bothered by crowds, still scans for suspicious persons and activities, and finds the noise irritating. But now there is no anger. "I'm much calmer than I have been."

Less fearful about his future, he began to see a life for himself. "I now have hope," he said, "that I will be able to function for my family and myself."

SESSION 4-5. Body temperature is normal during day and most nights. Sleep, energy, appetite, good. Now likes the foods he liked before Iraq. Mood good; anger replaced with "lots of patience." Blood tests showed that previously therapeutic doses of Tramadol and Percocet are now overdoses. Needed only one Percocet over the weekend to control pain of surgery.

Long-term memories that flooded back after Session 3 remain. "It was as if my brain opened and all memories came gushing out," including the ones he wishes he didn't have, hoped he would forget. But less intense—they are memories, not flashbacks. Wife lost way driving to office but suddenly Jay could see the route in his head and guided her. Increased energy: going to playground with children. Less volatile: wife reports he hasn't yelled at her for some time. Some changes uncomfortable for family. Wife must adapt to a husband now involved in their children's lives, discipline and family decisions, that had previously been hers alone.

SESSION 6-7. His doctor stopped Trazodone last week; he is sleeping well without it. No sweating at night. Physically stronger, even went into the water to play with his kids. Has been fearful about his future, but now that he can think and is beginning to remember things, he is hopeful that he will be able to function for his family. "Impatience is gone." He remembers phone numbers, what his wife tells him, and now is reading. Family moved into 4-room apartment. Slept 10 hours last night. Upbeat, conversation clear, energy very good. Items seen while unpacking brought back memories — excited that he could remember their histories.

Sessions 8-9. Mood excellent: "I'm getting back to my old self. Even my wife said so. She even told me she loves me, and gave me a kiss." Excited re trip for family visit. Wife eagerly scheduled appointments for after their return. In wheelchair because of leg pain from lifting furniture, doing repairs, playing outside with the kids during the move. More work than he has done in a long time. His doctor is tapering off lithium and Zoloft. Feeling clearer and memory continues to improve.
Sessions 10-17. Sleeping all night, good energy. Thunderstorms remind him of mortar fire setting him "on edge," but not panicked. No longer notices roadside rubbish. Began to talk about traumatic experiences in Iraq b/c emotional content not upsetting. OK in crowds.
Sessions 18-21. Depressed, but with good reason: he is losing vision in left eye, cause unknown. Doctors can't operate on his leg b/c might make it worse. Had just learned that another member of his group shot himself, the third person he knew at Walter Reed who had suicided. But also commented on his life before treatment: My wife hated me, I hated me, I hated my kids. Now my wife says she loves me, and I love her and my kids." Now feels good about himself and being "part of his family and society."
Sessions 22-23. Reported intense dream about Iraq, people he knew who died. Is in "medical limbo" b/c treatment plan is uncertain. Spontaneously[a] brought up suicides; three soldiers in Iraq had asked for help and were told to make an appointment. All suicided. Now feels good to talk about this with others.

a. Subjects are *not* required to discuss their experiences.

After his 23rd session Jay suffered an accident with concussion and possible skull fracture (see Color Section). Within the week he was also diagnosed with lung cancer. Before end of treatment, Jay had surgery, but memory remained good. Despite these stresses, on 6-month follow-up, Jay's symptoms had not worsened, a testament to the resilience that often appears with neurofeedback treatment.

Even more remarkable: improvements not only occurred but continued despite severe sleep apnea (untreated until after the study ended), the ongoing effects of toxic exposure during his service, and the stress of regular treatments to drain fluid from his lungs.

"The biggest achievement of treatment," said Jay, "is that it has given me back a feeling of being normal and human again. I can accept things that can't be changed, feel good about myself, and be part of society. If I hadn't gotten treatment I would be on the verge of divorce, kids hating me, and I not caring. Now I can be a dad.

"You have given me back my life," he said.

Paul: The Medic
PTSD, MIGRAINES, INSOMNIA, HYPERVIGILANCE, POOR CONCENTRATION, BACK PAIN

Q. How will you know you are better?
A. No expectations, but if only I could read without getting tired.

During Desert Storm, Paul endured long-term exposure to diesel exhaust, depleted uranium, and other toxins. On patrol in Iraq, they would bounce madly down a washed out dirt road at 60 m.p.h. with IED's exploding about every 5 seconds behind them. This was to outrun IEDs timed to target vehicles traveling at about 40-45 m.p.h. When an overloaded Bradley rolled, he struck his temple on an interior rifle mount and injured ribs, neck, and tailbone. Once, while he was eating breakfast, a rocket powered grenade blew overhead, so close that its wake pushed his head down. It hit 15 yards away.

> For two days we sat in the middle of a war zone, waiting for the Marines, who were going door-to-door and room-to-room, to catch up to us. The sound of rifle fire and breaking glass went on day and night. Nobody could sleep; wrestling matches to relieve stress were constant because our nerves were so charged. I don't think I slept for three days, and then when I did, it was only for a few hours. I couldn't stay lying down or even sit still.

At Walter Reed, signs and symptoms of PTSD included two severe episodes of extreme adrenalin rushes lasting two days. "I paced back and forth all night long, unable to sit still or lie down for more than five minutes, hearing the constant noise of breaking glass." If he shut his eyes he began to quiver. Night sweats were severe with daily migraines, inability to concentrate when reading, and a constant "busy feeling" in his head.

Sessions 1-3. For the first two sessions, symptoms got worse, especially headaches and sleep problems. Paul wrote: "By Session 3, I was feeling amazing beneficial effects. The busy feeling I had in my frontal lobe was the first symptom to go away, then my quick wit came back. The headaches went away next, then the night sweats and leg jerking, and finally my irritability with my peers and road rage."
Sessions 4-11. Sleeping 6 hours straight through the night, compared to 3-4 hours before. More relaxed around his peers, and "Back to my old self emotionally, socially, and mentally." Sleep continued to improve. Could study more efficiently and remember material better.

In a letter to the Deployment Health Clinical Center at Walter Reed, Paul wrote: "My medical background teaches me that when a patient is more relaxed, the healing process goes much faster. It is my opinion that this treatment should be available to every patient coming from the war in Iraq or Afghanistan, and recommended for all PTSD and TBI sufferers."

At end of the study, he took a difficult national certification exam and passed on his first attempt. Paul is now married and continues on active duty.

Kyle: The Marine
LOSS OF EXECUTIVE FUNCTION, HEADACHES, BACK PAIN, MEMORY LOSS, INSOMNIA, READING
AND BALANCE PROBLEMS

> Q. How will you know you are better?
> A. Better mood, better memory, and not afraid to sleep at night.

Kyle had an active, athletic life with many falls in the course of skateboarding and surfing. As a child he had sinus surgery and suffered two Grade 3 concussions.

Over two deployments and 15 months in Iraq, Kyle was hit twice by explosions that destroyed two Humvees and threw him 30 feet through the air. The first time he landed on his neck, the second on his spine. Both times he was taken out by MediVAC.

Because of crushed discs and vertebrae, he was 1.5 inches shorter and walked with a cane (partly for balance). He also suffered 24/7 non-stop headaches; these were frontal, centered around the eye. His doctors prescribed Flexeril® (cyclobenzaprine), Mobic (meloxicam) and anti-inflammatory NSAIDs such as Motrin®, but he stopped taking them because they interfered with his thinking. Worst of all, they gave no relief. Neither did physical therapy or chiropractic. He was getting almost no sleep.

Once a quick learner, Kyle had signed up for two on-line introductory college courses but he had to drop them because he could barely read. Even menus were so difficult that he would go only to restaurants whose menus had pictures of the food, so he could point. His psychologist said his symptoms were all psychological.

While still on active duty, FNS neurotherapy began with Dr. Esty in March 2009.

Session 1-3. Almost no sleep, can't read long enough to get anything done but headache immediately dropped from a 9 to a 4 during first treatment.
Session 4-7. Headaches much better, throbbing pain has disappeared, with only a couple of short spikes. Headache returned after a trans-Atlantic flight, but dropped from 10 to 3 with treatment. A sudden urge to write appeared after Session 4. "I got some paper and started writing" (both prose and poetry). Reading still difficult, but wants to write a screen play.
Session 8-9. Back is "killing me!" — because he mowed lawn and cleaned house. Despite the back pain, balance is better.

During a treatment break in early summer, Kyle phoned to report that headaches and back pain were much better. By July, he had the energy to drive over 600 miles in 12 hours to go jet skiing. Unfortunately, this resulted in two new hits to the head. First he hit a pothole; the shock slammed his head into the car's ceiling. Later, he tumbled off his jet ski, hitting the water so hard that his face was swollen.

Session 10-12. His back is still painful after jet ski accident but cognition better. Headache up to 5, but better after treatment. He is walking without a cane. "Not sure why I feel better" but *feeling so much better* that he now wants to go to Officer School and to a "brick-and-mortar" (not on-line) university for a degree in Journalism. Headache down to 2.
Session 13-15. Memories of the war and his concussions are returning. Not flashbacks; just memories. Headaches gone. Body temperature now normal. Running again (3 miles in 25 minutes and 10 seconds), and passed the Marine Corps physical. Recommended for promotion. Back in the online school, and getting A's on tests. Working towards Associate in General Studies but wants to try for higher degree.
Session 16-23. Many stresses but improvements continue. Designed his own program for Wounded Warriors. His stiff neck and arm have been relieved by a chiropractor at National Naval Medical Center.
Session 24-25. When Kyle started, all symptoms were rated as 9s and 10s — now zeroes.

Writing began after Session 4. "I couldn't, never did before, and I couldn't read when I came in. Now I am reading books. I knew I could get my back fixed but I didn't know about my brain. My life is a thousand times better than before I started treatment."

After treatment, Kyle was so improved that he passed the physical and was redeployed.

Kevin: The Mechanic
SEVERE COGNITIVE AND MEMORY PROBLEMS, SEIZURES, PTSD, NIGHTMARES, PAIN, NUMBNESS, MALNUTRITION, POOR HANDWRITING, DIFFICULTY READING, LOSS OF SPATIAL MEMORY, SUICIDAL

Terrible things had happened to Kevin, long before he went to Iraq.

As a toddler Kevin had fallen down stone steps, hitting his head hard enough to raise a memorable goose-egg. As a child, he was hit by a car while riding his bike. As a teenager, he crashed down the side of a mountain riding a bike while drunk. He lost consciousness several times due to hard hits during football and soccer games, but graduated high school with average grades. As an adult, he was again hit by a car while bike riding and thrown to the pavement. He had several blackouts due to alcohol, multiple concussions from fights, mixed martial arts, and water skiing. And then he went to war.

In Iraq, he was regularly exposed to blasts and toxins from burn pits, vehicle maintenance and armaments. Because the money for the planned maintenance facility vanished, the facility was never built. Teams worked in sealed shipping crates, without safety gear, in terrific heat with no ventilation for solvents and diesel fumes. In one blast, he lost consciousness long enough that the Marines who rescued him found him still unconscious.

After returning home, seeing his children triggered terrible flashbacks. He suffered severe memory problems and extreme difficulty maintaining a schedule or getting anything done. He needed all day to wake up, usually becoming alert by 4 pm, but back in bed by 8 pm, a pattern explained as "lack of motivation." Weekly seizures usually lasted 2-5 minutes, but some continued for up to 7 minutes. After being put on anti-seizure medication, he experienced lost stretches of time accompanied by dizziness, drowsiness, and muscle weakness. When his wife asked for a separation he went to live with his mother.

Then one freezing December dawn, Kevin walked out of the house wearing only a T-shirt and jeans. He had intended to commit suicide but was found and taken to a psych unit where he was diagnosed with major depression and PTSD. There was no mention of concussion contributing to his condition, however, an MRI revealed a temporal lobe lesion, thought to be the cause of his seizures. A SPECT scan found significant abnormalities possibly representing serious cortical atrophy. Diagnosed with ADD and a learning disability, he was admitted to a day program with intensive traditional therapies, but showed little improvement. A psychiatrist who specializes in PTSD referred him to BWB.

At intake, Kevin was on multiple medications, including lithium for depression, Lamictal®) for seizures, Buspar® for anxiety, Remeron® and Celexa® for anxiety. His diet was phenomenally bad, consisting mostly of chips, chocolate, and ice cream. He especially liked Hostess Ho Hos and ate 20 at a time while complaining of poor appetite. He felt his best, he said, at 160-170, but weighed 210. Exercise was extremely limited due to pain and fatigue. His skin had an unhealthy quality.

He could not sleep without medication. When sleep did come, it was poor, with terrible nightmares. Thoughts were scattered, tangential, incomplete. His memory was so poor that his wife would not permit him to drive. He also had body pain, comparable to sore muscles, but feeling more as if his skin was being stretched. Reading was difficult, and he practiced handwriting, forming letters as slowly and laboriously as a child learning to write cursive.

FNS neurofeedback treatment began in March 2012 in the USUHS study.

Session 1-3. After first treatment, no nightmares. Could remember more of what he read. After 2nd session his wife let him drive a bit. After third, pressure in head went away for short time.
Session 4-6. More control over hand; writing and reading continue to improve. On stroking rough fabric on arm of treatment chair, he realized that fingers were less numb. Thinks his comprehension and processing are improving. He did some "pleasing" things instead of sulking, watched TV in order to laugh, and fell asleep without meds at a reasonable hour. Mother is pleased, says "He is softer and gentler with me," talking more, making plans, coordinating better with other people. To diet of Ho Hos, has added baby spinach and apples.
Session 7-10. Pain is less. Can now read and remember sentences; when he copies things (practicing handwriting) not copying word by word. Suicidal thoughts are down. Long-term memory returning. Wife now more comfortable with his driving. More feeling in thumb. Has started a commercial driving course, and a home repair course and is able to apply what they are teaching. Can be with children now without flashbacks.
Session 11-13. Took his children to a movie. In classes can process more quickly. Muscles sore from exercise. Applying for jobs. Has "done some cooking", so eating less junk and fast food. More positive long-term memories in talking with his wife.
Session 14-19. Fewer nightmares. Thinks driving back to pre-Iraq levels. Much more coherent and fluid in conversation. Suicidal thoughts are gone. "Skin-stretch pain" and short-term memory ratings dropped from 10 to 2. Anti-seizure meds down to 200 mg from 300 mg. (Had already stopped Remeron, Buspar, and Celexa.) Improved feeling in all fingers. Eating only 6-9 HoHos *every other day*. What he was calling "fast food" is actually *burgers and salads rather than junk*. Now he eats out only once a week because he is able to organize, shop for groceries and cook meals. Skin looks much healthier than when he started.
Session 20. Diet now green salads, fruits and vegetables, more protein and *much* less sugar. His geographic memory of the area has returned.

At 6-month follow up: Kevin regularly takes his children to museums, something they used to do a lot. His mother is thrilled with his changes; he is doing a beautiful remodel of her house and getting more jobs from neighbors who see his good work. On the downside, he and his wife are divorcing, but his social world is steadily expanding. Previously isolated, he is reconnecting with others.

David: The Communications Tech

HEADACHE, BODY PAIN, PTSD, EXPLOSIVENESS, INSOMNIA, DRUG ABUSE, SEVERE DEPRESSION

> Q. How will you know you are better?
> A. When I can be in a crowd for an extended period.

David joined the Army after 9/11, and served in combat areas and on border security. He survived multiple concussions (three in 2004 alone), multiple blasts from IEDs and ammo dump explosions, plus back and knee injuries with shrapnel and torn ligaments. After a 2006 explosion, he began to suffer severe insomnia. A medic gave him a handful of pills but when friends found them, he was sent to the Army's Landstuhl Regional Medical Center. There he drank heavily, took any drugs he could find, and was repeatedly arrested for fighting. After a particularly wild night, he found himself facing four assault charges.

David gave away his belongings and cleaned out the room. When a friend saw this classic pre-suicidal behavior, he was sent to the Inpatient Psychiatric Ward. There he was diagnosed as bi-polar with PTSD and Post-Concussion Syndrome. Sedation with Trazodone caused severe depression, which was treated with Effexor®, which kept him from sleeping at all. It also caused seizures, "so they gave me *more* Trazodone; instead of getting better, I got worse." Back in the US and in the psych ward for PTSD and substance abuse, he complained again about seizures from Effexor®, and again the dose was *increased*. Drugs now included:

- Naproxen and nortriptyline for headaches with lithium to counteract the side effects from nortriptyline (insomnia, agitation, anxiety),
- Trazodone which produced depression and Effexor® to counteract Trazodone,
- Vistaril® and Seroquel® for anxiety, PTSD, insomnia, and bi-polar diagnosis[1].

Eventually, all traditional methods of treatment had failed. To call my prognosis "unhopeful" was an understatement. I was aggressive, paranoid, angry, depressed, and nihilistic, unable to focus enough to take part in conversations, unable to read more than a few sentences. "Sleep" was an hour or two in 48 hours. I would leave my room only when forced to, for appointments, or (rarely) for food. Drug abuse and violent behavior continued. And I was still suicidal.

David was referred to Dr. Esty by his therapist. FNS treatment began in September 2007

---

1. Seroquel® is prescribed off-label for sleep problems and nightmares related to PTSD.

Sessions 1-3. After first session felt "wired, floaty, as if I had taken Sudafed," feeling lasted the rest of day. Began sleeping at night, six straight hours of uninterrupted sleep. Went to Borders and found it relaxing. Less vigilant, able to read a magazine. Cleaned room. Headache returned briefly. Usually a pack / day smoker, he hasn't a cigarette in 48 hours.

Session 4-6. Remembering dreams (including one nightmare). Less anxiety even on flight home. Airports hard but startle response less, did not need anti-anxiety med. Still irritable but temper under control. Now leaving his room at WRAMC and going out more — grocery shopping, to the movies.Some headaches, but less frequent.

Session 7-9. Going out for pleasure. "Besides, dammit! I have to feed myself!" Previously he would call someone to bring food. Emotional after last treatment, some songs brought tears. Less noise sensitivity, startle response, and situations where once he would have blown up but didn't even get angry. Memory improving. Memory more "present, "not flashbacks."

Session 10-19. Everything good and holding. Slept 7 & 8 hours on weekend. Woke once with recurrent war-related nightmare. These started in 2004, less frequent now. Less fatigued, less light and sound sensitive. Walked several miles alone along busy highway ("I just felt like being *out*"), without sunglasses or headphones. Continues to go to mall and be comfortable. 5 hours at bookstore & no headache. Any headaches are sharp but short (15-20 minutes). Crowds no longer bother him. Can even sit by windows and has stopped taking anxiety med.

Session 20-24. The day before Session 20 was the anniversary of the Feluggia Fest, the day he lost half his platoon. "Now I remember so much. I'm not numb now. I have a life now. It still hurts, but not the searing pain and anger. It feels good to talk." Went to a military ball. Good mood. Has written 40 pages about his war experiences. "Other people noticing that I'm less scattered in my speech." In an argument, he was able to articulate his thoughts, something he had been unable to do since the 2007 VBIED. "Now I can just brush things off. I'm not angry anymore."

Session 25. Pleased at having "No explosiveness." Feels that his memory is better than before deployment. Anxiety is completely gone. At a bar, had been able to socialize with no anxiety at all, and talk about experiences without getting upset. He is moving back home with goal of going back to school for a degree in psychology.

A few weeks after finishing the FNS series, neuropsychology testing was repeated while David was ill and on cold medication. The examiner noted *"mild difficulties* with extended concentration and variable processing speed, most likely exacerbated by the antihistamines he took to treat the cold." Still, most of his scores were "Above Average" or "Exceptional."

But most importantly, I felt like *me* again, the *me before* all the deployments, before the physical and emotional trauma of war, but more mature than I was before it all. I had a real future, something to look forward to. I couldn't wait to get out and find a way to help other veterans who had found themselves in situations similar to mine. I wanted to study neuropsychology with a specialty in PTSD.

David was discharged from the Army with 30 percent disability, a low rating. Medical paperwork states *zero* deficits after the FNS treatments.

That is: *no* remaining PTSD or cognitive deficits.

Since then, the VA has officially amended his record to state that symptoms leading to diagnostic labels of Bipolar Type 2 and Borderline Personality Disorders were actually side-effects of Effexor® and Trazodone[1].

Back at school, majoring in chemistry with a psychology minor, he was declared Psychology Student of the Year and inducted into an academic honor society. "Academically," he said, "my biggest problem was deciding what to do next. The neurofeedback treatments didn't just *change* my life, they *saved* my life."

Today, the wounded warrior with disabling insomnia and PTSD, whose goal of community college was viewed with such skepticism, has gone on to advanced medical studies.

---

1. On the other hand, the psychiatrist dismissed any positive effects from neurofeedback.

Mike: the War Correspondent

DRIVING PHOBIA, POOR MEMORY FOR CONVERSATIONS, LOSS OF TECHNICAL SKILLS, IRRITABILITY, HYPERVIGILANCE, FATIGUE, POOR FOCUS, PROCRASTINATION, PROBLEMS FINDING WORDS IN SPEAKING AND WRITING, FEELING STUCK AND FLAT

The journalists who cover war zones endure many of the same conditions and stresses as the actual soldiers. Anyone who comes back from war needs time to adjust to "normal life" when, for too long, *normal* has been *war*. The big difference for journalists is that when they return, they have no job-related support system waiting to help.

At age 22, Mike was assigned to report on the Bosnian War only to find the experience so terrifying that he could not function. He lasted just one day, heading for home on the first plane out of Sarajevo. Two years later, he returned, reporting on the continuing fighting in Bosnia, Croatia, Macedonia, and going on to the Sudan and other war zones around the world. A good journalist and a good cameraman, Mike went on to work in music and sports, producing high-end documentaries, but his specialty remained war reporting. It was fearful work, but Mike did it very well.

From 2002 he worked, usually without military protection, filming and interviewing, working 19 hours a day, without a break for weeks at a time, while dodging IEDs, kidnapping attempts on journalists, and some of the most gruesome casualties he had ever seen.

In 2004, the truck was hit and Mike was hurled into the air, landing on his back. He was 3 weeks into a 6-week tour before he could get treatment for severe back pain. Eventually the pain eased somewhat, but other problems remained.

One was driving, often a major problem with veterans returning from Afghanistan and Iraq where wild driving was a technique to survive attacks by snipers and IEDs.

By 2005, Mike was having extreme difficulty driving on highways, especially through tunnels and over bridges. When he returned to the US in 2011, he drove no faster than 25 on the local streets. Every traffic light, every stop sign was a relief, time to catch his breath. But on driving through a tunnel, he had a sudden terrifying feeling that he could not control the car and an inexplicable urge to crash the car into the wall. His wife took over all driving. He had a short fuse with people in general, but was terrified of police[1].

Unable to drive and feeling that he was no longer a nice person sent him to a psychiatrist who diagnosed "fight-or-flight syndrome" and prescribed beta-blockers. They didn't help.

Meanwhile, the thought of applying for a job was hopelessly overwhelming and intimidating. He was afraid to pick up the phone, afraid to call, afraid to speak with people. Only

---

1. "Perhaps," he muses, "that was due to having so many guns pointed at me by people in uniform throughout my career."

sheer desperation — rent and bills to pay — drove him to approach a new company. Thanks to his extensive experience he was hired on the spot, but on his first shoot, he could not remember how to operate the camera he had used for 12 years.

> Some mornings I came in hours ahead of schedule just to practice with the camera. Even then, the film looked terrible because I was shaking so badly. I could not write or focus and was barely able to compose a single e-mail per day. I couldn't believe how badly I was doing and spent most of my time trying to hide my fears and challenges.

Because of continuing back pain, Mike had seen a physician who knew of Dr. Esty's study. Initial testing and evaluation by USUHS researchers revealed that he could not multiply or remember numbers, "and I failed the memory tests so miserably, even *they* were shocked."

Then FNS treatment began in Oct 2012 in the USUHS study.

Sessions 1 - 3: "I did feel quite a bit of pain in my back and ribs but it lasted only that evening." Next morning, pain not as strong as usual. Couldn't remember what wife said in a political discussion but wrote a new proposal and many e-mails. Energy "Great" and felt rested. Finished all goals. Surprised by vivid memories of traumatic events in Iraq. After Session 3: Drove fast on assignment, 84 m.p.h., without panic. "I see progress, big changes. Energy levels skyrocketed."
Sessions 4-9. Nervous but no panic attacks even in a difficult driving situation. Huge job stress. Cleaned up over 1,000 e-mails that had been meaning to do for a year. Taught at a conference, nervous but went well. Vivid feelings about Iraq lasted ½ hour after talking with soldier who drove over an IED. Still short term memory lapses but per energy: "I feel fantastic."
Sessions10-11. Extremely productive. Clearer thinking. Writing long concept e-mails and worked 40 hours in 2 days on a job. Going on overseas assignment.
Sessions 12-14. Fear of police gone. Handled press conference ("used to be the worst fear next to death") without fear for first time ever. Now can drive over bridges but with no fear. Still forgets whole events. After Session 13, described the trauma of seeing a friend killed by a blast 200 yds away. [Session 13 is often when clients bring up a detailed description of some trauma.]
Sessions 15-18 [done over 3 months]: Teaching overseas. Much calmer and making smarter decisions, able to think more strategically. Not afraid anymore. "I was weak, afraid, terrified of myself. My disability was handling life. Able to operate some complicated equipment had never seen before and did a superb job. Couldn't have done that in the past. "I can't comprehend how I was able to become that frail, weak, person that was so afraid. I can't tell you how my life is different."

By December, Mike was back to working on political campaigns, sports, and high-end documentaries. He has now returned to life as a high-powered full speed professional, in high demand for his excellent skills and high quality professional productions.

And he is driving at safe speeds.

Why Haven't I Heard of This Before?

PARADIGMS AND PRIORITIES, DRUGS, DENIAL AND INSURANCE COMPANIES.

N eurofeedback works, but its effects are often denied because it does not fit the paradigm. What is a paradigm? A belief set; an accepted idea of how to do things. If observations match the accepted pattern or template, we keep them. If not, we throw them out.

This process underlies much squirming about in search of a "logical explanation" for things that don't fit the current paradigm[1]. Sometimes "logical" has little to do with actual *logic,* more to do with desperate attempts to shove observed but awkward facts into (or out of) the existing pattern box. Those that don't fit are *anomalies*, things "against the law" of the existing pattern[2]. Blips in the data may be dismissed as "the exception that *proves* the rule," implying that exceptions somehow make the existing rule even stronger[3]. But too many will eventually require a different box, or trigger a "paradigm shift," a new pattern or model.

In 1848, Dr. John Harlow's report on the injuries of his patient, Phineas Gage, was received with frank disbelief that anyone could survive such a severe brain injury and still walk and talk (Neylan TC, 1999). Gage was later examined by Dr. Henry J. Bigelow, a classically trained professor of surgery at Harvard Medical School. Bigelow pronounced Gage fully healed, then used this case as proof against *phrenology,* at that time, the only field that considered the possibility of localized brain functions.

---

1. From Greek *paradeigma*, "a pattern, model or example that we follow. At root the word means to compare or "show" (things or ideas) "side by side." The idea of a *paradigm shift* originated with philosopher-physicist Thomas Kuhn in *The Structure of Scientific Revolutions* (1962).
2. From Greek *a* (not or contrary to) + *nomos*, the system of laws and measurements associated with a field (such as astronomy, economy, or taxonomy).
3. Originally, the phrase actually had the opposite meaning: the exception *tests* the rule, from Latin *probare*, to test. In English, this sense still survives as "proving ground" a place for *testing.*

In contrast, Harlow was interested in phrenology and had witnessed Gage's sufferings first hand. After Gage's death, Harlow had Gage (and his tamping iron) exhumed. With Gage's damaged skull in hand, he wrote a second, more detailed report that radically changed medical perceptions. Crude though phrenology may have been, Harlow's view of the case was a better fit with emerging theories of brain function (Barker FG, 1995).

We are all the product of our paradigms, but our biggest problem is in recognizing them. The current medical paradigm is generally high tech, highly interventional, delivered by white coat specialists with prescription drugs, and, of course, sadly expensive.

Drug Traditions

One reason neurofeedback isn't more familiar is that our medical system is so heavily based on medications. Drugs are easily stacked, stored, and prescribed in seconds. They are extremely profitable. In contrast, neurofeedback is a hands-on service that takes time and training and effort, and does not lend itself to huge profits. That issue aside, drugs are often given simply through custom. It is what is done. Even if a physician doesn't want to over-medicate, many patients feel cheated if they leave the office without a prescription.

Drugs Prescribed for TBI

Several drugs are often prescribed to treat individual side effects of TBI. Unfortunately, they often fail to help and can bring on dangerous or frightening side effects.

- AMBIEN® (ZOLPIDEM), prescribed for insomnia, has caused sleep-walking; users may awaken enough to get out of bed, but are not fully conscious. Incidents involving the drug have ranged from binge eating, conversations and shopping trips in the middle of the night, to falls, assaults and traffic accidents — of which the patient has no memory[1] (Kolla BP and Others, 2012).

- SEROQUEL® (QUETIAPINE) has been used to quell nightmares but has possible side effects of valve flutter and sudden death due to heart failure.

- AMANTADINE, originally approved as an anti-flu drug, was later used for Parkinson's and MS. In severe TBI, studies showed good results (Giacino JT and Others, 2012). But rate of improvement slowed after treatment, dropping below placebo so that the ending average improvement was similar in the two groups. It causes hallucinations if taken with other Parkinson's drugs.

Citicoline, long used worldwide for TBI, was recently tested in a randomized double-blind trial of 1,213 patients with mild to severe TBI. Not only did it fail to improve survival, there were no significant differences between those who received the drug and those who

---

1. The morning after David (page160) took an Ambien®, he learned that he had left his room at WRAMC, talked to other patients, and had long conversations on Yahoo, but with no memory of doing so. "Worse than a bottle of Jack," said his doctor.

were on placebo (Zafonte RD and Others, 2012). An editorial accompanying the report notes one obvious reason for failure: *too many kinds of injury.* No one drug can address hematomas, edema, clots, bullet wounds, tears, inflammation, depolarization, breakdown of the blood-brain barrier, and diffuse axonal injury. In conclusion, writers Ruff and Riechers stated a hard truth, still accurate in 2014:

> There are currently no effective treatments [medications] to reduce the severity of TBI-related deficits among patients with complicated mild or moderate TBI.
>
> —Ruff R and Riechers R II (2012)

Nevertheless, we keep trying existing drugs or waiting for new ones that one day, we hope, will work better. One may be the natural hormone progesterone.

The suspicion that progesterone might blunt the damage of TBI began with Dr. Donald Stein, neuroscientist and professor of emergency medicine at Emory University in Georgia. In the 1980s, he noted that female rats were better than males at memory tasks after induced brain injuries; *pregnant* females did best. Stein found that *progesterone*, a hormone high during pregnancy, reduced inflammation and appeared to aid neurogenesis and recovery. If given within four hours of injury, it blocks brain swelling and appears to protect against damaging free radicals while promoting repair of white matter (Stein DG, 2013). In human females, the degree of damage and likelihood of healing after TBI may depend on where they are in their menstrual cycle (Wunderle K and Others, 2013).

Long dismissed as "merely" a female hormone, progesterone (like estrogen and testosterone) is present in both men and women. Like many other hormones, it may have multiple functions including protecting the brain.

In a trial of 100 TBI victims, the death rate in the placebo group was 30 percent after 30 days. In vivid contrast, death rates dropped to 13 percent for patients given progesterone within 4 hours of injury and these patients also showed greater functional improvements (Wright DW and Others, 2007). Another study of 82 patients showed that higher function continued at 3- and 6-month follow-up (Xiao G and Others, 2008)[1].

So there may be an effective drug for TBI (one that we've had all along), coming sometime in the not-too-distant future. In the meantime (especially if your injury is more than four hours old), it may be time to try neurofeedback.

---

1. New research is underway in 15 states. For details, see www.clinicaltrials.gov. The studies are ProTECT III (funded by NIH) and Synapse (funded by BHR Pharma, LLC). Sites that are actively recruiting participants include: Arizona, California, Georgia, Kentucky, Michigan, Minnesota, Missouri, New York, Ohio, Oregon, Pennsylvania, Tennessee, Texas, Virginia, and Wisconsin.

Reducing Drugs in TBI

One interesting result of neurofeedback is reduction in the need for medications to treat symptoms. This allows physicians to reduce drug use in TBI and PTSD.

Table 9-1 shows the reductions in prescription drugs ordered by physicians at Walter Reed Army Medical Center (WRAMC) for their patients who were treated by Dr. Esty using FNS in the study with Iraq/Afghanistan veterans (Nelson DV and Esty ML, 2012).

Table 9-1. Drug Reduction in Veterans During Neurofeedback Study		
Prescription Drugs Being Used by Veterans at Beginning of Study	**Prescriptions Reduced or Eliminated by WRAMC Physicians in Course of Study**	**Physician-Prescribed Drugs Remaining at End of Study**
1-01[a] May 18, 2007 Ambien® 10 mg Lithium Percocet Phenergan® 25mg x 6 Tramadol® 150 x 3 Zoloft® 100 mg x 2	6/1/2007: Phenergan® Tramadol® 6/18/2007: Ambien®, Lithium Percocet®, Zoloft®	Lithium Zoloft
1-02 None reported	NA	NA
1-03 Depakote® and "Alcohol supplement"	Depakote®	None
1-04 Nortriptyline Vistaril®	Nortriptyline Vistaril®	None
1-05 Celexa® 40 mg. Effexor® Neurontin®	Effexor® Neurontin®	Celexa® (20 mg)
1-06 Abilify® Ambien® Klonopin® Trazodone Zoloft®	Abilify® Klonopin® Trazodone	Ambien® Zoloft
1-09 Celexa® 40 mg Prazacine 5 mg Seroquel® 700 mg	None	Celexa® 40 mg Prazacine 5 mg Seroquel®700 mg
1-11 All meds stopped pre-study. Subject said they didn't help, and hurt cognitive function.		

a. This subject is Jay the Driver whose story begins on page 151.

For physicians to be able to reduce medications (and disturbing side effects) in their patients is only part of the story. Consider also the improvement in quality of life that comes with return of the ability to function as a parent, a friend, a team member, as *yourself*.

When you can again participate in all levels of living, then you are *alive*.

Research Priorities

I have had the opportunity to visit the laboratory of Dr. Mary Lee Esty and reviewed the method as well as experiencing the (FNS) method on myself, and I have no hesitation in saying that this is a minimally invasive, non-traumatic technique, which certainly caused no discomfort whatsoever in the process of my experience with the FNS stimulation. Because of the lack of any formal treatment currently available for the treatment of the post-TBI symptoms, I would certainly recommend that this research be completed in order to define more closely the efficacy of this method.

—Dr. Ayub Ommaya (1997)

All agree that more neurofeedback research should be done, but despite the enthusiasm and recommendations of highly respected researchers, it is extremely difficult to get funding for biofeedback and neurofeedback in the US. Most studies have been small clinical studies. Larger ones (such as Monastra V, 202) have shown a persistent pattern. AD(H)D children improve with either drugs or biofeedback. But when the drugs are stopped, the children treated with drugs revert to their previous condition. When biofeedback is stopped, those children keep their improvements and continue to improve over time. Nevertheless, in the U.S., drugs are preferred for treatment -- and research.

When the American Academy of Pediatrics (AAP) declared biofeedback to be a Level 1— Best Support for ADD (page 118), equivalent to drugs, they based their evaluation on the German and Canadian studies below[1].

- Gevensleben H and Others (2009), Is neurofeedback an efficacious treatment for ADHD? A randomized controlled clinical trial. Study done at the Department of Child & Adolescent Psychiatry, University of Göttingen, Germany.

- Levesque J, Beauregard M and Mensour B (2006), Effect of neurofeedback training on the neural substrates of selective attention in children with attention-deficit/hyperactivity disorder: Done at the Centre de Recherche en Neuropsychologie Expérimentale et Cognition (CERNEC), Département de Psychologie, Université de Montréal, Canada.

- Beauregard M and Levesque J (2006), Functional magnetic resonance imaging investigation of the effects of neurofeedback training on the neural bases of selective attention and response inhibition in children with attention-deficit/hyperactivity disorder. Done at the Centre de Recherche en Neuropsychologie Expérimentale et Cognition (CERNEC), Département de Psychologie, Université de Montréal, Canada.

The following website provides the history of the decision, supporting studies, and links to journal articles.

www.braintrainuk.com/wp-content/uploads/2013/07/How-AAP-reached-conclusion-other-recent-evidence-July-2013-V3.pdf

1. www.aap.org/en-us/advocacy-and-policy/aap-health-initiatives/Mental-Health/Documents/CRPsychosocialInterventions.pdf.

Insurance Benefits

> 1.5 years after moderate TBI: I have serious questions whether [he] will be able to resume his usual work. It may be better to train for a different, less complex type of work.
>
> —Neurologist's prediction for recovery in Gregory's medical record (1984)

As insurance companies discover that neurofeedback treatment is effective, as they find they can save money, some are adding this treatment to their policies.

As a child, "Gregory" was hospitalized after a roll-over vehicle accident and after falling from a second-story window, but had never thought of these events as involving concussions. As an adult, he worked as a computer progammer, but in 1982, at age 26, he was accidentally hit in the head by a large rock thrown by a landscaper who was horsing around on his lunch break.

The result for Gregory was daily migraines so severe that he would lose vision suddenly. He could no longer work, did not dare to drive, and at least twice every month, he landed in after-hours care at Kaiser Permanente.

Table 9-2. Pre-Treatment Charges of Kaiser Permanente	
Desipramine	175 mg
Imitrex®	(as needed)
Inderal®	80 mg
Midrin	(as needed)
Ritalin®	500 mg
Demerol®	100 mg
Phenergan®	(as needed)
Charges for ER:	$2,100
Medications:	$ 544
3-month Total:	**$2,644**

Before starting FNS treatment in January 1998, the many ER visits over the previous three months cost Kaiser close to $900 per month (Table 9-2).

The day after his first FNS treatment, Gregory was once again in the ER with a migraine, but this one was unusual; it lacked the aura and vision loss that had accompanied his migraines for over 16 years. The next migraine, appearing after five treatments, was so unusually mild that he did not go to the ER at all. After eight sessions Gregory had not had a migraine for over a month. By the last of 25 treatments, he was able to resume full-time study for a technical computer certification. He returned to work at his previous level of employment. As of August 1999,

> I am rarely ever in after-hours care at all. I have been able to control my migraines with little intervention by Kaiser because they are far less frequent or severe. Migraines occur occasionally but are now so mild that they can be handled with OTC meds.

While this story shows clear benefits to a patient, it also shows benefit to his insurance company. Coverage depends on condition and on the individual policy. Aetna, Cigna, and sometimes Blue Cross cover biofeedback and neurofeedback for some conditions.

Others do not.

Figure 9-1 is a scan of an insurance company letter denying coverage for biofeedback / neurofeedback treatment for another client. (The Mayo site referenced, but poorly visible in the letter, is: **www.mayoclinic.com/health/post-concussion-syndrome/DS01020**.)

The letter is interesting from several standpoints.

---

regarding the appeal process, please feel free to contact us at the number listed below. Authorization has not been certified for the following clinical reason(s):

Rationale / Source of Determination:

According to the Mayo Clinic, there is no specific course of treatment for post-concussive treatment, but rather treatments for the specific symptoms experienced by each individual. Although the Mayo Clinic clearly does document that the best treatment for cognition and memory problems is "time," stating that most cognitive and memory problems resolve by themselves within weeks to months after the injury. Secondly, the Mayo Clinic also advises that cognitive therapies based on teaching compensatory memory strategies, such as utilization of calendars and/or relaxation strategies, can be helpful in treating post-concussive syndrome [1]. While it is possible that relaxation strategies were involved as part of the neurofeedback procedure, there is no documentation of this in the notes. There is also no documentation of the date of onset to determine if enough time elapsed to allow for the body to heal over time. There are some articles found that do lend some support for neurofeedback to treat post-concussive treatment, but they appear to generally involve very small numbers of test subjects and are thereby inconclusive.

The standard of medical necessity for the neurofeedback treatment provided does not appear to be met for several reasons. The initial intake reveals that the patient was, at the time of intake, able to drive, work and study, and maintain close relationships, so it is not clear from the documentation in the file in which major functional domain this patient was experiencing clinically significant impairment requiring such treatment. Also, the clinician submitted a letter dated 7/20/13 suggesting that justification for neurofeedback was at least in part related to failure of other treatments, which does not justify a course of treatment. The peer-to-peer call did not change the determination.

References:

1. Mayo Clinic. Post-concussion syndrome. Available at:
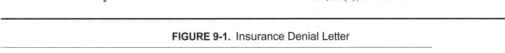 http://www.mayoclinic.com/health/post-concussion-syndrome/ DS01020. Accessed on 12/12/13.

2. Duff J. The Usefulness of Quantitative EEG (QEEG)and Neurotherapy in the Assessment and Treatment of Post-Concussion Syndrome. Clinical EEG and Neuroscience. 2004; 35(4); 198-209.

FIGURE 9-1. Insurance Denial Letter

The writer bases denial on a brief website overview, then misquotes it.

[The] Mayo Clinic clearly does document that the best treatment for cognition and memory problems is "time," stating that most cognitive and memory problems resolve by themselves within weeks to months after the injury.

In fact, the website does *not* document "time" as the best treatment. It says that after TBI:

Time *may* be the best therapy for the treatment of cognitive problems . . . as *most* of them go away on their own in the weeks to months following the injury.

What about the ones that don't go away? Clients seeking neurofeedback for cognitive problems do so because symptoms have *not* resolved, and because (as Mayo's website *does* state): "*No medications* are currently recommended specifically for the treatment of cognitive problems." It is precisely because drugs have worked so poorly that we must rely on innate body processes to heal over time. Approaches that support those processes are proving to be the most effective for problems that have lingered on for years. Only after neurofeedback did Carol recover suddenly after 7 years, Ben after 12, and Bill after 17 years of disability.

The only test mentioned in the Mayo Clinic overview of Post-Concussion Syndrome is a CT scan (normally done in the ER). In place of drugs, it suggests cognitive therapies.

Certain forms of cognitive therapy may be helpful, including focused rehabilitation that provides training in how to use a pocket calendar, electronic organizer or other techniques to work around memory deficits and attention skills. Relaxation therapy may also help.

But learning to use a pocket calendar does not heal TBI; Mayo clearly recommends this strategy specifically as a "work around" to deal with continuing memory problems. Strangely, the Duff paper, cited to support denial of the insurance claim, *directly contradicts* statements made in the letter. For Duff's actual words, see www.pubmed.com/15493535:

Post-concussion syndrome has been used to describe a range of residual symptoms that persist 12 months or more after the injury, often despite a lack of evidence of brain abnormalities on MRI and CT scans (Duff J, 2004).

Duff further notes that "Post-Concussion Syndrome" is not a matter of a few weeks or months. Physical evidence of memory, headache, and other problems may not appear on CT scans, the only test mentioned on the Mayo website. Sufferers need more. Duff goes on to say:

While cognitive rehabilitation and psychological support are widely used, neither has been shown to be effective in redressing the core deficits of post-concussion syndrome. On the other hand, quantitative EEG has been shown to be highly sensitive (96%) in identifying post-concussion syndrome, *and neurotherapy has been shown in a number of studies to be effective in significantly improving or redressing the symptoms of post-concussion syndrome, as well as improving similar symptoms in non-TBI patients.*

The insurance company writer appears aware only of studies with "very small numbers of test subjects." This is unfortunate considering the many studies of neurofeedback and AD(H)D, which is increasingly recognized as symptom of post-concussion syndrome[1].

It is perfectly reasonable for a company to deny payments for a problem that doesn't exist. The denial letter notes that at intake, the patient was able to drive, work, study, and maintain close relationships, so he must be Fine. Once again, the problem may be the words, which so often do not mean what we think they mean. When *Fine* is a point of etiquette (rather than real information), when *mild* TBI can end a life, one should be suspicious of other words such as *driving*, or *work* or *relationship*, or even *yes*.

Can you drive? Nearly everyone says "Yes!" But Ben could not deal with a four-way stop, Morgan had to be directed — block by block — by phone. Brian drove off with all four car doors open. All got lost. There is more to "driving" than sitting in the driver's seat.

Can you work or study? "Yes!" Many work and study very hard, with little result. Those unwilling to "give up" (as they may see disability payments) may insist that of course they *can* work, they're just having a few problems right now.

Can you be in a relationship with someone? "Yes!" Because they are, even if it isn't a good one. Marie and her husband were about to divorce; he was certain that her supposed symptoms were deliberate attempts to annoy him. Steve's marriage was on the rocks because his wife thought he was purposely rejecting her. Bill's fiancee left him. Just like Henry, Edweard, Mary, Howard and Elvis, all of these people were *in relationships with someone* — until that someone was gone.

So what do these words and questions really mean to the patient? *It is important to find out.*

It also matters what words mean to insurance companies and the words *biofeedback* and *neurofeedback* may present problems. *Biofeedback* (coined in 1969) was used through the 1970s. In the 1980s, as researchers targeted brainwaves, the name changed to *EEG neurofeedback*, then to *neurofeedback*. All of these may be used interchangeably. The research papers supporting APA recommendations of "biofeedback for AD(H)D" actually use the term *neurofeedback*. The older (as in "back to the 60s" word) *biofeedback* may be perceived seen as "relaxation," that is, something nicer than "tense," but of no great value. In contrast, the newer and less familiar *neurofeedback* may be interpreted as "new and untested."

In fact, *biofeedback* and *neurofeedback* are the same thing: an attempt to help the brain / body *system* return to a balanced state. The impact of that can be life changing.

Meanwhile, the insurance denial letter (Figure 9-1) offers several useful lessons.

---

1. Duff J (2004) further states: *The core deficits of post-concussion syndrome are similar to those of ADHD and mood disorders.* See Table 3-2 on page 41.

- Keep up with available information. There have been enormous advances in brain research over the last few years.

- Use *good* resources. The Mayo Clinic website is a reliable *general* source but offers little detail. For original research, see www.PubMed.com and page 260 for directions).

- Be aware that there is a serious time lag between research and application and even its availability. As of this writing (March 04, 2014), the Mayo Clinic page has not been updated since September 29, 2011. Newer or more complete information[1] (by organizations and researchers that specialize in brain research or its application) is not included.

As client or as clinician, be aware of the issues and be prepared to keep very good notes. Why? Because one day, you or a friend or a family member *will* suffer a TBI.

It may be anything from cartwheeling down the stairs to a slip on the ice, a fall in the tub, a deceptively gentle rear-end collision or crashing and rolling in or from a vehicle. Maybe there will be blood and broken bones, maybe not. Maybe just a bit of bruising, or no visible injury at all so that it seems, in the beginning, that nothing is wrong. And while you may feel a bit shaken, a little wobbly, surely all will be better soon. Well, maybe.

Hope for the best in terms of recovery, but assume and plan for the worst.

If symptoms appear, waste no time dismissing them as imagination, especially when they begin to impact life and function. Track them, write down and document what is happening and what is being done. Notice their effect on your job, what the boss says, what co-workers say, surprised comments or complaints by family and friends. Notice how life is different.

If you are unable to work, don't count on getting any kind of insurance compensation. Insurance examiners will not be looking at symptoms in your favor; their job is to protect themselves. And, in our experience, most neuropsych tests miss very real functional changes. Insurance companies are not required to cover rehab through *vocational recovery*[2]. They only need to cover enough to get victims *out of the hospital and home*, and only as long as the facility can document improvement. Keeping *very* good notes can help.

So can neurofeedback. Although claims of "no research" continue, there are decades of clinical research reports in the medical and psychological literature. Much new research is now appearing. Unfortunately, average readers never see it. When they do, they find reports that are purposely dry, stripped of any emotion, written in a conscientiously professional monotone. In the world of scientific writing, this is intended to present at least the appearance of objectivity, to avoid undignified screaming matches and to fit more data into less space in journals. Readers would scarcely know that, behind the statistics, there are live human beings

1. Such as the American Academy of Pediatrics (AAP) statement on Biofeedback / Neurofeedback in 2012. See page 169.
2. Personal communication, Maria Romanas, M.D., Ph.D., February 14, 2014.

tortured by nightmares, haunted by the past and fearful of the future. These are real people who have lived too long and too hard in head injury hell, whose husbands and wives and children are terrified for them or of them.

Larger studies are needed, but in the U.S., funding has been elusive. Studies are usually evaluated in terms of possible return on investment. Neither Wall Street nor drug firms wish to back research that may reduce or eliminate profits (Jim Robbins, personal communication, 2012)[1]. This is true despite the promise for the entire health care field and for many conditions long considered to be life-long problems or disabilities, even those starting in childhood.

If every school had neurofeedback available to every child who began to show problems in learning or behavior, it is possible that a lifetime of poor academic achievement, special services, and inability to work and earn might be avoided. This would save society — and even insurance companies — millions.

Physicians report that, in patients given neurofeedback treatment, they have been able to reduce or eliminate their patients' medications. Neurofeedback providers report that clients are able to return to work, finish school, stay out of trouble with the law and to live contented lives as productive family and community members.

What is the return on that investment?

What exactly is that worth to society?

---

1. Dr. Esty had a telling experience while giving a presentation at a Johns Hopkins lunch meeting. One slide showed reductions in prescription medications in veterans after neurofeedback treatment. On seeing this, the drug rep got upset and left quickly. The lunch her company provided was very good though!

Denial

Biofeedback and neurofeedback address the enormous power of the autonomic nervous system, which is, itself, much too wonderful to be true. So are the senses of sight, hearing, and smell, especially to those who have lost them. Getting them back again is *not* too good to be true, it represents truly good *healing*.

One problem is a long cultural tradition of Good versus Evil, and the assumed Free Will of heart and mind and spirit to choose between them. For many, it is difficult to accept the idea that choice of behavior is not necessarily under a person's control, that the ability to choose can be altered by illness or injury.

One of the oddest problems is denial of healing by patients themselves. Such terrible stigma is still attached to any mental problem that few are willing to admit to ever having had a brain injury — and therefore, cannot admit to having recovered from one.

Or, after repeated disappointments with high-tech traditional therapies, some refuse to believe that neurofeedback could work. It's just *too* easy, *too* simple. Just as there is no model for explaining the appearance of symptoms (other than "laziness") there may be no model for their disappearance (other than "Just going through a phase" or "It must not have been as bad as I thought").

Or, a return to normal is just *normal*.

Years after a car crash, Bobbie, a once-excellent athlete, had the usual post-TBI symptoms of depression, killer headaches, explosive anger, and such sensitivity to light that she could only listen to TV and never went out without dark glasses. Sequencing problems? "Anything more than *one* is too much" she said. Severe fatigue made simple household chores, such as washing a few dishes, an ordeal. She spent most of her time on the sofa. One day she needed to use her computer, but realized that it was upstairs: "I'll have to use it *tomorrow*." That is, after she dragged up to bed, after a night of poor sleep disturbed by nightmares, she would be in a position to bring the computer downstairs with her the next day.

Three sessions of neurofeedback brought many "little changes." Light sensitivity dropped after mapping alone and after the first treatment it was gone. Chores were *easy*, and she was running errands in town without exploding in rage at the driver in front of her. Headaches dropped in number and severity, she no longer thought twice about running upstairs when she needed to, and when she went to bed she was now sleeping through the night.

These are *"little"* changes? "Well yes," said Bobbie.

Look at what I'm saying: "I get up in the morning. I do my work. I wear dark glasses only if it's really bright out. And then at night I go to sleep. It's just . . . *normal*.

Normal is not the sort of thing we write home about, or announce to others. Especially to those whom we prefer to *not* know that there was a brain injury in the first place.

Others, regardless of obvious healing, see themselves as forever damaged. When a client's injuries are severe, when the standard drug therapies did not improve cognitive function and neurofeedback *did*, inability to recover *all* function, *all* of life before the TBI, may be seen as a treatment failure.

After his severe TBI, Bill (page 49) was unable to hold any job, or do his own work well; it took him nearly a week to do laundry. Body temperature was extremely low, he had vision loss and slowed speech. He could not stay awake more than 2-3 hours at a time, but sleep was poor and haunted by nightmares of the car crash. After neurofeedback *done 17 years after the injury*, he was suddenly and happily and busily awake all day. Body temperature and vision were back to normal, speech had improved greatly, laundry was done in just a few hours, and he was sleeping well with pleasant dreams. He was asked to write something about his neurofeedback experience.

"Oh, but I can't!" he said. *"I'm not cured."*

Others deny any changes at all. After many treatment disappointments it can be easier to assume that nothing, including neurofeedback, will ever help. If one points out obvious changes, or repeats those reported by the clients themselves, they may be dismissed as imagination or coincidence, or on the grounds that because there have always been Good Days and Bad Days, those things must have happened on a Good Day.

Changes may be marveled at by others but still fiercely denied by the client, who suddenly removes the clutter and trash piled three feet deep in the back of the van and has cleaned out the garage. He may notice nothing more than mysteriously sore muscles and complain that treatment is doing nothing except causing "terrible fatigue."

"What is the nature of this fatigue?" you might ask. And often it turns out that after years of being unable to sleep more than *two to four* hours per night, he is now "so tired" that he is suddenly sleeping *seven or eight*. Meanwhile, he has broken off a bad relationship, finished taxes three months early, and this week he painted the entire upstairs. What if you point out that the paint cans have been sitting there for three years?

"It was just *time!*" he retorts, swearing that nothing is different, this isn't working. But the terrible depression has lifted and the reason there has been no time to smoke pot or take drugs is simply that he has just been "too busy."

And then one morning, the guy who couldn't get out of bed before 3 pm and couldn't stand sunlight or motion or human company, calls to say that he won't be coming back because the neurofeedback wasn't helping anyway, and besides, on this brilliantly bright and beautiful July day, he would rather play golf with his friends.

It is helpful for clients to have outside observers, watchers, people who have known them well before and after the accident. It is important for therapists to keep good session notes, and if at all possible, for the client to keep a journal of how things are. Only then can they see how things used to be and how much better they have become.

Healing from a brain injury can be like sitting in a rowboat in the middle of the ocean, far from land. What do you see? Only the horizon.

Imagine that a giant wave passes under your boat, raising it higher. What do you see?

Only the horizon. But there may be a whole new world ahead.

If you have symptoms of brain injury, don't just assume they are things that you "must expect at your age." Check them out. You may get your life back, an easier, more productive life, sometimes better than ever before.

Neurofeedback may be resisted on the grounds that it is just too *simple*, too quick and easy to address serious physical and psychological symptoms. But neurofeedback does not replace appropriate medical care, counseling and psychotherapy. It is hands-on treatment, person-to-person and it takes time. It won't teach you to spell or do your math homework, but it makes it possible to learn again.

It does not do marriage counseling, or teach strategies to deal with the playground or office bully. All it may do is give you a better functioning brain and body that makes it possible to do things you may have thought you would never be able to do again.

Sometimes that can be everything.

Sometimes more is needed.

Part 3

Coming Home

CHAPTER 10 When More Is Needed

BASICS THAT MAY NEED ADDITIONAL ATTENTION AND TREATMENT. ASSOCIATED INJURIES, HEADACHES, PAIN, AND DEPRESSION. ON BUILDING A TEAM (AND A POINT OF VIEW) TO HELP AND HEAL.

There is no rule that limits injuries to one condition only, especially in concussion which often includes blunt trauma. Broken limbs are easily seen but more subtle strains may go unrecognized with enormous impact on the rest of the body.

When the cause of symptoms is unclear, some may dismiss them as imaginary. Others lump them with Post-Concussion Syndrome. But a *syndrome* is a group of symptoms observed to "run together." It is not a diagnosis or specific disease; at best it is a work in progress and more information is needed. TBI often causes injuries that are not normally considered — or treated — but should be. Continuing symptoms deserve a complete medical, neurological, and dental exam.

Common possibilities include problems with or damage to:

- Basic physiological processes or requirements.
- Sleep, including apnea.
- Muscles and connective tissue (page 186),
- Inner ear (page 194),
- Bones (including but not limited to neck and skull).
- Teeth including infections and breaks.
- Autonomic Nervous System (page 199).

The Basics: Food and Water, Light and Air

If you don't eat, can't sleep and can't breathe normally, you can't heal.

Basic, yes, but basics are often overlooked. There is no magic pill, no therapy, no high-tech intervention that can replace them.

Most of us know the importance of food, water, sleep, light and air. Deficits in any or all of these can contribute to one of the worst side effects of TBI: depression.

Nutrition

A dozen or more vitamins and minerals have "depression" as the first sign of deficiency. The cure for that is not anti-depressant drugs, which oddly enough, can actually perpetuate symptoms of depression[1].

The hardest time to eat well is when it is needed most, when too injured, too sick, too weak, too depressed, in too much pain or too confused to function. If may be hard to eat at all, especially if the injury involved teeth or jaw or abdominal injuries. When it is too fatiguing or painful to get up or to move, it is easier to avoid food or drink entirely. The result may be dehydration, which leads to slowed metabolism, which in turn causes constipation which can cause new and terrible symptoms including nauseating headaches.

Fast foods (such as a daily diet of pizza and soda or beer) are tempting, but cause more problems than they solve. Other seemingly healthful choices, such as commercial soups, are high in salt. They are also high in MSG which is blatantly harmful to an injured brain.

One of the best ways to help a person with TBI is with healthy food and fluids, possibly featuring home-made soups and broths, most conveniently done in a crock-pot.

Light and Dark and Depression

Light is a nutrient. It controls mood, wake and sleep cycles, all commonly disrupted in TBI. Bright light produces mood-elevating serotonin which is the raw material for the sleep hormone melatonin. Autopsies have revealed lower levels in persons who died in winter compared to those who died during the summer (Carlsson A and others, 1980). The same pattern was verified in live humans. Regardless of the season, levels varied with hours of sunlight exposure on the day samples were taken (Lambert GW and Others, 2002).

PET scans have also measured changes in serotonin synthesis occurring while subjects simply *thought* about positive or depressing things (Perreau-Linck E and Others, 2007).

---

1. Some drugs deplete B vitamins needed for energy metabolism. Others, containing fluorine, replace the iodine required to make thyroid hormone. Low thyroid alone can cause depression, fatigue, weight gain and often lower nutrient intake. . . and the cycle continues.

Up moods? Higher serotonin. Down moods? Lower serotonin. The findings suggest a two-way flow, with serotonin influencing mood and mood influencing serotonin (Young SN, 2007). This may explain why Cognitive Therapy can be as effective for depression as drugs (DeRubeis RJ, 2005). It matters what we think about, what we dwell on.

But light sensitivity is common in TBI; it does not encourage exercise in bright daylight that could help relieve many symptoms. Another possibility for more light exposure is through the Philips GoLITE, a small portable LED light that emits a specific wavelength of blue light, typical of early morning light. The intensity can be raised or lowered depending on sensitivity. For many people, the goLITE is like flipping a switch on depression.

Sometimes there is the opposite problem — not enough *dark*. For some people, if they can see any movement at all during sleep hours, there's too much light. If impossible to darken the room, a sleep mask can be a great help. At the very least, for two hours before and then during sleep hours, avoid bright light, especially blue light, the high-energy wavelengths that promote wakefulness in the morning. Sleep-destroying blue LED lights may appear on your computer screen (avoid late-night surfing!) or other electronic devices[1].

Also consider a daylight clock. It will wake you up slowly by gradually increasing the light level. It gives you time to finish a dream and to awaken gently and naturally with no screaming alarms or beepy noises[2].

Why can't we just take serotonin pills? Because serotonin does not cross the blood-brain barrier[3]. But serotonin is made from tryptophan, high in turkey, even higher in milk[4], hence the classic home remedy of a cup of warm milk with a pinch of nutmeg as a sleep aid.

---

1. www.webmd.com/sleep-disorders/news/20110119/light-exposure-may-cut-production-of-melatonin.
2. Bio-Brite has been around awhile and worked out most of the bugs. Philips has several models but stick with basics. Check reviews at www.Amazon.com.
3. Serotonin is carefully controlled in the body; too much can be deadly (as in serotonin syndrome).
4. And in chick peas. Levels in domesticated peas are almost twice that of wild varieties, suggesting that seeds have long been selected for higher tryptophan content (Kerem Z and Others, 2007).

Sleep Disruptions and Apnea

Good sleep is as critical as good food and good air. Sleep deprivation alone can trigger migraines, seizures[1], and eventually death.

Sleep disruptions are common after TBI, but sleep can be disrupted even in uninjured brains by noise and light. Some people go from a glowing computer screen straight to bed or leave the TV on all night in the bedroom. But light suppresses melatonin, the sleep hormone, which in turn interferes with the body's ability to regulate temperature, blood pressure, blood sugar levels, and weight (Hendricks B, 2011). In nature, morning light trends towards blue (the high-energy end of the spectrum); by late afternoon, towards red. Bright high-energy light at night can disrupt natural rhythms. To avoid this, consider the following.

- Incandescent bulbs towards the warmer red frequencies are less disruptive than "cool" (i.e., more "blue") lights which trend towards higher frequencies.
- Best night lights are red, not bright white, never blue.
- The room should be dark. If not, a sleep mask can help.
- The room should be quiet. If not, earplugs or a white-noise generator can help.

If there is no problem going to sleep, but you wake repeatedly during the night, there may be sleep apnea. Or maybe not. But if you suffer headaches and fatigue and never seem to get enough sleep, it's always worthwhile to check.

Apnea is named for interrupted breathing during sleep. Pauses between breaths (known as *a-pneas*, or periods of "no-breathing") may last from 10 seconds to several minutes, occurring up to 30+ times per hour. Or, breathing may be so slow and shallow that it qualifies as *hypopnea* ("under-breathing"). The person is breathing regularly, but getting inadequate oxygen (*anoxia*) which starves (and injures) the brain. Sleep apnea is strongly linked to headaches and linked so very strongly to heart problems that multiple studies have found some form of apnea to be common in heart failure patients (Krawczyk M and Others, 2013).

Sleep apnea is tested with an overnight sleep study (a *polysomnogram*). Clinicians look for 5 or more episodes of either apnea or hypopnea, neurological arousal, 3 per cent or greater drop in blood oxygen, or a combination of both arousal and low oxygen.

What is meant by *neurological arousal*? Essentially it means that your brain realizes it is suffocating and struggles awake, out of the deep slow brainwaves of sleep to deal with the situation. The constant arousal blocks deep, restorative REM sleep, contributing to hypertension and daytime fatigue.

---

1. When soldiers returning from Viet Nam with gran mal seizures were evaluated, the initial belief that most would be alcohol related was found to be incorrect; it was really sleep deprivation (Gunderson CH and Others, 1973).

Sleep apnea is categorized as two types: Obstructive Sleep Apnea (OSA) and Central Sleep Apnea (CSA). The two can occur together as complex or mixed sleep apnea. The obstructive form, with its snoring, choking, and sputtering, gets most of the press. It is caused by physical blockage to the airway, by overweight or floppy tissues, or by simple congestion or inflammation.

Central sleep apnea is rarely mentioned but even more insidious. It isn't a matter of blockage, there is no snoring. Breathing just stops, as if the brain simply *forgets* to breathe.

The primary muscle of breathing is the *diaphragm,* controlled by the phrenic nerve which tunnels out from between the cervical vertebrae (C3-C5).

What happens if the nerve that stimulates breathing is compressed? Uncertain, but we do know what happens if it is *stimulated*. In a study involving 13 heart failure patients with central sleep apnea, stimulating the phrenic nerve decreased apnea symptoms by over 90 per cent and increased oxygen uptake by 55 per cent (Ponikowski and Others, 2012).

Apnea may be due to obstructive tissues including weight gain. In children, enlarged tonsils or adenoids may be an issue and the result can be years of anoxia, impaired brain development and learning disabilities. Snoring in a child is not cute. It is a sign of blockage and needs immediate medical attention, possibly a sleep study, but these can take months to schedule. Anyone can do a basic "study" by collecting basic data. A parent, a spouse, a friend can sit by the sleeper with a watch and a note pad, to count breaths per minute, to time the interval between breaths, to listen for snoring and choking. A sound-activated recorder by the bed can record snoring or gasping episodes during the entire night.

Another issue is sleeping *posture*. The first step to easy breathing is a clear airway. Be sure that neck and airway are not contorted by too many pillows or awkward positions.

Apnea is usually treated with Continuous Positive Airway Pressure (CPAP) machines. These can be very effective, but it is important to realize that they do not provide oxygen; they simply *pressurize* the air available. This may be an issue in extremely energy efficient homes with poor air exchange, especially during in combination with gas stoves, dryers and other combustion appliances, especially during the winter.

Open a window or get out and get some air!

Soft-Tissue Injuries

The most common injuries are to muscles and connective tissue.

Muscles and Fascia

Even if there is minimal damage to spinal cord, brain, discs, spine and nerves, there may be significant injury to the cervical (neck) muscles producing pain and headache.

—Peter Dunne, M.D., Neurologist[1]
Professor Emeritus, University of South Florida, College of Medicine

Muscles alone can cause severe pain. And, specific muscles have specific pain patterns. Pain from the trapezius muscle of shoulders and back is often diagnosed as cervicogenic tension headache, migraine, and bursitis (Figure 10-1). One muscle, three diagnoses.

Pain also comes from fascia (*fash-uh*). This is the first nervous system of the developing embryo; it provides structure and communications long before nerves appear (Meyers T, 2008). Fascia is also *piezoelectric* ("pressure-electric"). That is, under pressure or strain (due to injury or poor posture) it can send signals to points far from the origin. Because the fascial net runs from head to toe and back again, stress anywhere along the path can show up as a pain signal somewhere else.

The trapezius muscle alone can produce pain variously diagnosed as tension headache, migraine, and bursitis. *One muscle: three diagnoses.*

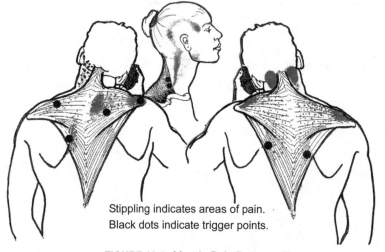

Stippling indicates areas of pain.
Black dots indicate trigger points.

FIGURE 10-1. Muscle Pain Patterns: Trapezius

1. Peter Dunne, personal communication (2013).

The combination of dysfunctional muscles and fascia (including trapped blood vessels and nerves) results in what is known as *myofascial* pain. *Trigger points* are areas of shortened tangled fibers able to "trigger" pain to distant areas along myofascial pathways[1].

One of the most striking examples of referred pain is from the soleus, a *calf muscle that sends pain to face and cheek*. No single nerve or muscle runs from calf to head. What does? *Fascia*.

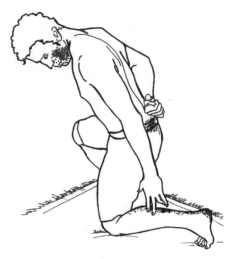

Pain of myofascial origin is often thought of as less serious, less "real" than other pain, but it includes labor pains and angina. In reality, pain from these organs is not necessarily separate from "organic" pain. Fascia enfolds individual muscles and organs like sheathing, or a shrink-wrap leotard. Nerves, blood vessels, and most pain receptors travel along, between, and through fascial layers so that tight muscles and fascial adhesions can entrap nerves and blood supply resulting in brutal pain.

FIGURE 10-2. Muscle Pain Patterns: Soleus

Myofascial pain appears in specific (or overlapping) patterns and is commonly involved in post-traumatic pain of all kinds.

---

1. Myofascial pain and dysfunction was a field largely pioneered by Dr. Janet Travell,

Post-Traumatic Headaches and Migraines

The most common continuing problems after TBI are headaches and migraines.

Migraine and TBI have many overlapping symptoms. Unfortunately a diagnosis of migraine, especially with an undiagnosed concussion, may result in inadequate treatment with migraine drugs and no further investigation. Migraines should never be explained away simply as "genetics" or something you have just because your mother had them — especially after a whiplash injury to the neck.

HEADACHES FROM THE HEAD

Saying that "*some* headaches come from the head" sounds a bit circular, but in fact, not all headaches start there. Those that do are often very different from those coming from the jaw, neck, back, and shoulders[1].

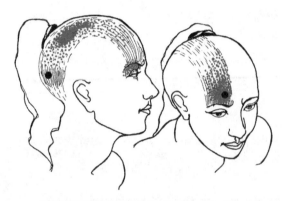

FIGURE 10-3. Pain Patterns: Occipito-Frontalis

Figure 10-3 shows a pain pattern typical of the occipito-frontalis muscle which runs from the occiput (at back of skull) to the front of the head.

This pattern appeared in a client who struck the top of his head on the corner of a kitchen cabinet producing a small puncture wound in the scalp. Pain at the point of impact was gone within minutes, but he suffered days of blinding pain in his eye, forehead, and at the back of his head.

The tissue he injured was the fascia connecting front and rear of the muscle, the same area that would have been damaged by Edweard Muybridge when he flew headfirst into a boulder and by Howard Hughes when he slammed into a ceiling instrument panel, gashing open the top of his head. Even in otherwise uninjured heads, the fascia can be strained by a tight ponytail, or compressed by tight wigs, hats or helmets.

---

1. For more on headaches and migraine, see Shifflett CM (2011).

HEADACHES FROM THE JAW

Jaws are commonly injured in whiplash and other automotive accidents. Muscles of the jaw[1] are heavily involved in headaches, especially migraines.

All jaw muscles have characteristic pain patterns (Figure 10-4). These muscles include:

- (A) Temporalis (portions of which are now known to connect to the sphenoid bone),
- (B) Pterygoids: lateral or external (left); medial or internal (right).
- (C) Masseter (for its size, the most powerful muscle in the body),

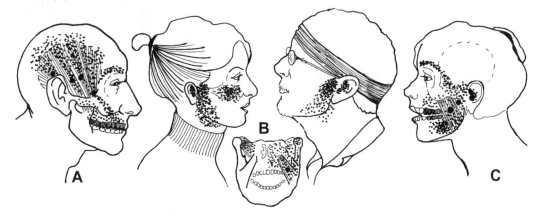

FIGURE 10-4. Pain Patterns: Jaw Muscles

Jaw muscles (plus teeth, sinuses and dura) are supplied by the trigeminal nerve (CN V) which can trigger symptoms of both sinus and migraine headaches.

All of these muscles are supplied by the "three-branched" trigeminal nerve, the cranial nerve that produces the vascular symptoms that make a headache a "migraine." It does this by controlling vasoconstriction and vasodilation (tightening and swelling) in the blood vessels of the brain. The trigeminal nerve also supplies the dura, the sinuses and the teeth.

Traditionally, women get migraines while men get "sinus" headaches, a more manly diagnosis. The trigeminal nerve is why sinus and migraine headaches, seemingly different:

- May actually be the same thing,
- May hurt right down to your teeth,
- May come with odd neurological symptoms (especially with strain on the dura, especially in combination with the spinal accessory and vagus nerves).

---

1. Technically known as "muscles of mastication," that is, the muscles of *chewing*.

HEADACHES FROM THE NECK

Head pain, *including migraine and sinus headaches,* can be *cervicogenic,* meaning "generated by the neck." When 10-year-old Krissy tumbled down the stairs at school, she injured both head *and* neck. It was hard to see improvement in TBI symptoms when severe pain clouded her mind and sapped her energy. Some pain was attributed to anxiety, but a scan (Figure 10-5) revealed clear loss of neck curvature.

The body is a system; bones do not move alone. One cause of straight or reversed neck curvature is a set of deep muscles hidden behind trachea and esophagus, attaching to the *front* of the neck vertebrae. The *longus capitis* and *longus colli* muscles are tough enough to oppose the powerful trapezius but commonly strained in whiplash and other injuries.

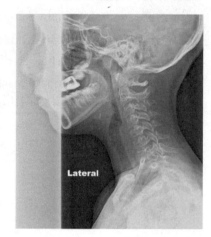

FIGURE 10-5. Neck Injury in Child

Besides pain in eye, ear and throat, victims may feel a lump in the throat and have difficulty swallowing. These muscles can also contribute to Thoracic Outlet Syndrome (by helping to raise the first rib) and cause chronic tightness in other neck muscles.

Two other muscles heavily involved in headaches are the trapezius (of upper back and shoulders) and the sternocleidomastoid (or more simply, the SCM, the powerful muscle pair that forms a V at the front of the neck). Both are commonly injured in whiplash along with other neck muscles. Pain patterns for *some* of these are shown in Figure 10-6. Headaches from this source are generally dismissed as "tension" but they can cause frightening neurological symptoms and convert to full-fledged migraines. A powerful link between muscle and migraine is at the base of the skull where a small but powerful muscle (rectus capitis posterior minor) connects directly to the dura of brain and spinal cord.

The "dural bridge" has been in the medical literature for nearly 20 years (Hack GD and Others, 1995). It has been demonstrated via dissection, MRI, and plastinated cross-sections of the upper cervical region. This direct anatomic link between the neck muscles and the dura of the brain has staggering implications for the care and treatment of chronic headache. And yet, not only is this critical piece of information missing from popular books and articles on migraine, TBI, or whiplash, it has yet to appear in any of the anatomy textbooks or dissection guides commonly used in American medical education (Kahkeshani K and Ward PJ, 2012).

These tough fascial connections are the link between muscle tension and migraine.

That is, *tight neck muscles can pull directly on the lining of the brain and upper spinal cord.*

Would that cause pain in the brain? Very likely.

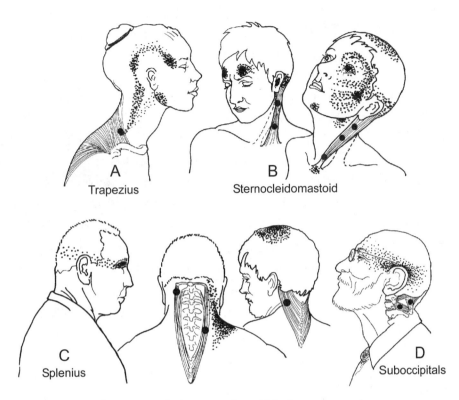

Some of the pain patterns that appear after whiplash are shown above.

FIGURE 10-6. Pain Patterns: Neck Muscles

(A) Trapezius and (B) Sternocleidomastoid (SCM) muscles are supplied by the spinal accessory nerve (CN XI) which shares fibers with the vagus nerve (CN X) which talks to all the organs, stomach, gut and autonomic nervous system. Vagus is one reason why straining these muscles can cause nausea and other neurological symptoms.

(C) Splenius sends pain through the neck and top of the head, through the head and into the back of the eye. (D) Suboccipitals send a vague persistent pain *through* the head.

(D) A direct muscular link (not shown) between muscles and migraines is found in the dural bridge formed by rectus capitis superior minor and obliquus capitis inferior (Pontell ME, Scali F and Others, 2013). These connections are not rare anomalies. When they are looked for, they are found.

(E) Longus capitis and longus colli are deep anterior vertebral muscles found behind the trachea and pharynx. They stabilize the neck by opposing the powerful trapezius; when tight, they can eliminate normal cervical curve. Commonly injured in whiplash from rear-end collisions, pain patterns extend from neck to head with pain in ear, and eye. Symptoms can include sore throat, a feeling of a lump in the throat, difficulty swallowing and pain on attempting to lift head while lying on back. These muscles are deep; palpation and treatment is for experts only.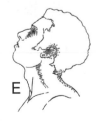

PAIN FROM THE BRAIN

It is commonly believed that brain tissue does not feel pain. It is true that neurons do not, but other tissues do, including blood vessels and especially fascia. There are several pain-sensitive fascial structures in the brain (Figure 10-7).

One is the dura mater, the tough fascial membrane just inside the skull and surrounding the brain. If you think of the skull as an eggshell, the dura is like the tough membrane just inside the shell and surrounding the yolk and white inside. Despite its name ("tough mother") some areas of the dura mater are exquisitely sensitive to strain and pain as are the falx and tentorium. These structures can produce severe headaches (Wolff HG, 1950). These can continue for years or forever . . . or until the root problem is corrected.

But the dura doesn't stop at the skull. Neither does the brain; it narrows into the *spinal cord* that travels through the *foramen magnum* ("big hole") at the base of the skull. The dura comes too, enfolding the cord like a glove or a tube. On reaching the spine, the dural tube anchors to the top three cervical vertebrae. If these are out of alignment, they too pull on the dura, its nerves and blood vessels, causing nauseating pain and frightening neurological symptoms typical of meningitis[1].

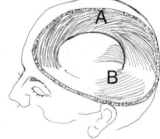

- The *dura mater* surrounds brain and spinal cord like a tough Mylar wrapper attaching to the top three bones of the neck (C1-C2-C3) and the tailbone (coccyx).

- The *falx* (B) which arises from the crista galli of the ethmoid bone, divides the brain into two distinct halves (hemispheres). See Figure 4-6 on page 85.

- The *tentorium* (C) sits like a "tent" over the cerebellum, dividing the "little brain" from the big one.

Dura, falx, and tentorium are all sensitive to pain. So are some blood vessels.

FIGURE 10-7. Pain-Sensitive Fascial Structures in the Brain

For most of the trip, as dura and cord travel down the spinal canal, both structures can (ideally) move freely. At the end, the dura attaches firmly to the tailbone (*coccyx*), *not* a useless appendage, but a critically important attachment for muscles and fascia. Anyone who has damaged it knows all too well that this seemingly minor injury can be followed by years of pelvic pain and *headaches*.

---

1. In the head, the cell bodies of these pain-sensing neurons report to the trigeminal nerves, those for the rest of the body report to the spinal cord.

Surgery can disrupt relationships between the separate fascial layers. When individual layers can no longer slide smoothly past each other, they form adhesions. A problem with surgical removal of anything, is that fascia and scar tissue fill the empty space possibly causing problems for years to come. This is true of appendectomies and Caesareans. It can also be true after brain surgery that may follow TBI or removal of tumors.

As if the post-traumatic headaches weren't enough, adhesions between suboccipital muscles and the dura of brain and spinal cord are strongly linked to post-operative headache. Integrating pathology and anatomy "into a unified theory of headache production," Hack GD and Hallgren RC (2004), reported a patient relieved of chronic headache after surgical separation of the dural bridge from the suboccipital muscles of the neck.

Another source of post-operative adhesions and headache is *removing and not replacing* the bone that normally separates neck muscles from the brain (a crani-*ectomy*). Removing the adhesions can relieve the headache but may also require repeated follow-up surgeries. When the first surgery is done by *replacing* the bone (a crani-*otomy*) or inserting a plate to block growth of adhesions in the first place, there is a far lower incidence of head pain compared to craniectomy patients overall (Soumekh B and Others, 1996; Koperer H and Others, 1999).

Ear Injury and Perilymphatic Fistula

An amazingly common but under-recognized issue behind many post-TBI symptoms is damage to the inner ears[1].

 Primary symptoms are sudden or fluctuating hearing loss or deafness, problems with balance, vertigo, nausea, and even with vision. There may be rushing or roaring sounds or a sensation of dribbles or stuffiness in the ears. These symptoms may be lumped under post-concussion syndrome or attributed to a sudden coincidental onset of Meniere's Syndrome without investigating the actual cause. Because inner ears *and* the eyes are so heavily involved in balance, vision may also be severely impacted; the brain diverts visual systems in an attempt to do what the ears would normally handle.

Normally, the *middle* ear is filled with air. The *inner* ear is filled with fluid (lymph). The two are never intended to mix, but blunt trauma (or even pressure changes from sneezing) can blow a hole in the delicate membranes that separate these areas. Fluid from the inner ear can then enter the air-filled space of the middle ear. The break, the hole that allows this abnormal communication is known as a *perilymphatic fistula*. Figure 10-8A shows a common area of breaks near the stapes bone. A similar (but rarer) condition is *superior canal dehiscence*, Figure 10-8B, a break in abnormally thin bone above the upper canal.

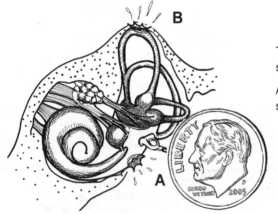

The stapes ("stirrup") bone is about the size of the letters "LIB" on a dime.

A break large enough to cause disabling symptoms is far smaller.

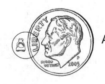

Actual sizes.

FIGURE 10-8. Structure of the Ear

A tear (fistula) is mostly likely at two especially delicate areas: A. the *oval window* (near the stapes bone) and the *round window* just below. Another possibility is a weakness or break (a *dehiscence*, meaning "to yawn or gape") in the temporal bone overlying the upper canal (B).

---

1. Dr. RJ Grimm wrote the definitive article on perilymph fistula in 1989. It is well worth reading, if only for the alarming variety of activities that led to the ear damage.

After whiplash, *with or without a head strike*, a fistula is especially common in *women*.

In subjects with neck injuries only, the number of women was disproportionately high (23 of 32 subjects) compared to men[1]. Of 65 women, 23 (35 percent) developed the condition in association with neck injuries alone, compared to only 9 of 37 men (25 percent). Of neck injuries in women, 87 percent came from vehicle collisions, compared to a only 28 percent in men (Grimm RJ and Others, 1989). The different injury rates between the sexes is due in large part to the heavier musculature of male necks compared to the more delicate female necks.

A perilymph fistula is difficult to diagnose because of its extremely small size. The injury often occurs near the *stapes* ("stirrup") bone of the ear. Figure 10-8 on page 194 shows this tiny bone compared to a dime. An injury large enough to cause symptoms need be little more than a pinprick, too tiny to be seen on X-ray, CT, or MRI. Symptoms must be evaluated by a specialist with special techniques and tools.

Sometimes fistulas heal spontaneously. Aids to non-surgical healing involve:

- STRICT BED REST FOR 1-2 WEEKS. Elevate head of the bed to 30°.
- NO HEAVY LIFTING. Nothing greater than 10 pounds.
- NO PRESSURE-INCREASING ACTIVITIES. These include sneezing, coughing, straining (childbirth) pressure changes (diving or subway / airplane rides) or nose-blowing and ear-popping to clear stuffed ears[2].
- STOOL SOFTENERS. To avoid strain due to constipation.

For many people, extended bed rest may be impossible or ineffective. Another option is surgical repair, done by closing the hole with a tiny tissue graft. Properly done, relief can be almost immediate. Untreated, symptoms can be unbelievably disabling.

---

1. Special vulnerability to whiplash also appears in female soccer players. See page 233.
2. All of these activities can *cause* a fistula; they must be avoided while a repair heals.

Bones

Neck Injury

The neck is the area where the brain becomes the spinal cord *and* where it is most exposed to injury. While the rest of the spine is inside the torso, the neck hangs out on its own, subject to the strain of bad posture or trauma of whiplash, while supporting an 8-12 pound weight in the form of a head.

Poor posture can cause an amazing amount of pain, in part by requiring muscles to provide support and never relax, to do the things that bones are supposed to do. One outstanding example is the head-forward posture (which strains muscles of back and neck). Skeletal misalignments are common after trauma, but many victims try to relieve or protect themselves from pain by distorting their posture still further, never realizing that they are actually perpetuating the problem. In the case of Bridgett (page 132) her poor posture (an attempt to guard against pain), was actually making her pain worse. Imbalances were found in the trapezius, sternocleidomastoid, and cervical paraspinal muscles. All contribute to head or back pain.

Injury or misalignment of neck (*cervical*) bones can cause a host of problems. When the normal cervical curve is lost (as often happens in whiplash), pain can be severe.

After such injuries, several of our clients have suffered severe and persisting body and head pain. It may improve with muscle therapies, biofeedback or neurofeedback, but improvements are temporary until structural distortions are corrected. Unfortunately, the impact of distortions — which can underlie chronic pain —may be overlooked or *actually rejected*, even though the person had no problem before the trauma.

When Sophia's physician saw films of her reversed cervical curve, he dismissed any link with her post-traumatic pain (page 207). "You were probably just born that way," he shrugged. He diagnosed arthritis, then prescribed Valium and Lyrica® to aid sleep.

Skull Bones and Cranial Distortions

Distortions of bony relationships don't stop with hips and knees, necks and shoulders. They can include the head itself.

The fact that skull bones move is still a relatively heretical idea. Orthodox medical thought has long said that sutures (joints) between individual skull bones ossify (fuse) by adulthood, but this is not necessarily true. Some do not ossify until middle age and later (see page 86.) So, what of children's bones, or the bones of young adults?

Anything that can move has some chance of moving out of place. A blow to the wedge-like occiput at the back of the head can shift other skull bones with painful and debilitating results. This is so not only because of the nerves that supply the sutures, but because these bones are attachments for the *falx* and *tentorium*, two pain-sensitive structures in the brain. Distortions between skull bones can strain pain-sensing fascial connections.

Most things that can move out of place may also be moved back into place again. This is the intent behind cranio-sacral therapy and its parent discipline, osteopathy. Skull bones and sutures can be jammed or distorted during birth or through traumatic injury. When bones go back where they belong, there may be remarkable changes in function and even *appearance*.

John, a superb high school athlete, suffered multiple head injuries. The most obvious was during a basketball game when he was knocked down and a large opposing player ran over him, stepping on his head. Soon after, severe migraines began to impact his life and academic performance. In just one semester (aside from the days when he was in pain but sitting in class), he missed 17 days of school. Migraine drugs offered little or no relief. He came for neurofeedback, but because his skull was so distorted, he was immediately referred out for cranio-sacral therapy.

To the casual eye, shifts in facial structure between John's before- and after-treatment pictures (Figure 10-9) may seem small. However, these small distortions were big enough to cause relentless pain and other symptoms that remained baffling as long as the source remained unrecognized. A small stone in the shoe can change gait and balance resulting in knee and back pain. Similarly, the misaligned temporal bones can shift the jaw and therefore the temporo-mandibular joint (TMJ). Every word, every bite of food involves the trigeminal nerve (CN V). Overstimulation, compression or damage sends confused sensory messages to the brain. This, in turn, can trigger alarms in the form of pain and migraine headaches, especially with pressure changes including changes in barometric pressure with oncoming weather.

After one cranio-sacral session, John's "barometer migraines" vanished. Easing cranial bones back into their proper relationships (done over six multi-hour sessions), restored the symmetry of ears, nose and nostrils, jaw, mouth, and head.

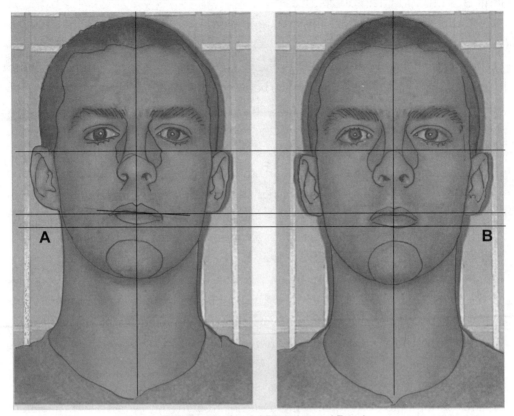

FIGURE 10-9. Cranial Distortion and Repair

Changes in a 20-year-old after 6 multi-hour sessions of osteopathic manipulation to restore normal relationships. See color section for original photographs.

A. (February 24) Pre-Treatment. B. (May 5) Restored symmetry.

> Ear: Raised and flared at left of (A) compared to the same ear in (B).When the temporal bone (which has the ear-hole) shifts, the ear must shift with it.

> Jaw and Mouth: The temporo-mandibular joint (TMJ) is the joint between the temporal bone and the jaw (*mandible*). Because the bone was shifted in (A), jaw and mouth went with it. The result was TMJ dysfunction, a major trigger for migraine that cannot be resolved until proper relationships are restored.

> Nose: Bridge of nose and even the nostrils are shifted and differently shaped between (A) and (B).

> Crown: Flattened in (A) with bulging in one temple (note hairline; in B note that there is a shadow behind the head which should not be confused with the head itself).

Traditional Biofeedback Techniques and More

At Brain Wellness and Biofeedback, passive and traditional neurofeedback are often combined with sEMG and HRV biofeedback. The reason is that any injury severe enough to injure the brain may also injure the body. These other techniques address physical problems including autonomic dysfunction. They can help correct life-long habits and chronic "stuck-ness," sometimes leaving clients even better than they were *before* the last injury.

sEMG and Muscle Retraining

Another source of pain is the strain of muscular imbalances. A first step is showing that these problems exist then training the body to release them.

Surface Electro-Myography (sEMG) is a painless, non-invasive method of observing and documenting muscle behavior, strength, and balance. A sensor on the skin picks up electrical signals as they are generated by muscles. Displaying them on a computer screen shows the actual muscle function and severity of the problem, making it clearly visible to the client, and in many cases, leading to immediate correction of dysfunctional patterns.

In the case of Robin (page 145), Emily Perlman's sEMG evaluation revealed that the previously prescribed hip exercises were actually *aggravating* her pain by forcing other muscles to fire unnecessarily; a muscle-releasing exercise relieved pain immediately. Without that information, available only through sEMG, a physical therapist can only guess at what intervention might be helpful. In Robin's case, a highly experienced physical therapist guessed wrong and his treatment actually increased the pain.

This is the essence of biofeedback: Information leads to correction of dysfunction.

Muscles behind headaches have long been ignored but sEMG can show that a problem actually exists, what it may be, and how to resolve it. Many terrible headaches, *including migraines*, start with muscles of the neck. Seeing muscle imbalances on the computer screen makes the problem clearly visible (Figure 10-10). Sensors placed on the shoulders of a headache client showed relative quiet on the left, but a storm of electrical overactivity on the right. The nauseating one-sided headaches were diagnosed as migraine but they began with imbalance in the trapezius, one reason why migraine meds failed to give relief[1].

---

1. Trapezius alone can cause the classic migraine symptoms of one-sided headache with nausea. Both trapezius and SCM muscles are supplied by the spinal accessory nerve (CN XI) that blends its fibers with the vagus (CN X), the nerve behind nausea and other autonomic symptoms.

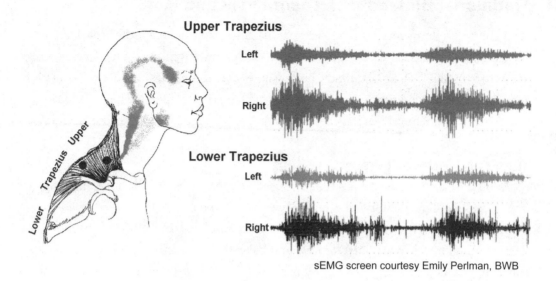

sEMG screen courtesy Emily Perlman, BWB

FIGURE 10-10. sEMG of a Trapezius Headache

Raw electrical firing of left and right trapezius muscles. Which side made the headache?

Muscle problems can be corrected through awareness, muscle retraining, guided imagery, and hands-on manual treatment. How do these problems and solutions differ?

Some improper muscle contractions are under the direct control of the client, who, if made aware of a problem, can correct it. Common instructions are to "Tense the muscles *more*, now relax them."

In contrast, sEMG offers more than "on" or "off. Clients are coached in how to make muscle pairs *work together* smoothly and correctly. Watching the computer screen, clients can *see* how their muscles work at the same time they *feel* the movement which provides wonderfully dynamic feedback. This makes it easy to change to pain-free body movements.

While some other contractions *are not* under the client's control, sEMG can reveal the difference. (See page 203).

Imagery, Handwarming, and Hearts

Along with spinal nerve stimulators . . . carotid baroflex stimulators, phrenic nerve stimulators for sleep apnea, and renal sympathetic denervation for resistant hypertension, valgus nerve stimulation for [heart failure] suggests that cardiovascular therapeutics are moving in the direction of devices that regulate or help to control autonomic balance.

—Moravec CS and McKee MG (2013)

The stronger the imagination, the less imaginary the results.

—Rabindranath Tagore

IMAGERY

Biofeedback uses a number of tools and techniques. One is imagery, not considered to be a biofeedback technique in and of itself, but an important aid in the process. People create images and sensations, or are helped to do so via "guided" imagery provided by a therapist, scripts, or recordings.

A common criticism of imagery is that it isn't *real*, it is just too *imagin-ary*, because what matters is real results. Very real results have been verified and documented with some of the most high-tech imaging equipment around but standard-issue human equipment offers valuable demonstrations. For example, at some time during nearly every human potential seminar ever held, attendees are invited to imagine . . . .

- Taking a fresh, juicy lemon from the refrigerator and holding it for a moment cool against your cheek. Feel its smoothness and texture.

- Picking up a razor-sharp knife, placing the lemon on a thick wooden cutting board, slicing into the smooth yellow skin. Smell the clean, fresh scent, see the spurt of juice as it is cut.

- Now pick up half of the lemon, and feeling it heavy with juice, raise it to your nose.

- Inhale the sharp lemon smell and feel it tickle your nostrils.

- Now put that cold, juicy lemon to your mouth, sink your teeth into it, take a big bite, and . . .

Did you notice a reaction?[1] It may be that muscles contracted and salivary glands went into action for no reason at all *except* the image that you created in your mind.

Changing real images changes the brain's perception of pain. When researchers asked chronic pain patients to view painful limbs through the wrong end of binoculars (making the limb look smaller), the pain and even *measurable swelling* decreased. The smaller the apparent size of the limb, the smaller the apparent pain. (Conversely, the larger the image, the greater the reported pain). Why this works is unknown, but it may relate to how the brain perceives danger (Moseley GL and Others, 2008).

---

1. In a similar exercise, a speaker facing an audience of fellow psychiatrists, skeptical and hostile towards the then-revolutionary concept of mind-body interaction, proceeded to read aloud a selection from *Lady Chatterley's Lover* — to the growing distress of his listeners.

At Stanford University Medical School, researchers taught chronic pain patients to reduce their pain by using visual feedback while inside a functional MRI (fMRI) machine[1]. Patients were shown specific brain regions responsible for the awareness of pain; they were then asked to *imagine* the painful area becoming smaller. Patients who learned to do this decreased their pain by an average of 44 percent on a visual analogue scale[2] and 64 percent on the McGill Pain Questionnaire (deCharms RC and Others, 2005). Using this extremely sophisticated (and costly) feedback, researchers confirmed what biofeedback therapists have known for decades: With fast and accurate feedback, people can learn to change brain function and physiology, to recognize and regulate brain states, to affect their own brains and bodies.

HANDWARMING

Learning to warm hands with the mind alone may seem irrelevant or trivial. It is not. It is an exercise in calming the entire autonomic nervous system. Brain waves change as the autonomic system shifts to a calmer state. It can be practiced at home with nothing more than a comfortable chair, a biofeedback thermometer (see Resources), and imagery.

HEART RATE VARIABILITY

Heart Rate Variability (HRV) is the most powerful predictor of mortality making it an essential biofeedback measure. HRV systems display multiple physiological measures including respiration rate, blood pulse volume, peripheral skin temperature, sEMG, and skin conductance. All of these are measures of arousal that show how well the autonomic systems (including heart and lungs) are working together.

HRV training teaches skills for dealing with stress-related problems, for return to a calm, balanced state. It can produce dramatic changes in panic/anxiety, hypertension, chronic pain, irritable bowel syndrome, and insomnia. Because cardiac function is linked to correct and efficient breathing, one of most important factors is breath training.

BREATH TRAINING

When offered breath training, clients often protest that they have already learned to Breathe Correctly in yoga or martial arts classes . . . even as they sit chest breathing, reverse breathing or visibly gasping for air. Sadly, the best measure of effective breathing technique is not the number of years spent in classes, but of *what is actually happening physiologically.*

---

1. A functional MRI (fMRI) updates every few seconds to show *ongoing* changes in brain function.
2. The McGill Pain Questionnaire is a survey form that measures sensory and emotional aspects of pain. The visual analogue scale is a series of cartoon faces, ranging from smiling to anguished.

This is done by measuring "end tidal carbon dioxide" ($ETCO_2$) during exhalation. This approach (*capnometry*) shows actual breathing efficiency. Combined with HRV, Galvanic Skin Response (GSR) and other readings, it reveals specific areas of physiological stress. Once this is known it is easier for a person to consciously achieve balance. Correct breathing can end panic attacks, chronic anxiety, and insomnia. It can reduce hypertension, irritable bowel syndrome, and some arrhythmias. Apparently it can even heal a failing heart.

In a pilot study at the prestigious Cleveland Clinic[1], investigators used breath training with patients so profoundly ill with end-stage heart failure that they were on the waiting list for heart transplants. Although transplants were thought to be their only hope, 2 of the 20 patients improved enough to be taken off the list; they were now "too well" to stay on. Most patients commented freely that they loved the training and thought it beneficial — as did several cardiologists and one psychologist who specifically commented on improved attitude and coping skills in the patients treated with this form of biofeedback.

In this group, data showed that hand warming and galvanic skin response were not a reliable therapy. But breath training improved the physiological HRV and also resulted in actual remodeling of the heart (Moravec CS and McKee MG 2013)[2].

Hands-On Bodywork

Some relaxation is beyond the client's control. For example, simultaneous but inappropriate contractions in adjacent muscles (*co-contractions*) that the client can't change with coaching and practice, suggests the presence of *adhesions*. That is, different layers of muscle are stuck together, unable to slide past each other as they must do for proper function. All the biofeedback and positive thinking in the world will not break adhesions or realign scar tissue. Drugs can't realign a distorted skull or pelvis. Direct hands-on bodywork *can*.

Practitioners with manual manipulation skills (such as osteopaths, orthopedists, rolfers, physiatrists, trigger point therapists, and physical therapists who emphasize hands-on techniques and therapeutic massage), can make enormous improvements in health and function, especially when different disciplines work together as a team. At Brain Wellness and Biofeedback, Ms. Emily Perlman coordinates sEMG and HRV biofeedback with a wide range of therapists.

---

1. Departments of Cardiovascular Medicine and Psychiatry and Psychology.
2. This included changes in beta-adrenergic receptor proteins of muscle cells with improved response to stimulation of those receptors thus increasing muscle contraction.

Case Histories: Thea, Honor, and Sophia

Thea: The Executive

HEADACHE, DIZZINESS AND NAUSEA, SENSITIVITY TO LIGHT, NOISE AND MOTION, SEVERE VISION PROBLEMS (DEPTH PERCEPTION, READING) LOSS OF MATH SKILLS, INSOMNIA, ANXIETY, IRRITABILITY, SLOWED SPEECH AND COMPREHENSION.

Thea was a department head at a large national organization. Her job description was long and complex, including program development, employee supervision, data collection, budgeting, and coordination with other departments locally and nationally.

In November of 2011, a speeding truck slammed into her car from behind with such force that an imprint of her hair clip was left in the headrest. After the crash, the left side of her face was numb, but when that faded the next day, she was assumed to be "fine." Two days later, Thea realized that although she could hear people talking, when she looked at their faces she had no idea what they were saying. Over the next few weeks this symptom worsened and more appeared. These included problems with:

- SHOOTING PAINS IN BACK OF HEAD. These followed any overstimulation, when she was trying to concentrate, and often randomly, for no obvious reason.

- VISION. Extreme sensitivity to light and motion. She needed dark glasses even in dim light, could not watch TV, or drive; as passenger, she had to cover her eyes. When trying to read, she could see only the first and last words of sentences. When trying to walk, she had to touch things before she could see them, often bumped into them, and was terrified of falling.

- SOUND AND SPEECH. Extreme sensitivity to sound and inability to follow multiple conversations. With any background noise, was unable to understand even a single conversation. Attempting to process sound affected vision. If she saw the motion of faces and hands, she could not understand what they were saying unless she closed her eyes. She could process short sentences, spoken slowly, but they had to be concrete, nothing abstract.

- SENSORY OVERLOAD. Too much light, sound, or movement triggered headaches and nausea. Crowds and busy environments were confusing, embarrassing, and terrifying. Inability to filter out sounds produced constant startle responses; she had to wear earplugs in public.

- MEMORY. Short- and long-term memory impairment. She would write "to do" notes and set a timer, but when it went off, she had no memory of what it meant. She burned herself using the microwave because she forgot that the food coming out would be hot.

- EXECUTIVE FUNCTION. Inability to identify parts of a task, to sequence, prioritize, or multi-task. Concentration was poor, she was extremely distractible. Even copying documents was too complex; she could do one page at a time, but no more, because she was unable to put the document together again. Math skills were now so bad that bank clerks had to help her count money and make deposits.

- MOOD AND SLEEP. Depression, severe insomnia, and low tolerance for frustration. Average sleep was three hours per night, but despite severe fatigue, she was unable to nap during the day. There was also a 12-pound weight gain despite poor appetite. Unable to work, read, drive, walk without a cane, or go out unaccompanied, Thea spent most of her time at home alone, descending into social isolation.

Despite this long list of symptoms, *her MRI was normal*. So apparently, was everything else. Thea's insurance claim required a neuropsychology exam, involving hours of tests that even functional people may find overwhelming (see "Neuropsychology Testing" on page 103). Examiners report not only the test results, but also the subject's level of *motivation*. Was the person really trying? Or trying to fail? When Thea did poorly on the exam, the neuropsychologist who gave the test wrote:

> [Her] overall performance raises serious concerns for motivation markedly limiting the validity of results. It can be said that her verbal and intellectual abilities and memory capabilities are at least average, with inconsistencies that confirm her failure on motivation indices.

That is, because Thea was (correctly) seen as intelligent, she *should* have been Fine.

Inability to do well on the exam *because of her injuries*, was seen as lack of motivation, an attempt to make her condition look worse than it really was. *Malingering*.

When Thea's neurologist received the report, he threw it on the floor and referred her to a more competent examiner. However, examiners are limited in how to score, based on gender, age, and educational level. There are restraints on defining outcome and effort.

"Another problem," notes neuropsychologist Angelo Bolea, "is that many examiners are inexperienced in recognizing complex cases or unfamiliar with the tests that would reveal the problems." (See Morgan on page 105.)

Thea was referred by her physician to BWB in June 2012. Dr. Esty quickly referred her to Dr. Dennis ("Dizzy Doc") Fitzgerald, an otologist and neurologist, who specializes in vestibular disorders[1]. Dr. Fitzgerald confirmed her vision loss and balance problems, diagnosed perilymph fistula in both ears and scheduled Thea for surgery.

Within a day after surgery, Thea could walk without holding on to a companion, and no longer suffered dizziness and vertigo. She could tolerate regular indoor lighting and no longer needed to wear sunglasses indoors. This is not the end of her story, but improvements in these most debilitating symptoms were huge, immediate, and would never have been achieved through any other therapy.

---

1. See www.DizzyDoc.com. Washington Hospital Center.

Honor: The Mathematician

NECK AND BACK PAIN, FATIGUE, VERTIGO, BALANCE AND COORDINATION PROBLEMS, MIGRAINES, COORDINATION, MUSCULAR WEAKNESS, AND NOISE SENSITIVITY.

Honor had degrees in math and marketing and worked as a business consultant. In August 2006, her car was rear-ended at a stop light and she was taken to the hospital on a backboard. A month later she had little memory of the accident but suffered severe pain and fatigue, sensory loss, migraines, loss of bladder control, sleep apnea, and severe arm weakness, problems with vision and hearing, nausea, vertigo, poor coordination and gait. Subway and supermarkets were disorienting, malls too much to bear.

Some symptoms were due to a herniated disc in the neck, with probable stretch injuries to her brainstem and spinal cord typical of whiplash. MRI showed small lesions in both sides of the frontal lobes. Physical therapy was attempted too soon, increasing pain to neck and back, making her feel worse.

Honor began FNS neurofeedback treatment with Dr. Esty in March 2007. At intake, symptoms ratings were 10 out of 10 for all activities of living: sleep, finding words, long and short-term memory, processing speed, balance and sensitivity to light and sound. By Session 11, only sound and light sensitivities had improved, so she was referred to Dr. Dennis Fitzgerald ("DizzyDoc"). Honor was unable to complete the usual battery of tests and diagnosed with probable perilymphatic fistulas in both ears.

The first surgery produced major improvements, but after the second, three weeks later, Honor was immediately able to stand and walk easily. She had feeling back on the left side and, for the first time since the crash, she could feel her left hand.

Honor went through a period of grief, because she could now remember what she had lost. As often happens, additional neurofeedback treatment brought back even more memories of her prior function and abilities. It was frustrating to have to re-learn old skills. Nevertheless, with additional FNS therapy, she reported return of function as exponential.

"I'm so grateful," she said, "to be off this roller coaster ride."

Sophia: Neck Injury and Fibromyalgia

FATIGUE, POOR MEMORY, FOGGINESS, FIBROMYALGIA, BODY AND NECK PAIN.

In 1995, Sophia, a college professor, suffered a motor vehicle accident resulting in a loss of normal cervical curvature, severe neck pain and fatigue, exacerbated by infection with Epstein-Barr, fogginess and poor memory. Attempting to relieve pain, she had undergone multiple epidurals and extensive myofascial trigger point therapy with no lasting relief.

Years later, she was diagnosed with fibromyalgia, and in 2009, accepted into a small study by Dr. Esty and Emily Perlman. Study design included eight sEMG treatments (with pre- and post-treatment evaluations of function[1]), followed by 20 FNS neurofeedback sessions. One study goal was to isolate effects of sEMG alone on muscle activity and pain. For Sophia, treating muscles was strikingly positive. Treatment with sEMG only resulted in:

- Quick reduction of pain in SCM and psoas[2]. By the third assessment, measurements of muscle tone in the 54445left shoulder and back (levator scapula, trapezius and paraspinals, Figure 10-11) were normal.

- Normalized muscle recovery measurements showing fast return to baseline, a significant change. Before treatment, muscles contracted, but never fully relaxed.

- Improved awareness of muscle tension and ability to reduce it on her own. Her massage therapist said that her muscles had never felt so relaxed, and she could take long car rides without developing severe pain.

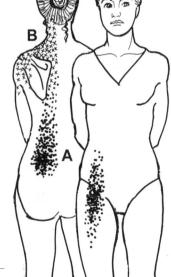

A. Psoas pain, front and back (indicated by stippling).

B. Levator scapula pain (indicated by x's), extends up to neck and can join with psoas pain.

FIGURE 10-11. Muscle Pain Patterns: Psoas and Levator

---

1. sEMG imbalances (differences in muscle firing 20% or greater between the left and right sides of a muscle pair) are a direct source of pain.
2. For trapezius pain, see Figure 10-1 on page 186. For SCM pain, see Figure 10-6 on page 191.

During the FNS neurofeedback that followed, Sophia noticed many improvements in executive function and energy. Now she could:

- Prepare lectures in less time and present them more easily, with good subject and word recall.
- Work and exercise longer with greatly improved energy, including walking more than a mile at a time — an impossible task before treatment.

Despite sEMG before documented and measurable changes, Sophia reported little functional improvement of her pain. Her *perception* of pain levels was essentially unchanged from when she began. Medications (Motrin, Klonopin®, and Lyrica.) also remained unchanged.

When pain demands all attention, subjective reports don't always match quantitative data. Patients may experience a sharpening of pain in localized areas; this gets most attention even if there is less pain overall. However, when pain does not respond to treatments we suspect neck injury.

Years later, on reviewing patient charts, Dr. Esty noticed the reversed neck curve had been documented in a scan; she called Sophia to suggest a consultation with osteopathic physician Frances Demmerle. By coincidence, exploratory surgery for continuing neck pain was scheduled in two weeks. After two osteopathic treatments by Dr. Demmerle, Sophia's pain vanished. Her physician cancelled the neck surgery saying he wanted to learn what Dr. Demmerle did to produce the changes. Sophia is now pain-free and off all pain killers.

This case illustrates the practical limits of neurofeedback and biofeedback in the presence of structural distortions. Neither neurofeedback nor drugs can shove misaligned vertebrae, compressed nerves or strained connective tissue back into position. Treatment must address the source of the problem.

In my opinion, the search for a single curative treatment for fibromyalgia is folly because so many body systems are involved, and they vary in intensity among individuals. There is no one Fibromyalgia Syndrome. Fibromyalgia is a complex condition that produces a great variety of symptoms. There are only people, all of whom suffer in their own unique ways, who struggle daily with pain, while continuing to hope for a simple answer or any substantial relief at all. Difficult problems often require multiple applications and biofeedback therapies should be a standard part of fibromyalgia treatment. —MLE

Functional Support

Recognizing the damage is the first problem. Dealing with it is another.

On Living in Hell and Getting Out Again

Positive anything is better than negative nothing.

—Elbert Hubbard (1856-1915)

If you have had a brain injury you may be living in hell. You may have been there for so long that your injury is all you can think or talk about.

Unfortunately, when you dwell on / focus on / build on the pain and disability, all you're doing is putting down deeper, stronger roots in hell. For starters,

- LEARN GENUINELY POSITIVE THOUGHTS AND WORDS. An excellent source is *Don't Shoot the Dog*, by Karen Pryor, a behavioral biologist.
- BUILD A TREASURE CHEST. List 10 things for which you are grateful. Dwell / focus / build on those.
- Focus on successes. List things you were able to do, even if it is only *one* thing.

Support groups are an excellent resource, but use with caution. They are useful for sharing information and skills, to appreciate that others are also struggling, and to help wherever possible. But be cautious about making these groups the focus of your life. If *all* your friends are there, getting better means losing all your friends. Some keep friends by staying stuck (or in AA for 20 years) because that's where all their friends are.

It is best to look for healthy, interest-based friends.

If you are a supporter, avoid being frightened away, avoid exhaustion, by setting clear limits and boundaries.

If you are getting support, take care not to frighten supporters away by making your injury the topic of every conversation. Doing so is an invitation to all to join you in hell.

But who wants to live in hell?

The point is not to enlarge your circle of hell, but to get out of it, to put mind and energy anywhere else but hell, not trying to drag friends and family in there with you or being disappointed or indignant if they don't come.

Placing your focus elsewhere is *not* fantasy. It does not trivialize what has happened to you. It is not a betrayal of yourself or your situation. *It is a way out of hell.* The easiest way out is with the willing and happy support of friends and family.

Unfortunately, very often, the most concerned helpers have no idea what is really needed or how best to help.

On Our Own

Annie knew she had fallen from the bump on her head. She couldn't remember how or why, or the last six months of her life. Surely by now she should be better, not worse. Light was painful, she suffered waves of nausea and vertigo with near-constant headaches. And, despite crushing fatigue, she could not sleep at night.

Her concerned family contacted a local Brain Injury Center for the first available appointment, months later. There, an intern took her for computerized ImPACT testing but left after brief verbal instructions. Within minutes, fluorescent lights and the stress of testing triggered a severe headache. When taken to talk with the psychologist, she opened her notebook with her list of symptoms but he cut her off to refer her to an Ear, Nose, and Throat (ENT) specialist and to a physician for a prescription for amantadine. But referrals were names only, no phone numbers or directions. "They're in the phone book," he said.

On the opposite side of town, she again took out her notebook, but the young M.D. cut her off and, with no further input or exam, wrote out the prescription for amantadine. The ENT was in another congested downtown area. Although native to the area, Annie had extreme difficulty finding the building. She failed to recognize signs, was confused by elevator buttons, and got lost in the hallway because the room numbers made no sense to her. When she finally found the office, she was asked to toss a ball from hand to hand. "After three tosses I was so dizzy and nauseated I thought I would vomit, and I was a 45-minute drive from home. The worst of it," said Annie, "was that this "brain injury center" was not a *Center*."

> It was staffed only by *psychologists* and appeared to exist only for computer testing. The sole purpose of the distant physician appeared to be to prescribe amantadine, apparently standard for all patients because I was never asked about my specific cognitive symptoms or pain, and I was cut off when I brought them up myself. No one ever touched me, no one asked for new tests or even copies of existing medical records. I saw no neurologist and no one even wrote down any notes on my condition.

There are many disturbing features to this tale. One is that this woman has an extremely close and caring family. Imagine the fate of someone who does not. But the overall issue is this: The injured brain needs help to do the things that it used to do, but can no longer do alone. It takes longer to figure out what and where something is, to find one's way, even around once-familiar areas, to make sense of information, and to handle stress.

Many well-meaning helpers ask "Are you sure you can do this? Will you be OK?"

"I'll be Fine," says the injured one politely, with no real reason to believe that is true.

MORAL: **When a brain is injured, do not leave the person alone to drive or solve problems of time and space, maps, bus schedules, or healthcare choices — no matter how Fine they may look. Find better ways to help.**

HELPING WHILE YOU WAIT

When I finally went and listened to the issues others were struggling with I was startled to find that I had all of the problems they talked about. Maybe I did belong there after all.

—Marie

It takes time, sometimes months, to set up appointments and begin therapy. Brain injury groups can provide information and support for the injured and for their families. The more family members and / or caretakers understand about the symptoms and challenges of TBI, the better they are better able to help reduce stress and anxiety.

Table 10-1 lists helpful strategies for helpers, caregivers, and therapists for easing the stress on persons with TBI. Notice, for example, that the stress and other challenges of driving through city traffic to an appointment violates nearly every suggestion on the list.

This list can also serve as an observational checklist for caregivers as healing takes place. And it can also help the patient to ask for help. For example, are symptoms getting worse? Or better?

Table 10-1. Accommodations for Cognitive and Affective Deficits[a]
Attention Deficits
<ul><li>Work only on one task at a time in session.</li><li>Limit auditory and visual distractions within testing room.</li><li>Provide scheduled breaks within planned treatment sessions.</li><li>Make sessions as interactive as possible to enhance patient's attention.</li><li>Redirect the patient when he/she becomes distracted.</li></ul>
Reduced Information Processing Speed
<ul><li>Speak slowly, stopping frequently to check comprehension.</li><li>Avoid speaking in a loud voice. Use a normal tone of voice.</li><li>Do not attempt to rush the patient with a task.</li><li>Allow additional time for the patient to formulate responses to questions.</li><li>Encourage family members to assist the patient with completion of written forms.</li></ul>

[a]Reproduced by permission from Table 1 in Suchoff IB, Ciuffreda KJ, and Kapoor N (2001, p. 46).

Memory Impairments

- Repeat information several times to ensure comprehension.
- Check the patient's understanding of new information by asking him/her to restate the information in his/her own terms.
- Do not assume a patient will remember new information between sessions. Inconsistency is the hallmark of brain injury.
- Provide written documentation, whenever possible, to augment verbal discussions.
- Present new information in small, concise chunks to maximize learning.
- Ask structured questions, as opposed to open-ended questions.
- Encourage the patient to write down instructions, home assignments, etc., for later review.

Executive Functioning Deficits

- Keep unexpected events to a minimum.
- Provide information in a factual manner, avoiding use of abstract concepts when possible.
- Prepare patient in advance when session focus will be shifting.
- Provide alternative solutions to a problem; empower the patient to select the best choice.
- Provide a written agenda of things to be accomplished in session.
- Provide a written outline which summarizes specific steps to be followed for completion of a home therapy program.

Communication Deficits

- Limit the use of open-ended questions during verbal questioning and on written forms.
- Use structured questions (yes/no; multiple choice) whenever possible.
- Redirect the patient when he/she wanders "off topic" in discussions.
- Cue patients who experience word-finding difficulties.
- Encourage appropriate eye contact and use of interpersonal space.
- Model use of nonverbal gestures when appropriate.

Affective Changes

- A flat affect should not be interpreted as a sign of lack of interest.
- Reassurance, education, and structure are useful.
- Encourage realistic assessment of the patient's current abilities.
- Avoid focusing only on the patient's deficits.
- Provide neutral, but directed, feedback when the patient behaves inappropriately.
- Suggest brief breaks whenever patient becomes irritable or agitated.
- Offer alternative activities when patient begins to show signs of agitation.

On Helping As a Team Sport

I'm either going to kill myself, or I'm going to turn this into a game. After the four most miserable weeks of my life, those seemed like the only two options left.

—Jane McGonigal (2009)

It looks like a solitary sport, but it takes a team.
—Diana Nyad, on swimming from Cuba to Florida on her fifth attempt at age 64 (2013)

When game designer Jane McGonigal hit her head on a kitchen cabinet, she got brain fog and headache and vertigo that wouldn't go away. Tests indicated that all was normal, but the normally bubbly Jane was anxious and depressed, symptoms that make it harder for the brain to heal. She couldn't work on the computer, read, or watch videos. She felt trapped and overwhelmed by an injury that was getting no better. The obvious way out was through a game. "A strange idea," she said, "but I literally had nothing else to do." In designing her game, she established three basic strategies:

- Stay optimistic, set goals, and focus on positive progress.
- Get support from friends and family rather than trying to do it alone.
- Notice where you are and gradually work up to more demanding activity.

To a gamer, this was just good multi-player design: a goal with progress tracking, ever higher levels of play, done while connecting with friends. And so was born *The SuperBetter Game*, a heroic journey to deal with an injury with less misery and lots more fun along the way. McGonigal began her game with five missions, ideally one per day.

MISSION #1: CREATE A SUPERBETTER SECRET IDENTITY. As hero of your own adventure, you can be any superhero you want. The point is to see yourself as powerful, not powerless, and heroic for carrying on in the face of illness or injury. Jane McGonigal became Jane the Concussion Slayer; (after TV heroine Buffy the Vampire Slayer). Symptoms became vampires, demons, and other forces of darkness. But even superheroes have helpers. They need other people. So do you.

MISSION #2: RECRUIT ALLIES. One of the hardest things about chronic injury is asking for help. McGonigal found it hard to explain, even to close friends and family, how anxious and depressed she was, how embarrassed she felt asking for help. But doing so prevents social isolation and disaster. It gives people who want to help something specific and genuinely helpful to do. It also avoids exhausting one helpful person. And so Jane the Concussion Slayer recruited:

- HER SISTER AS "WATCHER." Mission: To call daily for an update on slaying activities. "It was a huge relief to me when she accepted this role," says McGonigal, "because I didn't know how else to explain that every single day was really hard for me, that I really needed *daily* contact (not just checking in on the weekends), to get through it."

- HER HUSBAND AS "WILLOW." Mission: Score-keeping, record-keeping, and help with things she couldn't do without getting a headache.

- FRIENDS AS "XANDER." Mission: Comic relief, visiting once a week to cheer her up.

MISSION #3: FIND THE BAD GUYS. List things that suck life and energy, including triggers for fatigue and headache: caffeine, bright lights, crowded spaces, climbing stairs, trying to read, or dealing with people who are stressful under even normal circumstances. What makes you feel worse? or better?

MISSION #4: IDENTIFY POWER-UPS. Focus on senses unaffected by TBI and things that make you feel even a little bit good. Jane's touch was fine; she could cuddle her dog. Hearing was fine; she could listen to podcasts. Smell was fine; she collected perfume samples. Whatever you can do, however you can do it, celebrate the abilities that remain to break the cycle of stress and depression.

MISSION #5: CREATE A SUPERHERO TO-DO LIST. Make a list of goals. Small ones: the things you *could* do right now if only you put your attention on them. Big ones: things you might never have imagined doing before. Whatever the goal, take a step, even if it is the tiniest of baby steps, every day.

These 5 steps were the origin of what became Jane's SuperBetter Game. Did it really help? It wasn't a miracle cure for the headaches or the cognitive symptoms; those lasted for over a year, the hardest year of her life. But even while the pain and cognitive symptoms remained, emotional pain lost its grip. For the first few days McGonigal played, she felt better than at any time since her injury. One day she was miserable, the next day she wasn't, and she was never that miserable ever again. When the fog of misery lifted, symptoms improved, breaking the cycle of emotional pain and anxiety. This helps by:

- REFRAMING THE SITUATION. Reframing (seeing things from another point of view) is a key factor in cognitive behavioral therapy.
- REGAINING CONTROL OVER LIFE. Feeling better didn't require being *cured*, said McGonigal, it just required "making an effort to participate more fully in my own recovery process."

Participation is a critical issue for many athletes, military, and others who need to move, to *do*, to make things happen. They want something, *anything*, to jump-start the healing process, no matter how inappropriate it may be. This is why, when ordered off the field, the mat, the mound, they head straight to the gym. If they can't play or fight, they will lift weights. Does that help? Usually not. More likely it makes things worse. The SuperBetter Game approach provides, and makes it easier to ask for, *appropriate* help.

It saves us from simply sitting and ruminating about everything that's wrong: "I feel like crap, I can't play football, I can't go out because sunlight hurts my eyes, everything I used to do is gone, my life is over, nothing will be the same ever again, all is lost . . . what am I going to do?" Suddenly here is something to do. Even if The Game doesn't cure a head injury on its own, it allows you, once again, to take part, to re-engage in your own life. That is why it is so important.

—A Veteran

To see and play the game, go to **www.superbetter.com**.

On Flying

Dropping off my 4-year-old at preschool, I noticed how nicely all the other children were dressed. When I realized it was picture day and I hadn't even washed my daughter's hair, I fell apart.

—Marie

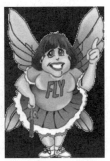

FlyLady.net is a group dedicated to freeing homes and lives from clutter and disorganization. It does not address TBI symptoms directly; it does address the problems of drowning in CHAOS (Can't Have Anyone Over Syndrome) and how to get out again.

Many Normals live chaotic lives almost by choice because they remember housework as punishment, or fear that organization and schedules will destroy creativity and spontaneity. But busy modern lives are tough enough on a normal brain; an injured one may have had all the spontaneity it can stand. A disorganized irregular lifestyle is harmful to all[1].

Dirty clothes and bad food all impact health and healing. So does the stress of unpaid bills that trigger late fees and penalties, frustration and fatigue. Even driving requires organization from gas and oil and legal papers, to adequate sleep and even proper clothing.

Imagine (or *remember*) having overslept again, frantically searching for the car keys then driving the children to school with no time to dress yourself, and running out of gas, but the AAA bill was never paid, and the cell phone battery is dead and now you are trudging down the highway with a gas can in pajamas and flip-flops. What a relief it is when the nice policeman stops to help! —until you realize that you're going to get another ticket because your tags expired months ago. When you finally get home, energized by anger and humiliation, you swear to finally put things in order, to deal with the piles of clutter and laundry, junk mail, late notices and dustballs the size of small dogs.

But the hard truth is this: the crush of too many things left undone is too much for a working brain, much less a damaged one. Never mind the strain of inventing yet another cover story, another lie, for family, friends, and employers as to how this happened *again*. So, after spending half an hour looking for the other shoe or a stamp, you may simply go back to bed, unable to deal with the mess that is your life. Today there is no time or energy to pick up a pen, pay a bill, to eat or shower or dress, but maybe tomorrow there will be. Tomorrow you *will* get a grip, get organized, get it all together. Or maybe *not*.

---

1. The term "regularity" usually refers to *elimination*, but there's far more to it. Disrupting rhythms of sleeping and waking, feeding and digestion causes ongoing stress responses, from weight gain to decreased immune function to disease. The injured brain needs *more* structure, not *less*.

Damaged brains can't function in the chaos that normal brains may be able to endure with passable functionality. They can't heal in an environment that does not support healing. Even for brains that do heal, problems may not be over. When an adult recovers function after 2 years or 20 years, chances are good that there are 2 to 20 years of clutter and confusion, from an impossibly disorganized house, to paperwork, financial and tax problems.

FOOD

Good food is critical to healing, but often ignored in favor of pizza delivery or a bucket of fried chicken. But what sends people to the drive-thru rather than cooking healthier (and more economical) foods at home? When *Consumer Reports*[1] surveyed readers, the answer was *too much time* required for planning, cooking, and clean-up. The surprise was that:

- The time seen as *too long* to cook a week-night dinner averaged 35 minutes.
- The time seen as *not* too long? 27 minutes.
- The amazingly tiny difference: *just 8 minutes.*

TBI victims may be simply unable to cook or prepare meals on their own. Easier to drink beer or gnaw on raw spaghetti than to face the complexity of finding a pot and boiling water. Anything else is hideously difficult. Besides the challenge of making a list, and fatigue too severe to organize or complete a shopping trip, there may be no money.

FINANCIAL TRAUMA

Financial advisor Gail Vaz-Oxlade marvels at the problems people get into with money.

"It isn't rocket science," she points out. Neither is driving or cooking, yet all these skills may be beyond the capability of injured brains. And even many Normal ones.

On her reality TV show, *Til Debt Do Us Part*, Gail delves into the finances of people who are deeply in debt — with no idea how they got there or how to get out again[2]. If normal brains see credit cards and payday loans as "income," and 30- to 80-percent interest rates raise no red flags, imagine the terrible trouble that injured brains can get into.

Money problems strain relationships even under the best of circumstances. The title of Gail's program reflects the painful fact that of marriages that fail, the vast majority fail because of problems with money. And nothing is more certain to impact finances than TBI.

---

1. *Consumer Reports Magazine* (2014), Save time in the kitchen. February, pp. 24-25
2. One episode even features a financial officer. Gail's website (www.gailvazoxlade.com) provides worksheets and tutorials.

A post-TBI brain may be unable to read or add a column of numbers, or to make sense of money *at all*[1]. Even when money is available, bills may be piled on a hopelessly messy desk, lost in the clutter, then overdue or unpaid, triggering late fees and cancellations.

These issues are not limited to the TBI *patient*. They also impact *care-givers*. When coping skills are already stretched to the limit, adding more responsibilities is a recipe for disaster.

CARETAKERS

> I am the wife and the husband, the mother and the father, the breadwinner, chauffeur, cook and nursemaid — and I am exhausted.
> —Spouse of a TBI victim

Imagine the adult who comes home from work one day to suddenly discover that he or she is now the primary caretaker, with no clue how to plan or cook meals or keep up with household demands. Even other adults who want to help may not know how. Life devolves into an endless series of emergencies and crises, lost sleep, fear, resentment, and exhaustion. *Now imagine that this person is a teen or a child.*

If the injured party can no longer work at an office, it may seem reasonable for them to stay home and run the household. We assume that is easier than a "real job." It can be far more difficult, especially with an injured brain. Schedules and routines crash, meals are random or based on expensive carry-out or junk food leading to stress and other health problems.

In theory, the few minutes between real food, calling out for pizza, or family melt-down and divorce are easily addressed through menu planning and by streamlining preparation and cleanup. In reality, these tasks may be too much even for "Normals," especially those who have never done it before.

Chaos and disorganization rarely resolve on their own. Outside help is usually needed. It may be too embarrassing to ask for help from friends or family, professional organizers are expensive, and most Do It Yourself plans for organizing are written by The Born Organized, the very people who are uniquely unqualified to teach the rest of us.

GETTING HELP

The FlyLady approach is a gentle but effective way out of darkness and confusion. It is applied cognitive therapy, a means of developing valuable life skills, a source of excellent high-quality organizational tools, and support from members world-wide.

---

1. In *The Lookout*, Chris hands the bartender a $20 bill for a bottle of beer. He does not find it the least bit odd when the man returns $3.00 in change.

A strikingly uniform refrain from many "flybabies" is a strange distortion of time (which can be another symptom of TBI). Real meals are never cooked, dishes are unwashed, laundry is never done or put away *because it will take too long*. A timer reveals a startling truth: that decent meals can be prepared and served in less time than it takes to park in the carry-out lane, that a mere 15 minutes (or less) may stand between a sink of dirty dishes and a clean kitchen, that a load of laundry can be put away in 5 minutes flat.

Flying starts with the simplest of baby steps:

- Shine your kitchen sink.
- Put on your lace-up shoes.
- Set your timer for the task at hand.

If you can do that, you're on your way. There is more, of course, a simple monthly habit and daily assignments based on the idea that we can do anything for 15 minutes. FlyLady's *Control Journal* and calendar provide the information needed to run a household or a life (especially if they are begun *before* a problem arises). There is help on how to *Face Your Finances* and get out of debt or to use existing income most efficiently.

There are also associated helpers. The House Fairy (www.HouseFairy.org) teaches organizational skills to children. The Dinner Diva (www.SavingDinner.com) shows that there is an enormous difference between *junk food* and nutritious *fast food*. She provides menus and shopping lists[1], with emphasis on easy crock-pot meals. A crock-pot can, for example, provide a continuous supply of broth and soup stock, made from bones and scraps, low cost and low effort but nutrient dense and a help to healing.

This may sound absurdly simple. But many who have approached the system with skepticism and disbelief now tell of surviving emergencies ranging from a boss dropping in unexpectedly for dinner to severe illness, floods, fires, and hurricanes — because simple but effective routines had been put in place for the first time.

With TBI, with pain and fatigue and disability, even 15 minutes may be impossible. But if you can only work or focus for 5 minutes, you can set your timer and change your world, 5 minutes or even 30 seconds at a time.

Things *can* get better and easier. Nevertheless, the best strategy is to prevent injury in the first place.

---

1. Grocery shopping can be enormously difficult after TBI but many stores offer assistance. Some will walk down the aisles with a customer and help to fill the cart. Others may fill an order sent by e-mail and have it ready for pick-up. Some community based stores will deliver. Obviously, any of these possibilities are easier with a regular menu or shopping list. Check with the store manager.

CHAPTER 11 Preventing Injury

THE PHYSICS OF INJURY, SURVIVING YOUR SPORT AND EVEN YOUR SAFETY EQUIPMENT. EDUCATING SELF AND OTHERS.

The laws of physics can be unforgiving. The rapid deceleration that occurs at the moment of impact increases an occupant's "crash weight" exponentially. A 60-pound child unbelted in the back seat of a car traveling at 30 miles per hour, will impact the windshield with the same force as a young elephant — about 3,700 pounds — if involved in a sudden collision.

—Richard Hamilton, Chairman, AAA East Central (2013)

I can no longer bear to watch "Funny Home Video" programs on TV.
They are mostly about children and adults risking or getting brain injuries.

— Dr. Mary Lee Esty

Besides avoiding dangerous situations entirely, the secret to avoiding or curtailing injury is to decrease acceleration. What does this mean?

Acceleration is a change in velocity (although slowing is usually called *de*celeration).

G refers to acceleration due to gravity, or about 32 feet per second per second[1].

If you are traveling in a car at 20 m.p.h. (about 30 feet per second) and crash into a concrete post, your velocity drops from 30 feet per second down to 0 over a very short time, perhaps 1/5 second, an acceleration (*de*celeration) of 150 feet per second per second, sending your head in the direction of the dashboard or steering wheel at almost 5 G's.

In any impact, a key concept is this: Even modest velocities with big changes over short times can produce powerful forces, inflicting serious injury on human brains and bodies.

Fortunately the opposite is also true. *Increasing* time and area *decreases* harm.

---

1. That is, a falling object picks up speed at a rate of 32 feet per second for every second it falls (until it reaches *terminal* velocity, the point at which it can go no faster).

The Physics of Injury

If you were hit, how hard were you hit?

The answer is defined by a basic law of physics:

Force = the mass of the object times its acceleration (F=ma).

This is true whether the oncoming mass is a small rock, a child, a truck, or the concrete or AstroTurf-ed surface of a planet. Falling from a horse, wall, or rooftop, is equivalent to being hit or punched by Planet Earth while moving at the acceleration of gravity (that is, moving faster and faster the longer and farther you fall).

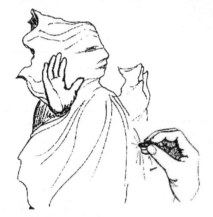

FIGURE 11-1. Increasing Time and Area

If you are hit, how likely are you to be injured? "Wounding energy," depends on speed and time and the size of the area of impact. A small but fast-moving force (such as a bullet or a five-year-old on skates) can cause serious injury. Wounding energy can be *decreased* by increasing time and area[1].

For example, slowly touching a bullet to the skin vastly decreases wounding energy compared to firing the same bullet from a gun.

Wounding energy is reduced if time is increased by mere fractions of a second. It is also decreased by increasing the surface area of impact.

Imagine that the same bullet is hammered into a huge flat sheet of lead and fired at you (in a vacuum where there's no air resistance) with the same velocity as a bullet leaving the muzzle of a gun. The flattened bullet will wrap itself like a sheet over your skin. Wounding energy is extremely low because of the increase in area. This is the point behind helmets and pads, crumple zones and other safety equipment. All are designed to increase time required to actually contact the body while spreading impact over a broader area.

Table 11-1. Physics and Injury	
The BIGGER the mass, or the FASTER it's moving, and the SMALLER the contact area, the MORE likely it's going to hurt.	The SMALLER the mass, or the SLOWER it's moving, and the LARGER the contact area, the LESS likely the damage.

1. Excerpted from Shifflett CM (2009).

A fall of just *one foot* can fracture an adult skull (Hodgson VR and Thomas LM, 1971; personal comm. Ziejewski M, 2013). Children's skulls are far more delicate. In general, if there is enough force to fracture, there is enough force to injure brain tissue. Even small bodies running into each other (especially on skates or skis), can generate hundreds of pounds of force. But what is the wounding energy? Was there a full-body "splat" into wall or mat or other player? Or did two bodies collide headfirst, channeling forces through neck and brain? If the latter, wounding energy is huge, even if everything else stays the same[1].

What if everything else doesn't stay the same? What if speed and mass increase? The sports "arms race" demands ever bigger, heavier, stronger players. In the 80 years between 1920 and 2000, the mass of the average pro football player has increased by 60 percent, speed by 12 percent; kinetic energy has effectively doubled (Fainaru-Wada M and Fainaru S, 2013, p. 72).

Many teams now require weights obtainable *only* through anabolic steroids. Although illegal since the 1990s, these drugs are used and abused by players from middle schoolers up to and including the professional leagues. To cover up, many users swear that their fantastic gains are merely the result of their dedication and long hours in the weight room[2]. Young boys (and some girls) who dream of making the team, any team, are tempted into their use, but they wreak havoc on bodies and brains — as do their results. Over the last 30 years alone, the average NFL offensive lineman has ballooned by 60 pounds; these refrigerator-sized bodies hit with several thousand pounds of force (Carroll L and Rosner D, 2011). No brain or body can survive such abuse unscathed.

Fortunately, physics also defines ways of *decreasing* injury. Increasing *time* makes the stop more gradual. Just as we bubble-wrap fragile items for shipping, we pad helmets, goalposts, and floors to increase the time it takes for a body to come to a complete stop. This increases the time over which an object changes velocity, lessens acceleration and reduces wounding energy. So does increasing the area over which these forces are spread.

The physics of time and area, safety and harm, are regularly demonstrated by the men of World Wrestling Entertainment (WWE). It is soap opera for guys. It is scripted. It is cartoon. It is the Three Stooges in spandex (although the Stooges never looked so good). But these men are real athletes. The physics are real, the falls are real and the risk of injury is real. The ability of a performer to increase time and surface area is a critical survival skill. Even milliseconds make a difference.

---

1. In football, blocking an opponent by ramming with the top of the helmet is known as *spearing*. It has long earned a 15-yard penalty. The NFL is now imposing fines and suspensions (page 243).
2. Compare these men (and women) with those on websites dedicated to *drug-free* weight lifting.

Crumple zones and padding lie behind standard WWE wrestling techniques and props including the mat, the table, and the steel folding chair.

THE MAT. Below the surface mat (too soft for boxing or karate), there is a "sprung mat" composed of multiple sheets of plywood mounted on springs[1]. The spring and bounce keeps players safe in falls, especially dives from the ropes. The same basic design protects dancers and students of other "falling" martial arts such as Judo and Aikido.

THE FOLDING STEEL CHAIR. The very icon of WWE "wrestling," but ignore the word *steel* (it's there to grab your attention). Focus on *folding* because that's what makes it somewhat safer; a hit with *non-folding* chairs (or a solid frame) would be a whole different matter. The classic chair hit to the head is done so the seat *unfolds* (Figure 11-2A), the equivalent of crumple zones in cars[2].

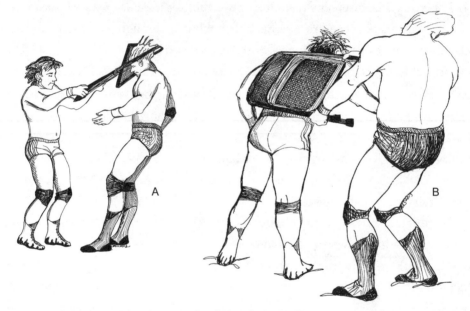

FIGURE 11-2. Pro-"Wrestling" with Chairs

Fun with Physics. (A) Hits with a steel folding chair are safer than with a non-folding chair of equal mass but *any* hits to the head are now banned. (B) Hits with the flat chair (not an edge or corner) are allowed to the upper back where they are likely to sting but unlikely to injure.

---

1. A microphone picks up the sound as the plywood sheets rattle together. Players stomp the mat when they feign a punch, to add to the illusion that something big is happening.
2. Receiving hits to the head was a specialty of the late Chris Benoit, believed to have led to his death from CTE. "Receiving hits" a *specialty*? Yes. WWF / WWE matches were and still are choreographed *performances*. Individual performers give permission (or not) for things that will be done to them. However, in 2010, WWE banned *all* intentional hits to the head, with or without partner permission. Violators now face fines, suspension or firing.

THE TABLE. The Throw-The-Opponent-So-Hard-Onto-A-Table-That-It-Breaks is a classic stunt but the tabletop is made of weak particle-board, unsupported in the middle. It is actually a door-sized crumple zone that slows the performer's progress to the (matted) floor below.

THE FALL. Pro *Wrestlers* are really Pro *Fallers*. Some of what *appear to be* the most dangerous stunts are actually techniques to protect the player, by increasing time and area. "Gaining height" before a fall is contrary to every natural instinct, but good physics. Better flat than pointy (Figure 11-3). In WWE you will see one performer help another vault off his back or thighs in order to spread out, get into position, to fall safely into the supposedly shattering (but mostly just noisy) slam to the mat.

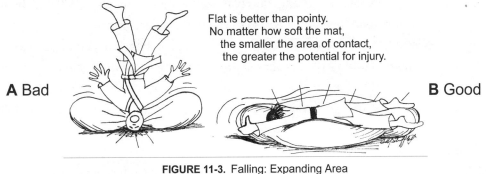

Flat is better than pointy.
No matter how soft the mat,
the smaller the area of contact,
the greater the potential for injury.

A Bad

B Good

FIGURE 11-3. Falling: Expanding Area

The actual application, the venue where these physical laws play out, does not matter. It can be a slide into the boards at the hockey rink, head-butting soccer balls, other heads, or helmets. It can be a vertical fall off a ladder, or a horizontal flight from horse, car or bike.

The same physical laws apply to injury and safety in all areas of physical life.

Make them work *for* you. And stop injury *before* it happens.

Home Injuries

Consider again the long list of household injuries on page 34, the millions of people killed or injured by the comfortable familiarity of throw rugs, socks, and bathtubs.

All throw rugs should have non-slip backs. Stairs and walkways should be clutter free with nothing to trip over in the dark. No papers, no boxes, no power cords.

Padding around the house in socks on bare wood or tile floors is also risky. If you prefer to keep outdoor shoes out of the house, then keep a pair of indoor shoes, or use socks with non-slip bottoms. "Slippers" should never be slippery!

Bathtubs should have non-slip bottoms or non-slip bath mats. Sturdy handrails tend to be thought of as something for handicapped users but they are equally useful for *preventing* a disabling injury. A child may survive a fall with a concussion. With or without concussion, a broken hip in an older adult is a common first step onto the downward path of disability and death. Loss of function and loss of life are all the more tragic when unnecessary.

School Injuries

When toddlers are learning to walk, when they tumble down stairs, when they suffer boo-boo's and dings, the assumption (especially by fathers of sons) is that little or no harm is done, because "kids bounce back" and kissing it may be enough to make it better.

When they start school, more injuries occur on the playground, in physical education classes, and even in the classroom. Many a bored child has pulled chairs out from under other kids, or tried to see how far he could tip his chair back without falling—only to fall, be sent to the nurse (or principal) then returned to class with an unrecognized concussion. When injury is recognized, the problems it can cause may still fail to be addressed by school staff.

Billy had suffered multiple concussions starting at age two when another child pushed him over in day care; he lay unconscious for two hours. In first grade, he was hit on the temple with a thrown basketball; on two separate occasions he hit his head when he fell or was pulled from the monkey bars. Later, he went down a slide headfirst then flipped head over heels, landing on the back of his head.

Then he dove into a pool and hit the bottom; this time the symptoms didn't go away. He was left with dizziness, nausea, headache and terrible fatigue that left him sleeping most of the day and unable to do homework. He was so sensitive to light that he closed all the drapes in the house and could not tolerate going outdoors. He was evaluated at a concussion clinic, but after missing weeks of school with little or no improvement, his parents brought him to Brain Wellness and Biofeedback. His first FNS treatment produced a bit more fatigue and headache, but 24 hours later he was off the couch, active, and opening drapes — no longer sensitive to light[1].

Billy returned to school, but tripped during gym class, falling backwards and hitting his head on a tree trunk. His pediatrician banned further gym classes. When classmates asked why, Billy explained that he had had too many concussions to risk more. The other children began teasing which escalated into taunting and bullying. When his mother asked the teacher to speak to the other children about the seriousness of the situation, she was told that the teasing was Billy's own fault, that he had created the problem himself by talking about his concussions to the other kids. There was no apparent understanding of the effects of concussion or the impact on students. Billy would love to be in class, but never again wants to feel so terrible, to live with such pain and dysfunction. Such lack of understanding points to a critical need for education — the greatest part of prevention — for educators and other school personnel.

---

1. Billy's parents were thrilled. "Neurofeedback was more effective than medication!" said his mother. She was eager to report his sudden improvement at his follow-up appointment at the concussion clinic. But the psychologist dismissed the possibility of improvement due to neurofeedback. "Billy just finally got enough rest," he said, then recommended that Billy return to hockey to get in shape.

Automotive Injuries and Equipment

In the US, yearly death rates from automobiles have sometimes been higher than the total death rate of the Vietnam War. In 1960, car crashes *killed* nearly 50,000[1]. Since then, thousands of lives have been saved by helmets and seat belts. Nobody loves them (especially the highest risk group: male teens), but they work. Meanwhile, other critical safety features — seats and headrests — are widely ignored or used in ways that actually *cause* injury.

Belts

When seat belts for passenger vehicles were introduced in the 1960s, they were widely viewed with suspicion. Girls would not wear them "because they will wrinkle my dress." Boys drag-racing or playing "chicken" on dark country roads would not wear them because, they solemnly agreed (often over beers), "Seat belts cause more injuries than they prevent." It was better to take one's chances, hoping to be "thrown free" — a notion far too trusting of fate and physics, rocks and trees[2]. The common romantic vision of this is:

The worst that can happen is that I die doing what I love.

But no. That is *not* the worst that can happen. Not even close.

The worst that can happen is to live on, able to remember who you were and what you could do — but unable to do it ever again, with no idea why you can't do the things you used to do, and no idea why you do the goofy things you do now, why bizarre and inept and stupid and embarrassing things blurt out of your mouth and mind.

The very worst is to watch a loved one slipping away with no idea of what is wrong or how to help it, or how to keep a relationship or a family together through the stress, the pain, and the often hellish expense.

The very best is to avoid all that or reduce the risk of damage.

---

1. In 2011, 32,367 were killed. In 2012, approximately 34,080. Source: National Highway Traffic Safety Administration (NHTSA, www.NHTSA.gov). In the US, traffic accidents are the leading cause of death for children aged 4 and for all ages from 11 to 27.
2. Recall Mary Lincoln and Edweard Muybridge. He flew headfirst into a boulder, she onto a rocky road. Muybridge's free-flying fellow passenger (who, like Mary, attempted to jump from the stage-coach) was killed outright.

Helmets

Captain! I canna change the laws of physics!

—Scottie (Star Trek)

Sports involving high speeds and risk of falls require helmets.

One of the most dangerous sports for TBI is horseback riding. It may combine an opinionated 1,000-pound animal, falls from one's own height plus height of the horse, sometimes at full speed in rough terrain. The traditional riding hat is actually a *helmet*. As horses gave way to bicycles, motor vehicles, and ever-higher speeds, helmets became even more critical.

Of bicyclists killed in 2010, 90 percent were not wearing helmets[1]. On the ski slopes, helmet use has more than doubled since 2003. Helmets are even recommended in *tornadoes* as most tornado deaths involve TBI and any head protection, from construction hard hats to motorcycle gear, is better than nothing (Oliver M, 2011)[2].

Motorcycles are great fun, but are involved in many head injuries and deaths. Michael Seate, a racing instructor and editor of Cafe Racer Magazine, notes that these are far higher in the US than in Europe, "because here," says Seate, "a motorcycle is seen as a *toy*."

In England, you must be over 27 before you can buy a high-powered bike and licensing involves a five-day test with an instructor. In the US, anyone of driving age can buy a bike of any size, speed, or power. And riders often refuse to wear safety gear, including helmets.

Why? "It's *fashion*," says Seate.

You can't be a Real Outlaw American Biker unless your hair is blowing in the wind. I have also seen a guy down 11 beers in an hour, climb on a bike and drive off through rush hour traffic dressed in cut-off jeans and running shoes. In case of a crash, many imagine they will simply step off the bike.

Or be *thrown free*?

"I hear it all the time," says Seate with a sigh.

Today, most states require seat belts while driving in a protective cocoon of steel but do not require motorcycle helmets. Many riders see helmet laws as an affront to individual freedom. Unfortunately, helmets have little to do with how free we *should* be to do what we want. They have everything to do with physics. Physics doesn't care if you ignore it; it will just shrug and leave you and your family with thousands in hospital bills.

Death rates for bikers are significantly higher in no-helmet states. Some states require youthful riders to wear helmets, but their rates of death and injury are about the same as in

---

1. Insurance Institute for Highway Safety, Fatality Facts: Bicycles - 2010. www.helmets.org.
2. And while you're at it, put on the motorcycle jacket too. Put small children in their car seats and cover with a mattress. http://blog.al.com/spotnews/2011/12/alabama_tornadoes_--_first_in.html.

states that require no helmet at all. Younger, less experienced riders won't wear them if they mark the wearer as "a kid."

In Pennsylvania, deaths from motorcycle crashes have risen steadily since the helmet law was thrown out. Following that act, insurance companies placed limits on insurance payments. This may be fair in a horrific sort of way, that is:

> If you're willing to die "doing what you love" in a foolish manner, but instead survive with disabling and expensive injuries, please don't expect us to pay for it.

In auto racing, a common cause of death has long been whiplash and basal skull fractures. Like seat belts in the 1960s, restraints to protect necks and heads were greeted with fears that they might actually cause more injuries than they prevented. And, as in earlier years, some racers declared their intention to take their chances, hoping to be "thrown free." After too many incidents, organizers rebelled. All major auto racing organizations now require Head And Neck Support (HANS) equipment to minimize head and neck motion in a crash.

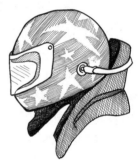

Helmets protect against fracture and abrasion, of wounding energies coming from *outside* the head; sticks and stones, twisting steel, blunt objects, sharp projectiles, concrete, and broken glass. But they also have their limitations. They do not change what goes on *inside* the head. They cannot, for example, keep the brain from bouncing off the inside of the skull during a sudden stop.

The notion of a helmet that will protect against all head injury is a popular dream (especially in football) but impossible. No one knows this better than Dr. Mariusz Ziejewski[1].

FIGURE 11-4. HANS

> The size and weight limitations of the helmet (due to potential for neck injury) restricts our ability to dissipate energy safely. The best way to deal with brain injury would be to link the head and neck to the upper torso. This would increase the effective mass (minimizing linear acceleration) and the radius of rotation (minimizing angular acceleration).
>
> —Mariusz Ziejewski Ph.D.[2]

Engineering the more protective helmet is *possible*, but the result would not be football. Better to ride safely and play safely, so you can continue doing what you love.

---

1. Professor of Engineering, North Dakota State University, College of Engineering, Director of South Dakota's Impact Biomechanics and Automotive Systems laboratories, and consultant to the Department of Defense in areas ranging from blast injuries to dynamics of ejection seats.
2. Personal communication, November 2013. See also page 245 on the critical relationship between neck and brain injuries (Goldstein LE and Others, 2012).

Seats and Headrests

Whether the stone hits the pitcher, or the pitcher hits the stone,
It's going to be bad for the pitcher.

—Miguel de Cervantes Saavedra, *Don Quixote* (1605)

Seats and headrests are often overlooked, both as safety features *and as sources of injury,* especially in whiplash. Mysterious injuries from rear-end crashes are all the more baffling when the victim did not hit her head on steering wheel or dash or windshield. How, then, can she possibly be (or claim to be) so badly injured?

Often the answer is that she was clubbed in the *back* of the head and neck — by the headrest. This is the automotive version of the "rabbit punch," the blow to upper neck and base of skull that regularly knocks out even Hollywood Super Heroes. They, of course, never suffer injury, but for Real Mortals in the Real World, this blow is so dangerous that it is forbidden even in "extreme" "No Holds Barred" martial arts competitions.

Cars are designed for the 50th Percentile Male. In practice, this means the average male in the US Army[1]. For shorter persons (teens, most women and many men) who must hug the steering wheel to reach the gas pedal, or for the passenger with head bent over a book, distance between head and headrest may be a foot or more rather than inches. If rear-ended so the head slams back, more force may hit the head/neck than hit the vehicle itself (Brown CR, 1996, p. 72).

Below the curve of the headrest, if there is nothing to support the neck, these forces can *hyper-flex* the neck (a reverse of normal cervical curve) forcing it to bend into the available space. That is, a headrest may guard against whiplashing of the *head*, but fail to protect the *neck* itself. Damage typically involves injury to the cervical spine and its supporting muscles and fascia, discs, ligaments and nerves and blood vessels. All of these can contribute to the brutally painful headaches and migraines that are so common after rear-end collisions.

Height brings other issues. A tall driver, who pushes the seat back, is protected from side impacts by the door pillar. Smaller, shorter persons who slide the seat forward to reach gas and steering wheel, are "protected" only by an expanse of window glass (Figure 11-5).

Other factors include age, health, bone density and musculature. A short woman with a slender neck is far more likely to suffer serious injury than a bull-necked male body builder, even if both are sitting with perfect posture. This is the classic crash-test dummy position, but real humans are rarely so ideally positioned[2].

---

1. A group often used for measurements but with size limits of its own: 60 to 80 inches (5' to 6' 8").
2. The same gender differences appear in soccer. Females are more subject to neck injury and breaks in the inner ear, often unrecognized (Fee GA, 1968; Grimm RJ and Others, 1989).

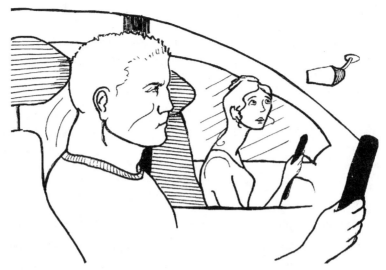

Posture is an important variable in injury. Two positions result in the most damage:

Head inclined, as when reading (leaving more space for head to slam against headrest) and head rotated, as when looking at mirrors (when neck bones are out of their strongest position).

When the vehicles above are struck from behind, *her* head will slam into the headrest. *His* will not. But neither is safe from a hyperflexion injury as their *necks* are forced to round into the empty air below the headrest. Meanwhile, his seat belt (not shown) may cross his chest as intended; hers may cut across her neck.

FIGURE 11-5. Drivers Large and Small

Air bags are intended to contact the upper chest of the 50thPercentile Male. In shorter persons (who also *sit closer* to the source) air bags may explode directly into neck or face causing severe injuries or death. The upshot: when males and females are passengers in the same car and in the same accident (and sometimes with minor injury to the vehicle) *he* may survive uninjured while *she* may suffer severe injuries and pain — a claim that may be seen as fantastical and fraudulent, in part because he is relatively uninjured, in part because there is little formal test data for females. *Female* crash test dummies were never *required* for automotive testing until 2011 (Newcomb D, 2012). Even now, engineers still tend to put males in the driver's seat, females as passengers[1].

For current safety information, see: **www.safercar.gov.** Katherine Shaver's *Washington Post* article (Shaver K, 2012) provides a historical overview and explains the new ratings.

---

1. See, however, Farnham A (2012) and vivid crash test footage.

Choice of Sport

"In 12 seasons, I believe I've had four documented concussions," said Mark Bruener, a tight end with the Houston Texans. Troy Vincent, a defensive back hoping to play a 16th year after being cut by the Washington Redskins, counted six: "Three that I know I was out . . . I was asleep," said Vincent, who said one of those hits appeared in a video clip at the meeting.

—Gary Milhoces reporting on the NFL concussion meeting (2007)

What if football is as dangerous to your brain as boxing? Would that change the way you regard the long-term risks of the game, or the way you parent your kids?

—www.SportsLegacy.org

Sports are important for physical development. It is important to have fun. But weigh the risks and the costs and realize that accidents happen. Choice of sport matters. Horses and dirt-bikes offer far more risk for brain injury than tennis, golf, or rowing. Recognize (and question) cultural attitudes and peer pressure. For example, many parents want their children on the field even after suffering a hit or other injury, and the players themselves want to be back on the field *rather than let their team down.*

It may be a matter of how the game is played rather than protective equipment or lack of it. The furious stampeding competition of basketball produces more injuries than the relatively calm and controlled environment of supposedly deadly martial arts. And although hockey produces many injuries, so does figure skating, especially pairs skating, especially for females as they are the ones who are tossed, flung, and thrown about.

Concussions aren't always noticed or tracked, but broken bones are. Records from the Mayo Clinic show that over 30 years, forearm fractures increased by over 40 percent largely due to inline skating, skateboarding, skiing, hockey, and bicycling (males); skating, skiing, soccer, and basketball (females) — all sports involving speed, potential falls or collisions (Khosla S and Others, 2003). A fall severe enough to fracture a forearm may also involve suffi-cient forces to cause whiplash or TBI.

Football, soccer, and rugby are the primary sports where athletes regularly receive sub-concussive brain trauma over 1,000 times in a season; high school football players have been recorded taking 197 hits to the head exceeding 15G in a game and 2,235 less forceful hits in the course of a single season (Broglio and Others, 2011).

Avoiding flagrantly and pointlessly dangerous damage is *not* about "wrapping a player in cotton wool," not the same, as some sneer, as putting the quarterback in a skirt. It is a means of protecting a player's brain, skills, abilities and *life*.

American Football

> As of 2009, only one dead NFL player tested for CTE did *not* have the condition — running back Damien Nash, who collapsed in 2007 while playing basketball at age 24, apparently too soon to have developed the disease.
>
> — Alan Schwarz (2009)

> Lectures about concussions in youth football tend to be a dull compound of science and moralizing. So instead of words, let's try a picture. Pick up a bobblehead and shake it—hard. Watch the little spring neck whiplash back and forth and hear the toy rattle, and imagine your son's 7-year-old brain inside the shell. That's why you need to hand him a flag instead of a helmet.
>
> —Sally Jenkins (2013)

In the U. S., 1.5 million boys play high school football; some 250,000 suffer concussions in the course of the season. The very few who make it to the professional leagues take huge risks for their paychecks[1]. Between 1988 and 1993, the 28 teams of the NFL reported 445 concussions, or about *four* acknowledged, documented concussions a week. Most go unreported.

Bennet Omalu identified CTE in six out of six of the following deceased NFL players.

- MIKE WEBSTER (D. 2002, AGE 50) in theory, of heart attack. But, death followed years of physical and cognitive decline, severe depression, dementia and drugs. He could not sleep, sometimes drinking multiple bottles of "night-time" formulas or tasering himself repeatedly in a desperate attempt to win a few hours of unconsciousness (Garber G, 2005).

- JUSTIN STRZELCZYK (D. 2004, AGE 36) in a fiery explosion after hitting a tanker truck at 90 miles per hour while driving against the flow of traffic. He was assumed to be DUI due to his past problems with drugs and alcohol, but toxicology showed none in his system.

- TERRY LONG (D. 2005, AGE 45) suicide from drinking anti-freeze after years of severe depression and multiple suicide attempts.

- ANDRE WATERS (D. 2006, AGE 44) suicide by gunshot wound. Tests showed that Waters' brain had degenerated into that of an 85-year-old man with characteristics similar to those of early-stage Alzheimer's. It was estimated that within ten years (by age 55), Waters would have been fully incapacitated.

- JOHN GRIMSLEY (D. 2008, AGE 45) of possibly accidental gunshot wound while cleaning guns.

- TOM MCHALE (D. 2008, AGE 45) of overdose of oxycontin which he used for severe shoulder and joint pain. Thought to be accidental.

Finding a condition that is incredibly rare in the general population in six out of six former NFL players, 50 or younger, would seem to suggest that football might be bad for the brain. However, Dr. Ira Casson, co-chairman of the NFL committee on brain injury, said

---

1. The average NFL career is about 3.5 years. A pension requires 4 years (Culverhouse G (2012). Meanwhile, many players who leave the NFL in less than that time, are too battered and broken to be eligible to buy health insurance on their own (Fainaru-Wada M and Fainaru S, 2013, p. 68).

he could have no reaction until the McHale case and other CTE findings appear in a peer-reviewed scientific journal. "It's very hard to react to things and to case studies that are not presented in appropriate, scientific form and have not gone through peer review" (Schwarz A, 2009). So is CTE associated with football? "I think that there is not enough scientific evidence to say that there is," said Casson, but CTE continued to be verified in other players, all young or relatively young men.

- CHRIS HENRY (D. 2009, AGE 26) after fall or leap from moving truck after a domestic dispute. He had played only 5 years of pro football but had years of problems with drugs, traffic offenses (including DUI without license or insurance), aggressive behavior and assault (Howard J, 2010).

- SHANE FRONETT (D. 2009, AGE 38) suicide after confusion, paranoia, and rage. Problems dating at least from 2006 ended with threatening his wife with a gun; he then shot himself.

- DAVE DUERSON (D. 2011, AGE 50) suicide, of gunshot wound to chest. He left a text message requesting that his brain be donated to CTE research.

We are less surprised by the deaths of older men, but these former players suffered years or decades of cognitive decline. It appears that CTE developed while they were still young.

- LOU CREEKMUR (D. 2009, AGE 82) following 30 years of cognitive decline.

- COOKIE GILCHRIST (D. 2011, AGE 75) following years of emotional problems. He was reclusive, estranged from friends and family, and so paranoid that he taped all conversations.

- OLLIE MATSON (D. 2011, AGE 80) from complications of dementia. He had been bed-ridden for years and had not spoken for four.

- FORREST BLUE (D. 2011, AGE 65) with symptoms of paranoia and dementia dating to the 1990s. Retired from 11 seasons in the NFL, Blue spent his last two years in an assisted living facility. Like Mary Lincoln he complained of "little people that lived in the walls" and hearing their voices. He was sure his phone was tapped by the devil (Carrol L and Rosner D, 2011, p. 227).

- JOHN MACKEY (D. 2011, AGE 69), after years of dementia.

- JOHN HENRY JOHNSON (D. 2011, AGE 81), with severe memory loss and Alzheimer's disease.

- Joe Perry (d. 2011, age 84) of complications of dementia.

- RALPH WENZEL (D. 2012, AGE 69), of complications of dementia. With serious memory lapses and other cognitive problems by 52, he entered a home for dementia patients at age 63.

- RAY EASTERLING (D. 2012, AGE 63). Symptoms of dementia began to appear in the mid 1990s, 10 years after his retirement from 11 seasons in the NFL.

Several players died in 2008 for whom CTE was not verified but is suspected: Wally Hilgenberg (66) of ALS (Lou Gehrig's disease) and Curtis Whitley (39) of accidental drug overdose or suicide. Another was Chris Mims.

The 6-foot 5-inch Chris Mims played 7 seasons for the San Diego Chargers as defensive end. He started at 270 pounds in 1992; team officials wanted him to play at 295. In 1993 he struggled up to 287. In 1995, he was suddenly 300 pounds; by 1998 he had ballooned to over 350.

While making millions with the NFL, he failed to pay bills for house and car, attorney fees, and child support (Schrotenboer B, 2009). He was taken to court over 20 times for unpaid bills and in 1996 was scolded by a superior court judge for writing bad checks. In 1999, he was convicted of refusing to take a blood alcohol test after suspected DUI, and of assault for beating a man with his belt. The Chargers cut him from the team.

In 2000, Mims joined the Chicago Bears, but never played a game. After being cut at training camp for oversleeping and failing to show up for practice, he retired that season at age 30. He spent his final years depressed and reclusive, surviving on disability payments and hiding from bill collectors. He died of heart failure in 2008 at age 38 At his death, Mims weighed 456 pounds.

Did Chris Mims have CTE? We can't know for sure, but in the downward spiral of a once beloved and kind-hearted man, we can see all the symptoms.

Soccer

Soccer is seen as less dangerous than tackle football, but this is not necessarily so.

High school soccer players sustained concussions at a greater rate than every sport except football. Rates for girls are 64 per cent greater than rates for male soccer players and greater than for (also male) football players (Carroll L and Rosner, 2011, p. 58).

One problem is heading the soccer ball. The weight of a regulation soccer ball (for players over 12) is about one pound. It may be moving at 20+ miles per hour. While female reflexes are faster than males, their neck strength is less, the same issue that predisposes women to whiplash at rates far higher than men. Some researchers find no difference in neurocognitive symptoms among low-, moderate-, and high-exposure header groups in boys and girls 13-18 (Kontos AP and Others, 2011). Others do. It may be that children and young women should not head soccer balls just as young boys should not play tackle football.

Female concussions can be complicated by culture. Through the 1960s, female basketball players were limited to a quarter court, three dribbles, three tosses in the air, and one roving forward who could move over the entire (half-size) court; basketball was considered too strenuous a game for women. Today, the notion continues that girls don't play hard enough to get concussions so their injuries may not be taken seriously. The most common symptom of concussion is headache, but because adolescent females are more prone to headaches than males, these may be dismissed as hormonal (Carroll L and Rosner D, 2011, p. 64).

Skateboarding, Snowboarding, and Skiing

Skateboard deaths are low, but brain injuries are common (Lustenberger T and Others, 2010). Injuries tend to be to long bones in younger children, but head injuries are common in all groups, especially blows to the tailbone then occiput from backward falls[1].

When summer skateboarders become winter snowboarders the same patterns appear. TBI is a common injury in both skiers and snowboarders, but snowboarders typically suffer the worst injuries, often to the occiput (Corra S and Others, 2012). For both groups, fractures are greatly reduced through use of helmets.

In Utah ERs, snowboarders had more head and spinal injuries than skiers, who tended to injure their lower extremities. Skiers landed more often in the operating room, but snowboarders more often in the intensive care unit (Wasden CC and Others, 2009).

Snowboard injuries are often due to jumping, especially by beginners. Injury to the occipital region is common and may come with subdural hematomas. Of 11 major head injury cases, 10 were caused by occipital impact (Nakaguchi H and Others, 1999). Wear a helmet and avoid jumping, especially as a beginner (Fukuda O and Others, 1999).

And learn how to fall safely.

---

1. See a mini-documentary on skateboard falls and helmets here:
www.skateboard.tv/video/22445/fractured-blake-johnston-jesse-ostroff-and-jason-segal.

Martial Arts

Martial arts are the arts of "war." They provide risks, but also benefits. Many see them as unnecessary violence. Others as training for the times when violence is necessary. In *Rodney Stone*, Sir Arthur Conan Doyle's Regency novel, Doyle presents prize-fighting (boxing) as key to winning the war against Napoleon[1]. Unfortunately, some practitioners lose more than they gain. There is a long tradition of instructors *(sensei)* who cannot bear noise or crowds, handle money, make change, or deal with time. They may explode in volcanic anger one moment and collapse into giggles the next. When students try to sneak up on them at night they are invariably found awake. A common explanation is that:

Sensei is functioning on a higher spiritual plane.

Perhaps. A more likely explanation is that, after years of injuries, *Sensei* is brain damaged. At least one famous historical martial artist reportedly tried to "toughen up" his brain by repeatedly smacking himself in the forehead with a rock. He shared many quirks and oddities with modern martial arts stars whose reputations (and obvious injuries) are based on how many cement blocks they have broken *with their heads.* Every style has its risks, but adding other techniques to the repertoire expands potential for injury.

Mixed Martial Arts (MMA) and events such as the Ultimate Fighting Championship were originally intended to remove the limits of different styles by *combining* them (hence Bruce Lee's "Style of No Style.) It allows punches and kicks (not done in real wrestling or judo) with throws and groundwork (not done in boxing or karate). But restrictions remain.

Contestants still can't gouge out eyes, rip out lungs or attack groins and kidneys. Biting and spitting are forbidden, as is "fish-hooking" (attacking the mouth), attacking eyes, ears, or other orifices or openings including open wounds. No hair pulling, no pinching, twisting, scratching or clawing[2]. No abusive language. *And no head butts.* The forbidden zone extends from neck and base of skull to top of the ears and includes the top of the head, hence no "pile drivers" staged (with protection to the actors) in WWE. And, as in all martial arts competitions, strikes to neck and spine are strictly forbidden, including the "rabbit punch" (a blow to the upper neck and base of skull)[3]. Another risk is falling.

---

1. Doyle presents parallels with modern-day "cage fighting." It sounds scary, but it's hype for those titillated by the fantasy of life-and-death matches. And despite breathless advertising, contestants still aren't allowed to murder their opponents on TV. In reality, the cage isn't there to keep competitors in, it's there to keep the crowd out. In "Rodney's" day, the line was kept with horse whips. Then as now, these were betting events where a lot of money could be made or lost.
2. Referees bring nail clippers and files to trim long or potentially scratchy nails. Rules are set by the Association of Boxing Commissions (ABC). See www.abcboxing.com/unified_mma_rules.html.
3. These organizations are more aware of TBI than some expert witnesses who dismiss automotive injuries. A blow with a headrest may be no less damaging than a blow with a boxing glove.

LEARNING TO FALL

> Whoa! Gravity is a harsh mistress.
>
> —*The Tick* (2001)

Safe falling is a first technique taught in acting classes to keep performers safe during the feint, the blow, the knockdown. On stage and film, the rolls and falls done by stuntmen to protect themselves from harm, are the most real part of the performance.

In martial arts, safe falling is the most practical, Real World self-defense there is, the one skill with the most immediate application. Few of us get into daily fights to the death "On The Street." All of us must deal with gravity and possible attack "*By* The Street."

Table 11-2. US Accidental Deaths	
Cause and Rate / 100,000:	**Deaths[a]**
Motor vehicles (14.9)	44,700
Poisoning (including drugs (8.5)	25,300
Falls (7.1)	21,200
Suffocation / Choking (1.4)	4,100
Drowning (1.3)	3,800
Fires, Flames, & Smoke (0.9)	2,800
Firearm accidents (0.2)	680

a. National Safety Council, *Accident Facts*, 2006 data on 120,000 accidental deaths.

We slip on ice, trip over curbs and our own feet. We land in the ER with broken wrists and heads. Sometimes we die. Yet despite the lurid headlines, more of us die from falls than from the combination of drowning, fire, choking, and gun accidents (Table 11-2). Someday you *will* fall. If you know how to fall safely may save your brain and your life.

Falling skills were fundamental in Asian martial arts, including various versions of karate. Traditionally, new students were assigned 1,000 falls. A beginner who has done this knows how to fall safely — and is no longer a beginner. In the US, falling skills were long avoided. "We aren't here to learn how to fall down," sniffed one instructor, "we're here to learn how to make the *other* guy fall down" [1].

In contrast, Judo and Aikido have always taught balance under extreme conditions and how to fall safely if you lose it. Some schools transform forces into a harmless roll and a return to standing position. Others emphasize *breakfalls*, full-body slams onto the mat, that maximize area to minimize damage. Some students hone technique by moving from the mat to the parking lot, or starting from ever greater heights. A handy skill, but if overdone, these techniques cause trauma. Some schools consider 300 breakfalls per night to be the lower limit of *serious* training; it should also be seen as *damaging*.

---

1. For years, this situation was gleefully exploited by the Gracie family (through their Judo-based Brazilian Jiu Jutsu) until the rest of the world caught on to what they were doing — taking down opponents untrained in falling or ground-work to the mat. This may be why many US karate and tae kwan do schools now teach these skills.

If you practice the arts of war, you're going to get hurt. Nevertheless, avoid potentially damaging activities that *are* under your control.

- TAKE A LONG HARD LOOK AT SENIOR PLAYERS / INSTRUCTORS.
  - Observe health and function. (Consider why the NFL Hall of Fame is too often referred to as "The Hall of Lame.")
  - Choose your sport accordingly.

- USE APPROPRIATE SAFETY EQUIPMENT.
  - No sparring without protection.
  - Is horseplay allowed? Are safety rules observed by students and instructors?

- DO NOT TRAIN ON AN UNSAFE FLOOR. REQUIREMENTS VARY BY STYLE.
  - Karate requires a floor that is firm and "fast" to allow quick movements.
  - Wrestling mats protect in falls and throws, but are too "slow" for karate spins and turns and can encourage tripping and knee injuries.
  - Judo requires a relatively fast mat combined with the shock absorbtion of a sprung floor (more likely found at a dance school than at a gym or garage[1].
  - Mixed styles requires a mix of mats. Students learning to breakfall need a crash pad (a big fluffy vinyl pillow) totally different from mats appropriate for stepping or spinning kicks.

It is important to play and have fun, and important to learn how to use a body, to face attack, to be able to apply these skills when defense is necessary. However, brain injury does not build better brains or bodies. It should never be seen as a badge of honor.

And taking steps to protect brain and body should never deserve contempt.

We need other humans and other humans need us. Don't let the things you bring to the table — the skills, the abilities, the knowledge — be lost to brain injury, lost to others, and lost to the world.

---

1. At www.YouTube.com, ignore the soaring judo throws. Focus on heads bouncing off the mat.

Educating Self and Others

Over the last few years, there has been a huge increase in awareness of concussion and its impact on life and health. Many studies are now available, more are planned, and while more research is always good, it is also good to apply what we already know on the field. Unfortunately, studies consistently show a serious problem: non-compliance.

Over 40 percent of concussed high school athletes return to action before the effects of the last injury have time to stabilize. Coaches in every sport ignore published guidelines that define or limit the time to return to play. Even more disturbing, 16 percent of high school football players who lose consciousness return to the same game in which they were injured. Loss of consciousness in concussion is relatively rare (only about 10 percent), but it is *obvious*. So consider this: if coaches don't sideline the players who were actually knocked out, how can they be trusted to sideline the ones with the subtler symptoms typical of the vast majority of concussions? (Carroll L and Rosner D, 2011, p. 34).

Pre-Play Testing

Athletes are notorious for ignoring or downplaying symptoms so they can stay in the game. So are some coaches. In the culture of sports and military, a player who doesn't charge back into play is "weak." Even worse is the notion that a brain should be banged around *more* to toughen it up. Unfortunately, every concussion increases the likelihood of more and more severe injuries, and any injury must be given time for the acute phase of the injury to heal, such as internal bleeding. Proper recovery is critical for preventing more damage and neurological and cognitive problems far into the future.

Meanwhile, symptoms of serious injury may not appear until hours or days later.

Baseline tests of cognitive function in athletes can be compared with tests done on the sidelines after injury. The final test scores can also *assist* in judging severity of injury and help predict how soon an injured athlete can return to play. This helps reduce the possibility of rare but deadly second-impact syndrome a second blow to damaged tissue before the first injury has stabilized. If there is no baseline available, scores can be compared to a normalized database of the athlete's peer group.

The tests below are stress tests for the brain. Some are amazingly simple, yet sensitive to subtle changes in function that may be missed by CT, MRI, or standard neuropsych exams. Subjects whose scores differ from baseline should be checked by a neurologist.

THE MEASURING STICK TEST

The simplest test for impaired brain injury reported in the research medical literature is this: catching a falling measuring stick weighted at the bottom with a hockey puck.

To start, the examiner holds up the stick; the subject rests an open hand on the puck

When the examiner drops the stick, the subject catches it as quickly as possible.

The distance the stick falls is converted into milliseconds of reaction time.

When concussed and unconcussed athletes were tested (at baseline and within 48 hours of injury), this simple test reliably showed significant differences in reflexes and reaction time (Eckner JT and Others, 2010).

THE KING-DEVICK TEST

The King-Devick (K-D) test was developed in the 1970's by optometrists Al King and Steve Devick to test eye behavior in reading and learning disabilities, including dyslexia. It is now used to identify TBI thanks to its ability to capture problems with eye movement, focus, attention, speech and other symptoms of impaired brain function.

Test I has guidelines and regular spacing.

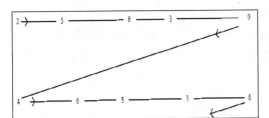

Tests II and III have no guidelines and the numbers are spaced irregularly.

These seemingly simple tests challenge 6 of the 12 cranial nerves and the muscles of the eye itself.

FIGURE 11-6. King-Devick Tests for Eye Movements

To test, the subject reads rows of single-digit numbers from left to right as quickly and accurately as possible. The numbers are unevenly spaced and become progressively more difficult to read in a flowing manner as space increases between them. This simple test gives an objective physical measure of a wide variety of functions. It evaluates visual recognition and reaction time by challenging the eye's rapid movements called *saccades*[1].

---

1. From French, originally meaning a quick strong jerk or pull, as on the reins of a horse. Here it refers to the quick movements of the eyes between fixed points in response to pulls from the muscles of the eye and the nerves that drive them.

Reading numbers tests proper eye tracking and focus which requires coordination of 16 different muscles and six of the 12 cranial nerves. Reading aloud requires focus and attention, visual pattern recognition, speech and language skills. It takes two minutes or less, is timed with a stopwatch, scored for speed and accuracy, then compared to a normalized database of subjects.

Poor scores? Poor brain function.

In boxers and Mixed Martial Arts (MMA) fighters, post-fight scores more than 5 seconds slower than baseline appeared *only* in fighters with head trauma, especially those who had been knocked out (Galetta KM and others, 2011a). These findings were duplicated in concussed college athletes who averaged 6 seconds slower than baseline (Galetta KM and Others, 2011b). Besides TBI, K-D can reveal neurological deficits in conditions ranging from Parkinson's disease and multiple sclerosis (MS), to hypoxia in mountaineers and pilots, and impaired function in sleep-deprived hospital residents and staff (Davies EC and Others, 2012).

To test, the subject simply reads numbers from cards or computer. Baseline is the fastest time (of *two* attempts) required for the subject to read the numbers aloud with fewest errors. After a suspected TBI, the test is administered *once*. If time or errors are greater than baseline, the athlete should be removed from play and evaluated by medical personnel. Test materials (including a stopwatch) cost about $40, can be purchased by anyone and used anywhere.

The NFL's first Summit meeting (in 2007), barely acknowledged and largely denied concussion in NFL players. The fourth Summit meeting (in 2012) discussed better testing and evaluation. This included the idea of adding the K-D Test to the NFL's existing SCAT2 test, but, according to a King-Devick spokesperson, the NFL concluded that the cost was too great at $1.75 per player. It is a comfort to know that almost any parent can do better than the NFL[1].

For more information, current pricing, and video demonstrations of the test, see:

www.kingdevicktest.com/about/

---

1. King-Devick, personal communication (July, 2013).

COMPUTERIZED TESTS

There are now numerous computerized tests available. Their focus is Return To Play. Several systems have been widely adopted.

- IMPACT (IMMEDIATE POST-CONCUSSION ASSESSMENT AND COGNITIVE TESTING).
- HEADMINDER CONCUSSION RESOLUTION INDEX (CRI).
- CONCUSSION SENTINEL.

Glowing reviews have been provided by developers but in 2007, independent reviewers found moderate to low reliability (Broglio SP and Others, 2007). ImPACT, the most widely used program was the least reliable; many subjects who repeated the test just days later showed lower scores, although none had suffered new injuries. The 2007 findings of moderate to poor reliability of ImPACT were replicated in a 2013 study showing false positives ranging from 22 to 46 percent (Resch J and Others, 2013). A history of false positives might tempt some coaches to dismiss results, to send concussed athletes back to play prematurely. In short, *computer-based concussion evaluations alone do not provide stable measures of cognitive function.*

One weakness of computer testing is the computer. Where milliseconds count, slowed computer processing can radically alter results. More development (with testing by independent evaluators), will improve programs, but coaches, clinicians and parents must not rely on computerized tests alone. A multifaceted approach is still best.

IMPACT SENSORS

The NFL and NFL Players Association have agreed to a limit of 14 full-contact practices during the season, less than one per week, primarily to limit exposure to brain trauma, and yet we are aware of youth programs practicing in full pads four days a week. The toughest men in the world, NFL players, have asked to be hit in the head fewer times because they recognize there is no such thing as a tough brain. Children, who cannot provide informed consent, have never been asked that question, but I believe their answer would be the same.

— Chris Nowinski, Sports Legacy (2012)

In 2012, the Sports Legacy Institute proposed a Hit Count modeled after the "Pitch Count" used by Little League and other baseball organizations. Young pitchers are limited to a specific number of pitches they can throw in one day with required rest periods. For example, children 10 and under are limited to 75 pitches followed by three days of rest after more than 61 pitches. Asks Dr. Robert Cantu: "If we go to such great lengths to protect the *elbows* of baseball players then heck, don't you think we ought to set limits to the number of times we allow a child to be hit in the *head*?"

Impact sensors provide the data to support this vision. These are the same devices (accelerometers) used in industry to track various kinds of damage. For some years now, sensors have been built into helmets, but there were drawbacks. The sensors measured impact to the *helmet*, not to the *head*. They stayed with the helmet (expensive) and could not be used in helmet-less sports such as soccer and rugby. Newer versions avoid these problems.

None of these devices test for concussion or eliminate the possibility that one exists. A series of mild hits can be as damaging as a single severe one, and other hits occur off the field. They do not replace medical evaluation before or after play.

On the other hand, they do provide basic data that can help protect players.

The simplest approach to reducing injuries may be simply reducing hits in practice (Cobb BR and Others, 2013).

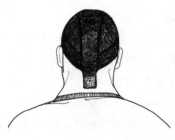

FIGURE 11-7. CheckLight

CheckLight

CheckLight consists of a mesh cap, lined with flexible sensors, worn under the helmet. It tracks number, force and focus of blows to the head (Gorman M, 2013). A tab with LED battery check and three warning lights hangs below the helmet: green for low, yellow for moderate, and red for a severe impact. CheckLight measures impact to the head, not the helmet. It can be worn under a helmet or by itself for soccer and other helmet-free sports. It also removes the issue of non-reporting of concussions; information is instantly available to team mates so that players can monitor each other, bypassing the issue of "toughness" or the temptation to return injured players to the field. See **www.Rebok.com**.

The Biometrics Mouth guard

Another possibility is an impact-sensing mouth guard. It contains a gyroscope and feeds wireless sensor data on jarring head motions to a sideline computer. The system has been tested on high-school athletes (in Middletown, NY) with additional testing planned on college players at Purdue University and University of South Carolina. From i1 Biometrics, **www.i1biometrics.com**.

The X-Patch

The X-Patch attaches directly to the player's head, under a headband or an adhesive patch. Data on any hits are sent wirelessly to sideline computers. From X2 Biosystems, **www.x2biosystems.com**.

Going With the Data — or Not

Knowing is not enough, we must apply.

Willing is not enough, we must do.

—Johann Wolfgang von Goethe (1749-1832)

After years of stonewalling and denial, there is finally progress in *recognizing* brain injuries in sports, especially football. The problem then becomes whether or not this information is taken seriously. Helmet-to-helmet hits have caused concussions, neck injuries, paralysis or death, in high school, college, and professional football players. For over 20 years, ABC's "Monday Night Football" opened with an image of two helmets crashing into each other then shattering. In 2010, the NFL began to make some changes (Thomas K, 2010). ESPN was asked to halt the helmet-crashing image, players began to be fined for head-to-head hits, and NFL Films began editing illegal hits from their films.

On December 8, 2011, Cleveland Browns quarterback Colt McCoy was stunned by a ferocious helmet-to-helmet hit. McCoy lay on the field for several minutes. From the stands, his father noted the rigidity of his body[1]. On the sidelines, trainers looked at McCoy's injured *left hand*, but he remained there (as timed by his father, a high school football coach), for just 3 minutes and 50 seconds, too short a time to properly evaluate the effects of such a severe blow. When McCoy returned to the field, he threw an interception. After the game, he showed the classic concussion symptoms of light sensitivity, nausea, and amnesia; he had no memory of being on the field after the hit.

The Browns were severely criticized for mishandling the injury. Within two weeks, the NFL (then facing over 4,000 injury lawsuits), began to try to limit damage.

- James Harrison, the Steelers player who made the illegal helmet-to-helmet hit, was the first to be suspended (for one game). Other players have since been suspended *and* fined.

- Concussion protocol was expanded and Certified Athletic Trainers placed in the press boxes. They have access to instant replay and can notify sideline personnel if they suspect a head injury (Reed T, 2012). Oddly, there are still no *neurologists* as required for boxing.

It's a start, but harmful behavior is far from over and will remain so long as concussion is seen as a point of honor, no matter how destructive it may be to players' own lives, and those of their friends and families.

---

1. McCoy was out for the rest of the season, then spent nearly a year on the bench as backup. He would never start again until his replacement, Brandon Weeden, suffered his own concussion.

Within two years of leaving the NFL, about 78 percent of players are unemployed, bankrupt, or divorced (Schrotenboer B, 2009). Often this is due to TBI suffered in the course of the game. Nevertheless, despite the increasing awareness of unrecognized and untreated TBI and their consequences, TBI is not necessarily a death sentence. Life goes on.

The problem is that a good life needs to involve more than One Thing. For many pro football players this has never been the case. High school was about football, college was about football. Today, football is about football *only*, a big change from how the game was played before. Until the 1970s, players had other jobs and interests during the off-season. Some worked construction, some sold insurance. Today, training goes on all year. If a life is only football, when the football is over, the life is over too. Part of having a life after TBI is having laid the groundwork for a life, and actually having a life to go back to.

Mike Reid played football at Penn State. In 1969, his senior year, he was a unanimous All-America choice, won the Outland Trophy, the Maxwell Award, and graduated from college with a degree in music. He went on to a stellar career with the Cincinnati Bengals. During the off-seasons, he performed as a concert pianist for the Cincinnati, Dallas, and Utah symphony orchestras. Then in 1974, at age 26, after four knee operations and— most ominously, *hand injuries* — he left football to focus on his music. Fans remember great distress:

"He could have made the Football Hall of Fame — *but he just quit!*"

In reality, Reid simply moved on to other life skills that were important to him and he left the game in time to be still be able to do these things well.

Through the 1980s and 1990s, Reid wrote 12 Number One hits and co-wrote the Bonnie Rait standard *I Can't Make You Love Me*. In 2005, Mike Reid was inducted into the Nashville Songwriters Hall of Fame. He may have missed the Football Hall of Fame but he won the NFL Alumni Career Achievement Award for success in his post-NFL career[1].

In theory, Reid left *before* he was too seriously injured.

What happens to those who do not or cannot stop?

---

1. The NFL awards a prize for this because so many of its former players do so very poorly, spiraling down into drugs, divorce, bankruptcy, and sometimes suicide.
   For industry estimates on just how long you can stay in your sport, see:
   http://www.ramfg.com/RAM-Financial-Group-Solutions-Professional-Athletes-Athletes-Services

Aftershocks

Clinical symptoms of CTE include progressive affective lability, irritability, distractibility, executive dysfunction, memory disturbances, suicidal ideation, and in advanced cases, cognitive deficits and dementia.

—Goldstein LE and Others (2012)

In 2002, when Bennet Omalu examined Mike Webster's seemingly normal brain, he saw the strange features that now define CTE. But that was not the first time he saw them. The first was while examining tissue from a woman in her forties who had been beaten into a coma by her abusive husband. It was her sadly broken brain, its clumps of torn and tangled neurons, that crossed his mind when he saw the same puzzling details once again under his microscope (Fainaru-Wada M and Fainaru S, 2013, p. 151). The NFL scoffed at his findings, but he would see them again and again in more athletes and in soldiers — as would others.

In 2012, Dr. Lee Goldstein (with 34 other contributors from a wide variety of disciplines), reported on research comparing tissue from normal brains with tissue from:

- Five soldiers with blast or multiple concussion injuries (ages 22-45),
- Three high-school / college-age football players (ages 17-21),
- One professional wrestler (age 27).

And mice. Attempting to reproduce the changes seen in the human brains, researchers exposed mice to a single blast emulating an IED. On autopsy, their brains, like the human brains, showed no external damage; *outside*, they looked perfectly normal. *Inside*, autopsy revealed damage identical to those seen in the human victims, the same broken nerve cells, the same autoimmune antibodies (see Color Section). "Blast injuries were indistinguishable from football injuries," says Dr. Goldstein, "the pathology was *identical*."

This study also showed the critical relationship between neck and brain injuries. Mice whose heads were free to move (think "whiplash" or "bobblehead") suffered far worse damage than those whose necks were restrained.

The implications of this study are staggering. So are the possibilities.

It reveals the overlap between different sources of injury. The uniform worn during injury — whether WWE, football, or military — does not matter. The results are the same.

It also suggests the possibility of healing. If clinical symptoms indicate CTE in blast-injured veterans and others, does it follow that reduction in or loss of those same symptoms via neurofeedback (as in Chapter 8) indicates healing?

We don't know, because we can't yet test directly for CTE in living patients, or track its progress. To date, direct validation of CTE can be done only on autopsy, much too late for some patients, much too soon for others.

More research is needed. And more healing.

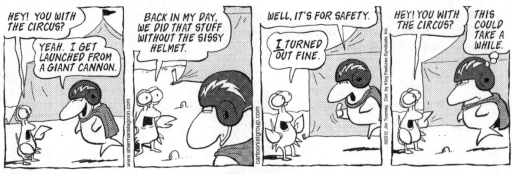

FIGURE 11-8. I'm Fine!

I Did X and I'm Fine

Despite the studies, regardless of the research, the real question after concussion is "*How soon can I (or my child or my star player) go back?*"

Statements such as "I had 17 concussions and I'm *Fine*!" have actually been part of serious family discussions on whether or not children should play sports, which ones and how often, and whether or not a high school boy should return to football after a five-day coma.

If you are Fine, great! But how is everyone else in your world? Some may have failed to survive long enough to make that claim. Some may think they are Fine but are far from it. And some are not Fine at all and never will be ever again.

Pro football players, in theory our most powerful and capable athletes, have a hugely increased risk of dying from neurodegenerative causes. "Speed players" are at special risk. These are the quarterbacks, running backs, halfbacks, and linebackers. Compared to the US population in general, they face three times the rate of mortality from all neurodegenerative causes, including four times the rate of Alzheimer's and ALS (Lehman EJ and Others, 2012).

Homeless groups and prison populations have extremely high levels of brain injury. Some of those same injured NFL and other athletes have ended in that company.

The best way to deal with brain injury, in children and adults, is to avoid it. When it does occur, know how to recognize it and how to deal with the consequences. Be aware that, very often, the terrible symptoms of TBI can be helped with neurofeedback.

This is shown by the case histories of past injuries and healing. It is also shown in the continuing life stories of these same people, many of whom were once believed to have no future at all.

The Rest of the Story

WHAT HAPPENED TO CHARLOTTE AND BRIDGETT, TO BILLY AND KYLE, TO KEVIN, GREGORY, DAVID AND CAROL.

T he success of a treatment isn't only a matter of what happens during treatment, but of what happens afterwards. The men, women, and children throughout this book suffered disabling symptoms for months, years or even decades.

Many modalities offer temporary relief, but the real test is *later*. What has happened to these people and how did their lives change (or not) after treatment ended?

Where Are They Now?

Charlotte

Charlotte (page 25) was knocked out on the playground in elementary school. Her grades fell, and by high school she needed detailed lists to remember the most mundane activities. College was a struggle, and her professional career a disappointment compared to what she felt she *should* have been able to accomplish.

After several FNS sessions at age 60, she was startled by profound changes in function, especially memory. Suddenly there was no need to write things down, the list was just *there*, in her head. There was also sudden improvement in ability to retain and apply professional material (old and new), to absorb and express ideas, to write and lecture, to communicate verbally.

> For decades, problems with academic, professional, and social skills were painful and frustrating. Now, social situations are fun and I continue to be surprised when the words flow. If only I had found this treatment years ago!

Bridgett

After a kick in the head during a soccer game, 10-year-old Bridgett (page 132) suffered steadily worsening head and body pain, dizziness, nausea, and sensory disruptions. Then she lost her ability to walk. After her ninth treatment Bridgett wrote the following essay.

When It All Went Clear

Before I went to Dr. Esty, I could not do any schoolwork. At first, I went to the office grumbling because I thought it was a waste of time and money. Then my six-month-long headache was gone. Right after that everything went clear, like the first time you put on glasses. I used to get a headache from the four-page *Henry & Mudge* books. Now, four weeks later, I have plowed through four book reports with no headache at all. No one wants to live life with a headache and if neurofeedback can heal me 100%, why can't it heal someone else at least 90%?

As of Spring 2014, Bridgett remains completely active with full cognitive function. She has returned to soccer, and is a formidable member of the debate team. She is once again a straight-A student, and an excellent competitive dancer. Her mother comments:

The treatment that abruptly ended our six months of misery can help many people as they struggle with concussions, learning issues and emotional traumas. This technology has turned my daughter's life around.

Bill

Bill (page 142) survived a horrific motorcycle accident and multiple surgeries. For years he lived with severe fatigue, memory loss, impaired vision and speech, terrifying flashbacks and nightmares. His story is a vivid contradiction to the popular notion that "How you are a year after the injury is as good as you're going to get."

Bill began FNS neurofeedback treatment *17 years after his crash*. Within 3 sessions, the terrible fatigue began to lift; within 10 sessions, he had lost the flashbacks and nightmares. By the end of 25 sessions, full vision and normal body temperature had returned, and speech was much more fluent.

In 2008, 10 years after initial treatment, Bill's vision and body temperature, remained normal, speech was fluent, and he could work through the entire day.

Bill described years of life after TBI as being like one heavy individual picture frame after another. There was no beat, no rhythm, just a grind.

"Now," he says, " it *flows*. Now it's like music. It's in motion and I'm in motion with it. Now I can breathe and think at the same time."

Kyle

After multiple injuries in Iraq, Kyle (page 156) suffered severe sleep problems and fatigue with non-stop headaches. He walked with a cane and was unable to read. These symptoms resolved so well that he was running again and on passing the Marine physical, he volunteered to return to combat. On a mission there, he was re-injured. In the hospital, he asked for treatment for TBI, but was told they had nothing. "These people know nothing about brain injuries!" he growled.

In March 2013, Kyle returned to BWB for additional FNS treatment for TBI and pain. Once again he responded rapidly: headaches disappeared and cognitive abilities returned. Kyle has now retired from the Marine Corps and begun full-time studies at a highly ranked university. He is making excellent grades and is on track to write professionally.

Kevin

Kevin (page 158) suffered multiple TBIs, with loss of consciousness and seizures. With sleep problems, reading problems, nightmares, and pain, he was depressed and suicidal.

Seven months after beginning FNS treatments at BWB, Kevin was in college, getting A's and recommended for a scholarship. On completing his courses, he plans to get an MBA and start his own company. He has a solid time line for his career.

Kevin also reports the return of full sensation in fingers. Before FNS treatment he couldn't feel a hammer blow; now he feels splinters. The man who once lived on Hostess Ho Hos now eats no sugar at all, has made a serious study of nutrition, plans to get a certificate in fitness training, and is teaching his children good eating habits. Meanwhile, he works three days a week as a team leader for a community organization and is thoughtful and gentle with others.

Gregory

Gregory (page 170) lost his career in computer programming to an idly thrown rock. He was on disability for 14 years, with little hope for recovery. The letter he wrote detailing his improvements after FNS should be of interest to taxpayers and insurance companies alike.

> Before the FNS treatments with Mary Lee Esty, I had migraines daily. I would end up in Kaisers' after-hours care at least twice a month for migraines so severe that they could be relieved only by a 100 mg shot of Demerol. Since the treatments, I am rarely in after-hours care at all. Migraines are far less frequent and less severe, I have been able to control them with little intervention by Kaiser.
>
> I highly recommend that Kaiser seriously consider using [this] for treatment for others like myself. I am back to work and attending technical computer classes. Neither would have been possible if not for the end of my migraines.

Thea

Thea (page 204) was injured when a speeding truck slammed into her car from behind. Her injuries were severe and problems continue, but so does healing.

After FNS neurofeedback and surgery for perilymph fistula, her function continues to improve. She is still hampered by visual distortions and reading problems, but can put on her own makeup, which, besides vision, requires fine motor control, and tactile sensitivity.

Extreme pre-treatment light sensitivity required her to wear dark glasses at all times. Now she never needs dark glasses indoors and outdoors only rarely. Noise is also less of a problem — only occasionally a restaurant will be too noisy. Although she is bothered by rapidly moving traffic, she no longer needs to hold on to a companion for balance; she is able to walk alone.

Executive and organizational skills have improved. Arithmetic is still a problem, but better. For the business she ran with her partner, she can now start and finish tasks that once would have been beyond her. For example, when 150 napkins had to be laundered then folded in a special way for a special event, she started and finished it all in one pass.

Sleep is still poor and weight is a problem — she needs to be checked for thyroid and pituitary function. She is beginning vision therapy, but because her insurance was cut off, she can no longer afford other treatments of any kind. However, she is no longer confined to the house as a refuge against light, sound, and sensory overload. Not only is she able to go walking downtown, she is willing and happy to do so. Despite the problems that remain, the terrible depression has vanished, her mood is upbeat, and friends and family observe that she is more and more coming back on-line.

David

After multiple concussions from IEDs and falls, David (page 160) was, in his own words, "aggressive, paranoid, angry, depressed, nihilistic, and suicidal." Things changed radically after neurofeedback. He writes:

One advantage that neurofeedback has over other treatments is the lack of effort. It was as simple as answering a few questions and a couple sensors on my head. Then I'd sit back, close my eyes and relax. In just a few minutes we were done.

Sometimes during the treatments, I could feel myself become noticeably more relaxed. Sometimes, my hands and feet would tingle, perhaps a sign of better blood flow. A few times after a treatment I felt noticeably "buzzed." This usually lasted only a few hours, but nearly every time, I left the clinic with a sense of well-being.

Suddenly I had no cravings for drugs or alcohol. Instead there was sudden concern about what I was putting in my body. After only a few visits, my anxiety subsided enough for me to be able to go out on my own to a shopping plaza to get coffee, shop for books, and eat at restaurants. I found myself in the coffee shop reading a book, my back to the door, something many veterans, with or without a diagnosis of PTSD, wouldn't or couldn't do.

I was also released from ASAP treatment early. My ASAP case manager was able to see my changes and felt I no longer needed treatment. I had lost the urge to drink to intoxication or to abuse drugs. Oddly, I became very sensitive to pain medication.

The schrapnel lodged in my knee can't be removed without risking more severe injury. For years, I was prescribed 28 5-mg Oxycodone pills a month for the pain. After FNS, I only needed one or two pills per month. In June 2011, I discontinued the prescription.

After completing FNS treatment with Dr. Esty, I had a real future, something to look forward to. I couldn't wait to get out and find a way to help others in situations similar to mine, but when I first presented my school plan to VA Vocational Rehabilitation, I was nearly laughed out of the office.

Because I had been diagnosed with PTSD, TBI, and Bipolar Disorder, and a host of other physical problems, they were unwilling to invest large amounts of money for academic training in someone who didn't look all that great on paper. I was restricted to community college and placed on probation for the first year, required to keep my GPA at 3.0 or higher. Over that first year, while taking chemistry and psychology courses, not only did I maintain a GPA of 3.8, I was also inducted into an academic honor society.

I went on to one of the top-ranked schools in my state. Later, I transferred to biochemistry at another university to be closer to my brother who has also been diagnosed with PTSD and TBI from Iraq. Academically, my biggest problem became deciding between medical school (psychiatry) or a doctoral program in biochemistry (with focus on drug mechanisms). Meanwhile, I'm in a stable loving marriage and have a beautiful daughter with whom I have a great relationship.

None of these things would have been possible with my aggressive and abrasive disposition before treatment. Neurofeedback not only improved my quality of life, it also gave me the chance to help others like me.

I'm not saying these things to brag, but because there are others out there, suffering from the physical and emotional trauma of their war experiences. I see my little brother going through the same things I went through. I have lost friends to suicide and drug addiction years after they returned from war. It hurts seeing them and it hurts knowing that we have a solution that's being severely underused. I firmly believe that if this treatment had been available, friends would still be alive today and the lives of my brother and many others would be dramatically improved.

I know this system can help others because it helped me. It more than helped me, it gave me a life that I could never have dreamed of while I was at Walter Reed. In the combined throes of PTSD, depression, and TBI, it's hard to see the light, hard to believe that anything will ever get better. Now I know that it does. Everything isn't perfect. Life still has its ups and downs, but now I can deal. Things that seemed so cataclysmic while I was caught in the web of PTSD and TBI have become the small things they should be. My hair-trigger temper and anger are gone, replaced by love and appreciation for life and just how precious it is.

I want others who are caught in pain, fear, depression and anger to have the same opportunity that I had to be cut free of the horrors they've experienced, to be able to view those experiences as just *experiences* instead of being haunted and tormented by them. I want them to have their lives back. I want them to be given back their futures and allow them the chance to appreciate the present.

I was given these gifts by the neurofeedback treatments performed by Dr. Mary Lee Esty. It is my hope that more will be able to benefit from this miraculous system.

———

Today, David works in a medical laboratory and is deeply involved in his studies. He has applied for Ph.D. candidacy" because," he says, "*now I know how to treat TBI and PTSD.*"

From the viewpoint of a wounded veteran, this is a striking story. But consider the same story of brain injury followed by drug abuse, assault, escalating crime, rage and despair from a civilian point of view[1].

Brain injury is now known to be extremely high among juvenile offenders and their adult counterparts in prison system. A growing movement is underway to actually test for TBI on intake, to treat and hopefully to heal what is broken, to rescue these lost ones, to save lives and families.

---

1. See page 24, "Concussion and Crime".

Carol

"How will you know you are better?" she asked.
"When I finish my book," I said.

I had the usual childhood falls, perhaps with a few extras. A fall backwards off a swing, onto concrete. A fall headfirst off a top bunkbed. Learning to bike and roller skate in a hilly neighborhood. My favorite toy was the stairwell. Running up and down, two and three stairs at a time, was my favorite game. Sometimes I lost.

As an adult, I collected more dings while skiing, caving and climbing. Soccer alone was responsible for multiple concussions, but a worse injury occurred at a dance.

It was the Halloween contra dance, the hall was packed, and the lines too close for safety. In the midst of a high-speed swing with my partner, the elbow of a very large man in the next line (who was rotating in the opposite direction) slammed into my left temple. The force of the blow threw me several yards onto my back and the back of my head. The headache lasted for days, merging into weeks, but as a life-long migraineur, I was used to that.

What I didn't understand was the fatigue and confusion, why it was so hard to get things done, or why I was suddenly "accident prone." In February, at Snowmass, where I used to ski the double black trails, I couldn't understand why I was falling on the beginner slopes. Skiing above the 10,000 foot boundary brought on mountain sickness and sleepiness. Meanwhile, pressure changes from flying became hideously painful; the last two times I flew, I was carried off the plane, barely conscious. I also noticed a difficulty learning new things which astonished me. Now I am astonished that I failed to connect these symptoms to a concussion only a few months earlier.

The final blow was in 1996, when I stepped off an icy curb and went airborne. When I came crashing down, my head hit the concrete curb. The result was basal skull fracture and the end of my life as I knew it.

Soon, the most basic skills were too difficult, too exhausting. Headaches that had plagued me all my life were worse than ever before, relentless waves of pain that came every three to five seconds; no one knew why. At the time of the accident, I had been doing doing software validation and programming distributed databases for the FAA. Now I couldn't even remember how to start the program and was unable to stay awake for more than three hours at a time. I lost my job and income. Eventually, I also lost my husband. It was years before I realized that I had lost him long ago to his own concussion, undiagnosed and untreated, from a bad bike accident on the day we were married.

Strangely, I could still write, so I wrote. I plodded through two book manuscripts, a few hours, a few minutes at a time. But reading was painful and difficult, cooking or organizing a meal or a shopping list almost impossible, and everything hurt, all the time.

After years in head injury hell, I stumbled across something called neurofeedback. I learned that Dr. Mary Lee Esty had treated injuries far worse than mine, but it was seven years after that last fall, long after I had done everything I was supposed to have done (to little or no avail), *far after improvement was no longer believed possible.*

But suddenly things got better. Suddenly I could stay awake for 5 or 6 hours, then 8, then 16, and when I awoke, I could remember my dreams. Suddenly I could shop for groceries, remember to put them away and even do something with them beyond standing in front of the refrigerator with a fork. I could recognize the can opener. And rather than eating all meals out on overloaded credit cards, I could remember how to cook, I could manage the steps to make an omelette, then a real meal. Losing the devastating fog, confusion, and the crippling ADD was miracle enough, but the real surprise was that life-long migraines began to disappear. So did some once-violent food sensitivities and other triggers[1].

Before treatment, my sure-fire migraine triggers included the classics: red wine, all the good cheeses, onions, weather and pressure changes. Bright light or glare was so deadly that I never went out without wrap-around dark glasses.

After treatment, these sensitivities began to disappear. I could drink red wine with my friends and enjoy the most ferociously aged cheeses. The change in light sensitivity was especially striking. Today, I will wear a hat in hot, sunny weather, but no longer own even a single pair of dark glasses. I no longer need them. On the other hand, changes in weather and barometric pressure could still trigger migraines, but the pain was *nothing* compared to what it had been.

In retrospect, it is astonishing that neurofeedback worked as well as it did. Apparently the last fall in the ice storm was just the final blow to the system. A year or two after Dr. Esty's FNS treatments, a cranial therapist commented on my oddly skewed head. Correcting those cranial distortions eliminated my extreme sensitivity to pressure changes. Overnight, I was no longer "Barometer Girl," at the mercy of changes in the weather. This seems to have been the final missing piece. Only a chronic migraineur can really appreciate the amazement of awakening to find two feet of snow on the ground with no previous warning.

When I started neurofeedback treatment with Dr. Esty, the manuscript I was trying to complete, the finished book that would show that I was better was *Surviving Martial Arts.*

---

1. I now think of these migraine triggers more as autonomic symptoms, dysautonomia, that has now resolved. They are usually attributed to genetics, but have the same genes and my eyes (which no longer need dark glasses) are still are blue as they ever were.

By necessity it included a section on concussion, but I never knew there were ways to heal a broken brain (or chronic migraine). Not really. Surely that information should be included! And so I went off to experiment on my brain.

It has been a long and twisty road from turning in circles trying to remember how to microwave a potato. Experiencing such amazing improvements made it impossible to *not* want to know more. On observing Dr. Esty and her clients, on training in this field, I have seen injuries that were painfully familiar and difficulties I had never imagined. I have seen adults and children get their lives back, sometimes reaching levels of function better than *before* their injuries (or as is often the case, before their last, most recently recognized injuries).

But I have never finished that book, at least not yet.

Meanwhile, perhaps this one will do.

Back when I was clearly suffering symptoms of hypergraphia, compulsively writing 500-page manuscripts and sending 5,000 word e-mails to my long-suffering friends, I remember defining a Real Writer as "Someone who couldn't *not* write." I still love the research, the discovery, the process and craft of writing, but I no longer leap out of bed at 3 a.m. to capture a phrase.

Nevertheless, it has been my very great pleasure to write down these stories, to have had the wonderful opportunity to tell just a few of the things that I have seen and learned and experienced.

It is my fervent hope that these case histories and stories will help to explain the many faces of concussion, why neurofeedback and other biofeedback therapies may be helpful, and to make the same possibility of help and healing available to others.

—Carol (C. M.) Shifflett

Glossary

ADHESIONS. Fibrous tissue that forms abnormal connections between tissues, often as a result of injury.

ADRENALS. Endocrine glands located atop the kidneys (Latin "*ad-*, towards the kidneys, *ren*"). Produce the stress hormone, cortisol. Work with hypothalamus and pituitary. See HPA axis.

AUTONOMIC NERVOUS SYSTEM (ANS). Also known as the involuntary nervous system. Affects heart rate, digestion, respiration, salivation, perspiration, pupil dilation / constriction, urination, and sexual arousal. Classically divided into two subsystems: sympathetic and parasympathetic and long believed to be outside of conscious control. Arises from the lower brainstem, controlled by the hypothalamus.

BLOOD-BRAIN BARRIER (BBB). A layer of tightly packed cells that separates circulating blood from the brain fluid. It is weak or lacking in some organs of the brain including the hypothalamus and pituitary and the *area postrema* (known as the "vomit center" due to its extreme sensitivity to toxins).

BMI (BODY MASS INDEX). The relationship between mass and height. BMI = kilograms divided by height in meters squared or, pounds divided by height in inches squared multiplied by 703. Waist-to-height ratio is simpler and more accurate (Ashwell M and Others, 2012). Measure waist one inch above belly button; divide by height. Calculator at: www.health-calc.com/body-composition/waist-to-height-ratio.

CRANIAL NERVES. The 12 pairs of nerves arising from within the brain. These enable sense of smell and taste (CN I), vision (CN II, CN III, CN IV, and CN VI), hearing (CN VIII), functions of the tongue and swallowing (CN IX and CN XII), and the jaw (CN V).

Three of these are strongly linked to headaches. The trigeminal nerves(CN V) control chewing, supply dura and sinuses, constrict and dilate blood vessels in the brain. The accessory nerve (CN XI) receives postural input from the neck. The facial nerve (CN VII) controls muscles of expression.

CEREBRAL SPINAL FLUID (CFS). A clear fluid that circulates through brain and spinal cord.

CHRONIC TRAUMATIC ENCEPHALOPATHY (CTE). Neurological deterioration of the brain as a result of traumatic brain injury. Currently, CTE can be positively diagnosed only on autopsy with samples of brain tissue, but seen in brains that have suffered traumatic injury from abuse, sports, or blasts.

DURA MATER ("TOUGH MOTHER"). The outermost (and pain-sensitive) layer of the three-part membrane (*meninges*) surrounding the brain. The *dural bridge* connects the suboccipital muscles and fascia of the neck with the dura of the brain.

ENDOCRINE GLANDS. Includes pituitary, thyroid, adrenals, gonads (ovaries in women / testes in men), and pancreas. These secrete hormones directly into the bloodstream.

HPA AXIS. The combination of hypothalamus, pituitary gland, and adrenal glands working together.

HYPOTHALAMUS. The major control system of the brain and autonomic nervous system. Links nervous system to endocrine system via the pituitary gland. Synthesizes and secretes hormones that stimulate or inhibit secretion of pituitary hormones. Different areas control temperature, hunger and thirst, fatigue and sleep, circadian rhythms and attachment behaviors.

NEURONS. Nerve cells. These transmit messages through electrical and chemical signals. Parts include *axon* (central stalk) and *dendrites*, the "tree"-like branches. Each neuron has many connections; damage to one neuron may damage thousands more. The drawing at left (by Santiago Ramón y Cajal, 1899) shows the delicate spiderweb network of neural connections to the cortex of a human infant.

PERILYMPH FISTULA. A break in the vestibular region of ear, allowing fluid to enter the middle ear from the inner ear. May cause hearing loss, vertigo, and visual problems.

SURFACE OR SURFICIAL ELECTROMYOGRAPHY (SEMG). A test of electrical activity of muscles, but done painlessly with sensors on the skin rather than with needles inserted into muscle.

SYNDROME (GR. *syn-*, TOGETHER + *dromos*, RUNNING). A group of symptoms appearing together.

TSH. Thyroid Stimulating Hormone, released by the pituitary, is a request to the thyroid gland for more thyroid hormone. If the HPA axis is damaged, the pituitary may release low or no TSH. Thus a TSH test alone may result in a diagnosis of normal or even *hyper*-thyroidism even in the presence of blatant *hypo*-thyroid symptoms.

Resources and References

BOOKS, MATERIALS, EQUIPMENT, AND MEDICAL ORGANIZATIONS.HOW TO FIND IINDIVIDUAL PRACTITIONERS AND WHAT TO DO IN THE MEANTIME.

Books and Websites

- *A Symphony in the Brain*, by Jim Robbins (2008).

- *The Healing Power of Neurofeedback* (2006), and *The Neurofeedback Solution* (2012), both by Dr. Stephen Larsen of Stone Mountain Center in New Paltz, NY.

- *LENS: The Low Energy Neurofeedback System* (2007) by Dr. D. Corydon Hammond.

- Doonesbury Books. Gary Trudeau's trilogy collection on war injuries (*The Long Road Home*, *Signature Wound*, and *The War Within*) feature B.D., Toggle, and caretakers. Compassionate, insightful and proceeds benefit Fisher House which supports soldiers and their families.

- For a bibliography of research papers on biofeedback and neurofeedback see:

    www.isnr.org/neurofeedback-info/injury-stroke.cfm.

- Research studies used by the American Academy of Pediatrics to support bio- and neuro-feedback in AD(H)D (with links to articles):

    www.braintrainuk.com/wp-content/uploads/2013/07/How-AAP-reached-conclusion-other-recent-evidence-July-2013-V3.pdf

- For a gallery of brain connections, see **www.humanconnectomeproject.org/gallery/**

- For crash test information: see **www.Safercar.gov**.

Film and Video

- For an extremely accurate film depiction of TBI, see *The Lookout*.

- See **www.YouTube.com**, for presentations by many neurofeedback experts.

- TEDTalks. These excellent presentations are available at **www.ted.com**; some are on **www.Netflix.com**. Shawn Achor presents *The Happy Secret to Better Work*; Amy Cuddy reveals *The Emotional and Hormonal Impact of Posture*; Jane McGonigal describes her Super-Better game, and neurologist Jill Bolte Taylor explains her stroke of insight.

- *The Hornet's Nest*. Eye-witness in Afghanistan. See **www.thehornetsnestmovie.com**.

Information Databases

DRUG INTERACTIONS

Because the many symptoms of TBI are medicated individually, interactions with food and other drugs can occur. Track the possibilities at: **www.drugs.com/ drug_interactions.html**.

CLINICAL TRIALS

Information on trials of drugs and other treatments submitted to the FDA can be found by topic or by study name at: **www.clinicaltrials.gov**. You can, for example, follow the trials of progesterone used in TBI (Ma J and Others, 2012).

The Cochrane Collaboration is a non-governmental and not-for-profit organization that attempts to review medical research without bias or outside influence. It looks for high-quality trials, then runs statistical analyses of the results. Cochrane Reviews include a "plain language" summary, usable by non-medical people: **www.summaries.cochrane.org/**

PUBMED

PubMed is the free database of references and abstracts (currently some 23 million) on life sciences and medical topics. It is maintained by the U.S. National Library of Medicine (NLM) at the National Institutes of Health (NIH). Online: **www.PubMed.com**. To find a topic or specific articles, type a keyword, title, or PMID number into the search box.

Organizations

ASSOCIATION FOR APPLIED PSYCHOPHYSIOLOGY AND BIOFEEDBACK

The Association for Applied Psychophysiology and Biofeedback (AAPB) began in 1969 as the Biofeedback Research Society, promoting understanding of biofeedback, methods and practice. See **www.aapb.org**.

AMERICAN ASSOCIATION OF COLLEGES OF OSTEOPATHIC MEDICINE

The following website includes a list of Motion Animations to Demonstrate Musculoskeletal Functioning. Movements (greatly exaggerated for visibility), are small in real life, but when blocked or jammed by trauma, tight muscles or scar tissue, the result may be pain and increasing dysfunction. **www.aacom.org/people/councils/Pages/MotionAnimations.aspx**

- FLEXION AND EXTENSION OF THE SPHENOBASILAR SYNCHONDROSIS. Shows normal motion at the joining of the occiput and sphenoid bones of the skull.
- SACRAL MOTION THROUGH THE GAIT CYCLE. Shows shifting of pelvic bones in walking.

CENTER FOR THE STUDY OF TRAUMATIC ENCEPHALOPATHY

Created in 2008 as a collaborative venture between Boston University School of Medicine and Sports Legacy Institute (SLI) to study CTE, its symptoms, risk factors, and ways to prevent its progressive dementia. The CSTE is looking for all types of athletes and military personnel for its research studies. See **www.bu.edu/cste/**.

BRAIN INJURY GROUPS

There are many brain injury associations, by state and city. Let them help.

Brain Injury Association of America
#608 Spring Hill Rd, Suite 110
Vienna, VA 22182 (800) 444-6443
www.biausa.org

To find affiliates, go to www.biausa.org/state-affiliates.htm and click on your state.

I waited many years to actually attend one of these meetings. I assumed that most of the people there would have had much more serious injuries than mine. After all, I hadn't been in a coma and to me, that's what "Brain Injury" implied. Many people who knew me didn't even know that I had a brain injury. At my first meeting, people started sharing the symptoms they found most troublesome. As each person spoke I said to myself "I have this too!" After about the fourth speaker I thought "Maybe I *do* belong here!" -- Marie

MEDICAL SPECIALTIES

- VISION PROBLEMS. Not every eye doctor is trained to deal with or even recognize symptoms from TBI. Find those who are via: Optometric Extension Program Foundation, (949) 250-8070 / **www.oepf.org**. Their book, *Visual & Vestibular Consequences of Acquired Brain Injury* by Suchoff IB, Ciuffreda KJ, and Kapoor N (2001), is one of the most comprehensive available on the many symptoms (not just *visual*) of TBI.

- PERILYMPH FISTULA. The specialist best trained to treat vestibular injuries is a neuro-opthamologist or neurotologist. Find specialists in your area through the American Academy of Neurology: **www.aan.com.**

SPORTS LEGACY INSTITUTE

As Harvard graduate turned pro-wrestler, Chris Nowinski appeared as the character that fans love to hate. "I'm Chris Harvard," he would roar. "I'm smarter than you are!" When his wrestling career was ended by a kick to the head, he dove into research on TBI in an attempt to explain and heal his own injuries. In 2007, Nowinski and Dr. Robert Cantu co-founded the Sports Legacy Institute (SLI), to further education and research on TBI in sports and military. In 2008, SLI partnered with Boston University School of Medicine to form the Center for the Study of Traumatic Encephalopathy. It is work that is changing the face of American sports. He really *was* smarter. See: **www.sportslegacy.org.**

Biofeedback

PRACTITIONERS

Different practitioners have different training and background, use different systems and different protocols. Results will differ.

The most important quality is concern for the patient, but all health care practitioners should also have a thorough knowledge of symptoms, neuropsych disorders, and know when to refer out.

- Traditional biofeedback practitioners: certified through Biofeedback Certification International Alliance (BCIA), **www.BCIA.org**.

- The International Society for Neurofeedback and Research (ISNR) maintains a a database of research on biofeedback and neurofeedback at:

  www.isnr.org/resources/comprehensive-bibliography.cfm.

- For information on military / combat injuries including TBI and PTSD treated with biofeedback / neurofeedback, see **www. brainwellnessandbiofeedback.com**. Dr. Esty's practice in Bethesda, Maryland, offers biofeedback, neurofeedback, and muscle retraining via sEMG.

EQUIPMENT

Traditional stress thermometers are available from biofeedback suppliers and scientific catalogs. Biofeedback programs for non-professionals are increasingly available. New "games" such as *Wild Divine* track temperature, heart rate, and galvanic skin response as well as did older professional systems once costing tens of thousands of dollars. It may be of most interest to adults, but the Inner Tube 3 Space Game Add-on is very popular with children. See **www.wilddivine.com**.

See also EmWave and Inner Balance from **www.heartmath.org** and Stress Eraser from **www.stresseraser.com**.

Sensors for temperature, Galvanic Skin Response (GSR), and even sleep patterns are appearing as apps for iPhone and Android.

They are limited, but can be a starting point.

References Cited

Achor, Shawn (2011), The Happy Secret to Better Work. *TED Talks* (May). www.Ted.com.

Adams JH, Graham DI, Murray LS, Scott G (1982), Diffuse axonal injury due to nonmissile head injury in humans: an analysis of 45 cases. *Annals of Neurology*, Vol. 12, n. 6, pp. 557-563. PMID: 7159059.

Adler LA, Kunz M, Chua HC, Rotrosen J, Resnick SG (2004), Attention-deficit/hyperactivity disorder in adult patients with posttraumatic stress disorder (PTSD): Is ADHD a vulnerability factor? *J of Attention Disorders*, Vol. 8, n. 1, pp. 11-16. PMID: 15669598.

Aglioti S, Beltramello A, Girardi F, Fabbro F (1996), Neurolinguistic and follow-up study of an unusual pattern of recovery from bilingual subcortical aphasia. *Brain*, Vol. 119 (Pt 5):1551-1564.PMID: 8931579.

Aimaretti G and Ghigo E (2007), Should every patient with traumatic brain injury be referred to an endocrinologist? *Nature Clinical Practice Endocrinology and Metabolism,* Vol. 3, n. 4, pp. 318-319. PMID: 17377615.

Altman J, Das GD (1965), Autoradiographic and histological evidence of postnatal hippocampal neurogenesis in rats. *J of Comparative Neurology,* Vol. 124, n. 3, pp. 319-335. PMID: 5861717.

American Academy of Pediatrics (2010), *Evidence-Based Child and Adolescent Psychosocial Interventions.* Vol. 125, S128, Appendix S2. The current update (2013) is online at:

www.aap.org/en-us/advocacy-and-policy/aap-health-initiatives/Mental-Health/Documents/CRPsychosocial-interventions.pdf. Studies used by AAP (with links to articles): www.braintrainuk.com/wp-content/uploads/2013/07/How-AAP-reached-conclusion-other-recent-evidence-July-2013-V3.pdf

American Psychiatric Association (2000), *Diagnostic and Statistical Manual of Mental Disorders (*4th Ed.)

Anderson SW, Damasio H, Damasio AR (2005), A neural basis for collecting behaviour in humans. *Brain*, Vol. 128 (Jan), pp. 201-212. PMID:15548551. Includes full article.

Ashrafian H (2012), Henry VIII's obesity following traumatic brain injury. *Endocrine*, Vol. 42, n. 1, pp. 218-219.

Ashwell M, Gunn P, Gibson S (2012), Waist-to-height ratio is a better screening tool than waist circumference and BMI for adult cardiometabolic risk factors: systematic review and meta-analysis. *Obesity Reviews*, Vol. 13, n. 3 (Mar), pp. 275-286. PMID: 22106927.

Association of Boxing Commissions (ABC). See the complete rule set at www.abcboxing.com.

Auble BA, Bollepalli S, Makoroff K, Weis T, Khoury J, Colliers T, Rose SR (2013), Hypopituitarism in Pediatric Survivors of Inflicted Traumatic Brain Injury. *J of Neurotrauma.* 2013 Nov 23. PMID: 24028400.

Austen, Jake (2005), *TV-A-Go-Go: Rock on TV from American Bandstand to American Idol.* Chicago Review Press, 368 pp.

Baker AJ, Moulton RJ, MacMillan VH, Shedden PM (1993), Excitatory amino acids in cerebrospinal fluid following traumatic brain injury in humans. *J of Neurosurgery*, Vol. 79, n. 3, pp. 369-372. PMID: 8103092.

Baker RR, Mather JG, and Kennaugh JH (1983), Magnetic bones in human sinuses. *Nature* Vol. 301, n. 5895, pp. 78-80. PMID: 6823284. Online: www.nature.com/nature/journal/v301/n5895/abs/301078a0.html

Barker FG (1995), Phineas among the phrenologists: the American crowbar case and nineteenth-century theories of cerebral localization. *J of Neurosurgery,* Vol. 82, n. 4, pp. 672-682. PMID: 7897537.

Barlett, Donald L & Steele, James B (1979), *Howard Hughes: His Life and Madness.* W. W. Norton & Co., 688 pp.

Barlow, John (1960), Rhythmic activity induced by photic stimulation in relation to intrinsic alpha activity of the brain in man. *Electroencephalography and Clinical Neurophysiology*, Vol. 12, pp. 317-326.

Bartsch A, Benzel E, Miele V, Prakash V (2012), Impact test comparisons of 20th and 21st century American football helmets. *J Neurosurgery*, Vol. 116, n. 1, pp. 222-233. PMID 22054210

Bazarian JJ, Blyth BJ, He H, Mookerjee S, Jones C, Kiechle K, Moynihan R, Wojcik SM, Grant WD, Secreti LM, Triner W, Moscati R, Leinhart A, Ellis GL, Khan J (2013), Classification accuracy of serum Apo A-I and S100B for the diagnosis of mild traumatic brain injury and prediction of abnormal initial head computed tomography scan. *J Neurotrauma*, Vol. 30, n. 20, pp. 1747-1754. PMID: 23758329.

Beauregard M and Lévesque J (2006), Functional magnetic resonance imaging investigation of the effects of neurofeedback training on the neural bases of selective attention and response inhibition in children with attention-deficit/hyperactivity disorder. *Applied Psychophysiology and Biofeedback.* Vol. 31, n. 1, pp. 3-20. PMID: 16552626.

Becker, Robert O (1998), *The Body Electric:Electromagnetism and the Foundation of Life.* William Morrow, 368 pp.

Beidler, Anne E (2009), *The Addiction of Mary Todd Lincoln.* Coffee Town Press, 180 pp.

Berger, Hans (1929) Über das Elektrenkephalogramm des Menchen. *Archives für Psychiatrie*, Vol. 87, pp. 527-570. [On the Electroencephalogram of Man]. PMID 4188918.

Bigler ED (2012), Symptom Validity Testing, Effort, and Neuropsychological Assessment. *J of the International Neuropsychological Society,* Vol.18, no. 4, pp. 632-640. PMID: 2305708.

__ (2009), Neuroimaging Methods that Define Structural and Functional Pathology in Traumatic Brain Injury. *North American Brain Injury Society*, Austin, TX.

Bishop, Gregg and Davis, Ray (2012) Junior Seau, Famed N.F.L. Linebacker, Dies at 43; Suicide Is Suspected. *The New York Times,* Sports, May 12, p. B1.

Blanchard, Ken and Brill, Marietta A (2004), *What Your Doctor May Not Tell You About Hypothyroidism: A Simple Plan for Extraordinary Results.* Wellness Central, 252 pp.

Blaylock RL (2013), Immunoexcitatory mechanisms in glioma proliferation, invasion and occasional metastasis. *Surgical Neurology International,* doi: 10.4103/2152-7806.106577. Epub 2013 Jan 29. PMID: 23493580.

__ (1996), *Excitotoxins: The Taste That Kills.* Health Press, 320 pp.

Blum, Deborah (2011), *The Poisoner's Handbook: Murder and the Birth of Forensic Medicine in Jazz Age New York.* Penguin Books, 336 pp.

Branch, Eric (2011), Forrest Blue dies after years of dementia. *San Francisco Chronicle*, Wednesday, July 20.

Branch, John (2011), Derek Boogaard: A Brain 'Going Bad'. *The New York Times*, Dec. 5, Sports.

Broglio SP, Eckner JT, Martini D, Sosnoff JJ, Kutcher JS, Randolf C (2011). Cumulative head impact burden in high school football. *J of Neurotrauma*, Vol. 28, n. 10, pp. 2069-2078. PMID: 21787201.

__, Ferrara MS, Macciocchi SN, Baumgartner TA, and Elliott R (2007), Test-Retest Reliability of Computerized Concussion Assessment Programs. *Athletic Trainer, Vol.* 42, n. 4: pp. 509–514, PMCID: 2140077.

Brown, Christopher R and Shankland, Wesley (2000), *Anatomy of Soft-Tissue Injuries.* TMData Resources, LLC, Albuquerque, NM.

Brown, Mark (2009), A life in armour: How Henry VIII grew from L to XXXL. *The Guardian*, 31 March 2009.

Brown NJ, Mannix RC, O'Brien MJ, Gostine D, Collins MW, Meehan WP 3rd (2014), Effect of Cognitive Activity Level on Duration of Post-Concussion Symptoms. *Pediatrics*, Jan 6. [Epub ahead of print]. PMID: 24394679.

Brown, Peter H and Broeske, Pat H (1996), *Howard Hughes: The Untold Story*, 482 pp.

Brown WA and Meszaros Z (2007), Hoarding. *Psychiatric Times,* Vol. 24, n. 13.

Buchanan, Christopher (2010), *In Search of the Lost Platoon.* www.pbs.org/wgbh/pages/frontline/woundedplatoon/journey/

Cantu RC (2012) Preventing Sports Concussions Among Children. *The New York Times* (Oct. 6). www.nytimes.com/2012/10/07/sports/concussion-prevention-for-child-athletes-robert-c-cantu.html

Carlsson A, Svennerholm L, Winblad B (1980), Seasonal and circadian monoamine variations in human brains examined post mortem. *Acta Psychiatrica Scandinavica. Suppl*ementum 280, pp. 75-85. PMID: 6157305.

Carroll, Linda and Rosner, David (2011), *The Concussion Crisis: Anatomy of a Silent Epidemic.* Simon & Schuster, 320 pp.

Carter JL and Russell HL (1993), A pilot investigation of auditory and visual entrainment of brainwave activity in learning disabled boys. *Texas Researcher: J of the Texas Center for Educational Research*, Vol. 4, pp. 65-73.

Cavendish, George (1524), *1524, King Henry VIII Has a Jousting Accident.* An eye-witness account at: www.Englishhistory.net/tudor/h8joust.html. Accessed: Jan 3, 2012.

Chen Y, Huang W, Constantini S (2013), Concepts and strategies for clinical management of blast-induced traumatic brain injury and posttraumatic stress disorder. *J of Neuropsychiatry and Clinical Neurosciences,* Vol. 25, n. 2 (Spring), pp. 103-110. PMID: 23686026.

Chrisafis, Angelique (2001), Rise in domestic mishaps puts strain on NHS: Accident survey shows home is hazardous place. *The Guardian*, 6 June. http://www.theguardian.com/uk/2001/jun/07/angeliquechrisafis1

Clegg, Brian (2007), *The Man Who Stopped Time:* The Joseph Henry Press, 266 pp.

Cloud, John (2012), Nightmare Scenario. *Time Magazine*, July 09. On nightmares as a symptom of sleep apnea.
http://www.time.com/time/magazine/article/0,9171,2118290-1,00.html

Cobb BR, Urban JE, Davenport EM, Rowson S, Duma SM, Maldjian JA, Whitlow CT, Powers AK, Stitzel JD (2013), Head Impact Exposure in Youth Football: Elementary School Ages 9–12 Years and the Effect of Practice Structure. *Annals of Biomedical Engineering*, Jul 24. PMID: 23881111.

Colten HR and Altevogt BM, Eds. (2006), *Sleep Disorders and Sleep Deprivation: An Unmet Public Health Problem. National Academies Press*, 424 pp.

Conboy, Sean (2012), Death by 1000 cuts: New research suggests that, despite safety claims from helmet manufacturers, athletes' brains may be stark naked. *Pittsburghmagazine.com.*

Corra S, Girardi P, de Giorgi F, Braggion M (2012), Severe and polytraumatic injuries among recreational skiers and snowboarders: incidence, demographics and injury patterns in *South Tyrol. European J of Emergency Medicine* , Vol. 19, n. 2, pp. 69-72. PMID: 21673576.

Cotsonika, Nicholas J (2012) NHL players to participate in ambitious concussion research project: *Yahoo Sports*, April 5, http://sports.yahoo.com/news/nhl-players-participate-ambitious-concussion-210500736--nhl.html.

Culverhouse, Gay (2012), *Throwaway Players: The Concussion Crisis From PeeWee Football to the NFL.* Behler Publications, 152 pp.

Dagi TF, Meyer FB, and Poletti CA (1983). The incidence and prevention of meningitis after basilar skull fracture. *American J of Emergency Medicine,* Vol. 1, n. 3, pp. 295-298. PMID: 6680635.

Dahlberg, Tim (2004), Bowe sees bright future in comeback, others fear brain damage or worse. Associated Press, 09-25-2004. http://www.boxingscene.com/forums/archive/index.php/t-290.html.

Damasio H, Grabowski T, Frank R, Galaburda AM, Damasio AR (1994), The return of Phineas Gage: clues about the brain from the skull of a famous patient. *Science,* Vol. 264, n. 5162, pp. 1102-1105. PMID: 8178168.

Damoiseaux JS, Seeley WW, Zhou J, Shirer WR, Coppola G, Karydas A, Rosen HJ, Miller BL, Kramer JH, Greicius MD (2012), Gender modulates the APOE4 effect in healthy older adults: Convergent evidence from functional brain connectivity and spinal fluid tau levels. *J of Neuroscience,* Vol. 32, n. 24, pp. 8254–8262. PMID: 22699906.

Daniel RW, Rowson S and Duma SM (2012) Head Impact Exposure in Youth Football. *Annals of Biomedical Engineering,* Vol. 40, n. 4 (April), pp. 976–981. PMCID: 3310979.

Davies EC, Henderson S, Balcer LJ, Galetta SL (2012b). Residency Training: The King-Devick test and sleep deprivation: Study in pre- and post-call neurology residents. *Neurology, Vol.* 78, n. 17. PMID 22529208.

Davies RC, Williams WH, Hinder D, Burgess CN, Mounce LT (2012), Self-Reported Traumatic Brain Injury and Postconcussion Symptoms in Incarcerated Youth. *J of Head Trauma Rehabilitation.* Vol. 27, n. 3, p. E21–E27. PMID: 22573045. See also the excellent Scientific American article by Katherine Harmon at:

http://www.scientificamerican.com/article.cfm?id=traumatic-brain-injury-prison

DCoE Clinical Recommendation (August 2012), Indications and Conditions for Neuroendocrine Dysfunction Screening Post Mild Traumatic Brain Injury. Defense Centers of Excellence for Psychological Health and Traumatic Brain Injury, 2345 Crystal Drive, Suite 120, Arlington, VA 22202. Online:

http://www.dcoe.health.mil/Content/Navigation/Documents/DCoE_TBI_NED_Clinical_Recommendations.pdf

deCharms RC, Maeda F, Glover GH, Ludlow D, Pauly JM, Soneji D, Gabrieli JDE, and Mackey SC (2005), Control over brain activation and pain learned by using real-time functional MRI. *Proc National Academy of Sciences,* Vol. 102, n. 51 (Dec. 20), 18626–18631. PMID: 16352728. Online: www.pnas.org/content/102/51/18626

Dematteo CA, Hanna SE, Mahoney WJ, Hollenberg RD, Scott LA, Law MC, Newman A, Lin CY, Xu L (2010), My child doesn't have a brain injury, he only has a concussion. *Pediatrics.* Vol. 125, n. 2, pp. 327-334. PMID: 20083526. Includes full article.

Demirtas-Tatlidede A, Vahabzadeh-Hagh AM, Bernabeu M, Tormos JM, Pascual-Leone A (2012), Noninvasive Brain Stimulation in Traumatic Brain Injury. *J of of Head Trauma Rehabilitaton,* Vol. 27, n. 4 , pp. 274-292. PMID: 21691215.

Diamond, Jared (2013), That Daily Shower Can Be a Killer. *The New York Times,* Jan. 13, Science.

Downs, Martin F (2006), To Sleep, Perchance to . . . Walk: Reports Raise Questions About Sleeping Pill Side Effect. Is Ambien Sleepwalking Understated? *The Washington Post,* March 14 (Tuesday), Health, p. 1.

Doyle, Sir Arthur Conan (1896), *Rodney Stone.* Interweaves a coming-of-age and mystery story with that of boxing, featuring famous bare-knuckle fighters whose names appear in Georgette Heyer's Regency novels. There is also a vignette of Lord Nelson and Lady Hamilton, whose relationship began after Nelson's war injuries, baffling and scandalizing England. Online: www.online-literature.com/doyle/rodney-stone.

Duff J (2004), The usefulness of quantitative EEG (QEEG) and neurotherapy in the assessment and treatment of post-concussion syndrome. *Clinical EEG and Neuroscience,* Vol. 35, n. 4, pp. 198-209. PMID: 15493535.

Duffy FH (2000), The state of EEG biofeedback therapy (EEG operant conditioning) in 2000: An editor's opinion. *Clinical Electroencephalography,* Vol. 31, n. 1, p. v-vii. PMID: 10638345.

Dwyer CA (1996), Cut scores and testing: statistics, judgment, truth, and error. *Psychological Assessment,* Vol. 8, n. 4, pp. 360-362.

Eckner JT, Kutcher JS, Broglio SP and Richardson JK (2013), Effect of sport-related concussion on clinically measured simple reaction time. *British J of Sports Medicine,* Jan 11. See also Eckner JT (2010). PMID: 23314889.

__, Kutcher JS, Richardson JK (2010), Pilot evaluation of a novel clinical test of reaction time in national collegiate athletic association division I football players. *J of Athletic Training,* Vol. 45, n. 4, pp. 327-32. PMID: 20617905.

Emerson, Jason (2007), *The Madness of Mary Lincoln.* Southern Illinois University Press, 256 pp.

Emori RI and Horiguchi J (1990). Whiplash in low speed vehicle collisions. SAE Technical Paper 900542., pp. 103-108.

Erichsen JE (1867). *On Railway and Other Injuries of the Nervous System.* Henry C. Lea, 103 pp.

The first full-length study on Railway Spine, the 19th-century diagnosis for whiplash in railroad accidents. As today, companies dismissed the injuries as imaginary. Also of interest are his records on treating brain and CNS dysfunction with mercury. His quote of Robert Liston (page 81) is the likely source of a similar quote commonly attributed to Hippocrates, who said no such thing. Online www.ncbi.nlm.nih.gov/pmc/articles/PMC2310448/.

Eriksson PS, Perfilieva E, Björk-Eriksson T, Alborn AM, Nordborg C, Peterson DA, Gage FH (1998), Neurogenesis in the adult human hippocampus. *Nature Medicine*, Vol. 4, n. 11, 1313-7. PMID: 9809557.

Expósito-Tirado JA, Forastero Fernández Salguero P, Cruz Reina MC, Del Pino-Algarrada R, Fernandez-Luque A, Olmo-Vega JA, Rodríguez-Burgos MC.[Complications arising from traumatic brain injuries in a hospital rehabilitation unit: a series of 126 cases] (2003), [Article in Spanish], *Revista de Neurologia*, Vol. 36, n. 12, pp. 1126-1132. PMID: 12833229.

Fainaru-Wada, Mark and Fainaru, Steve (2013), *League of Denial: The NFL, Concussions, and the Battle for Truth*. Crown Archetype, 416 pp. See clips from the film at www.PBS.com.

Fairclough SH, Graham R (1999), Impairment of driving performance caused by sleep deprivation or alcohol: a comparative study. *Human Factors*. Vol. 41, n. 1, pp. 118-128. PMID: 10354808.

Farnham, Alan (2012), Female Crash Dummies Injured More: What Car Should Women Buy? *ABC News / Good Morning America,* March 29, 2012. Video at:

http://abcnews.go.com/Business/female-crash-dummies-injured/story?id=16004267

Fee GA (1968), Traumatic perilymph fistulas. *Archives of Otolaryngology, Vol.* 88, n. 5, pp. 477-480.

Fields, R Douglas (2009), *The Other Brain.*Simon & Schuster, 371 pp.

Flaherty, Alice W (2004), *The Midnight Disease: The Drive to Write, Writer's Block, and the Creative Brain.* Houghton Mifflin Company, 308 pp.

Fleming, Mike (2012), CBS Rejects 'Three Stooges' Drug Spoof Ad On NCAA Hoops Championship Broadcast. (April 2). http://www.deadline.com/2012/04/three-stooges-drug-spoof-ad-cbs-rejects-ncaa-hoops-championship-broadcast.

Florida Museum of Natural History (2003), Annual Risk of Death During One's Lifetime. Online: www.flmnh.ufl.edu/fish/sharks/attacks/relarisklifetime.html. Accessed Dec. 2013.

Foa EB, Cashman L, Jaycox L, Perry K (1997), The validation of a self-report measure of posttraumatic stress disorder: The Posttraumatic Diagnostic Scale. *Psychological Assessment*, Vol 9, n. 4, pp. 445-451.

Fodor JA (1983), *The Modularity of Mind*. MIT Press, p.14, 23, 131.

Freeman John (2003), *The Changing World of Brain Injury.* Presentation at the Brain Injury Association of Maryland, 14th Annual Education Conference, March, 2003.

Frost, Randy O and Steketee, Gail (2010), *Hoarding and the Meaning of Things*: Houghton Mifflin Harcourt, 290 pp.

Fukuda O, Takaba M, Saito T, Endo S (1999) Head injuries in snowboarders compared with head injuries in skiers: A prospective analysis of 1076 patients from 1994 to 1999 in Niigata, Japan. *American J of Sports Medicine,* Vol. 29, n. 4, 437-440. PMID: 11476382.

Gainer R (2011), Sleep Disturbance and TBI. Neurologic Rehabilitation Institute. Onlinet: http://www.traumaticbraininjury.net/sleep-disturbances-and-tbi. Accessed Feb. 10, 2013.

Galetta KM, Barrett J, Allen M, Madda F, Delicata D, Tennant AT, Branas CC, Maguire MG, Messner LV, Devick S, Galetta SL, Balcer LJ (2011a), The King-Devick test as a determinant of head trauma and concussion in boxers and MMA fighters. *Neurology, Vol.* 76, n. 17, pp. 1456-62. PMID: 21288984

__, Brandes LE, Maki K, Dziemianowicz MS, Laudano E, Allen M, Lawler K, Sennett B, Wiebe D, Devick S, Messner LV, Galetta SL, Balcer LJ (2011b), The King-Devick test and sports-related concussion: study of a rapid visual screening tool in a collegiate cohort. *J of Neurological Sci*ence, Vol. 15, n. 309, pp. 34-39. PMID: 21849171.

Gania C, Birbaumera N, Strehla U (2008), Long term effects after feedback of slow cortical potentials and of theta-beta-amplitudes in children with attention-deficit/hyperactivity disorder (ADHD). *International J of Bioelectromagnetism*, Vol. 10, n. 4, pp. 209-232. www.ijbem.org.

Ganong CA and Kappy MS (1993) Cerebral salt wasting in children. The need for recognition and treatment. *American J of Diseases in Children*, Vol. 147, n. 2, pp. 167-169. PMID: 8427239.

Garber, Gregg (2005), A Tormented Soul. *ESPN.com,* Jan 24. A superb five-part series on Webster and the NFL. http://sports.espn.go.com/nfl/news/story?id=1972285.

García-Caballero A, García-Lado I, González-Hermida J, Area R, Recimil MJ, Juncos Rabadán O, Lamas S, Ozaita G, Jorge FJ (2007), Paradoxical recovery in a bilingual patient with aphasia after right capsuloputaminal infarction. *J of Neurology, Neurosurgery, and Psychiatry,* Vol. 78, n. 1, pp. 89-91. PMID: 17172568.

Gardner, Ava (1992), *Ava: My Story.* Bantam Books, 356 pp.

Garnick D (2009), 24-Hour Diary of a Pregnant Guy. Darren Garnick's Culture Schlock (Jan 24).

www.darrengarnick.wordpress.com/2009/01/24/bellydiary-1/

Gennarelli TA and Graham DI (1998), Neuropathology of the Head Injuries. *Seminars in Clinical Neuropsychiatry.* Vol 3, n. 3, pp. 160-175. PMID: 10085204.

Gevensleben H, Holl B, Albrecht B, Vogel C, Schlamp D, Kratz O, Studer P, Rothenberger A, Moll GH, Heinrich H (2009), Is neurofeedback an efficacious treatment for ADHD? A randomised controlled clinical trial. *J of Child Psychiatry and Psychology and Allied Disciplines,* Vol. 50, n. 7, pp. 780-789. PMID: 19207632.

Giacino JT, Whyte J, Bagiella E, Kalmar K, Childs N, Khademi A, Eifert B, Long D, Katz DI, Cho S, Yablon SA, Luther M, Hammond FM, Nordenbo A, Novak P, Mercer W, Maurer-Karattup P, Sherer M. (2012), Placebo-controlled trial of amantadine for severe traumatic brain injury. *New England J of Medicine,* Vol. 366, n. 9, pp. 819-826. PMID: 22375973.

Gilmore G (1956), *The Toledo Blade,* Nov. 5.

Goldstein LE, Fisher AM, Tagge CA and Others (2012), Chronic Traumatic Encephalopathy in Blast-Exposed Military Veterans and a Blast Neurotrauma Mouse Model . Science Translational Medicine, Vol. 4, n. 134, 16 pp. PMCID: PMC3739428. Full article online with superb color pictures per glial damage, immune response.

Goodwin, Doris Kearns (2005), *Team of Rivals.* Simon & Schuster, NY, 944 pp.

Gorman, Michael (2013), Reebok and mc10 team up to build CheckLight, a head impact indicator. Posted Jan 11.

Gould E (2007), How widespread is adult neurogenesis in mammals? *Nature Reviews, Neuroscience,* Vol. 8, pp. 481-488. PMID: 17514200.

__, Farris TW, Butcher LL (1989), Basal forebrain neurons undergo somatal and dendritic remodeling during postnatal development: a single-section Golgi and choline acetyltransferase analysis. *Brain Research / Developmental Brain Research,* Vol. 46, n. 2, pp. 297-302. PMID: 2470531.

Granacher, RA (2007), *Traumatic Brain Injury: Methods for Clinical & Forensic Neuropsychiatric Assessment,* (2nd Ed.), CRC Press, 584 pp.

Gregg C, Shikar V, Larsen P, Mak G, Chojnacki A, Yong VW, Weiss S (2007), White matter plasticity and enhanced remyelination in the maternal CNS. *J of Neuroscience,* Vol. 27, n. 8, pp. 1812-1823, PMID: 17314279.

Greve MW, Young DJ, Goss AL, Degutis LC (2009), Skiing and snowboarding head injuries in 2 areas of the United States. *Wilderness Environmental Medicine,* Vol. 20, n. 3, pp. 234-238. PMID: 19737041.

Grimm RJ, Hemenway WG, Lebray PR, Black FO (1989), The perilymph fistula syndrome defined in mild head trauma. *Acta Otolaryngologica,* Supplement 464, pp. 1-40. PMID: 2801093.

Gunderson CH, Dunne PB, Feyer TL (1973), Sleep deprivation seizures. *Neurology,* Vol. 23, n. 7, 678-86.

Guralnick, Peter (1999), *Careless Love: The Unmaking of Elvis Presley.* Back Bay Books, 768 pp.

Gursoy-Ozdemir Y, Qiu J, Matsuoka N, Bolay H, Bermpohl D, Jin H, Wang X, Rosenberg GA, Lo EH, Moskowitz MA (2004), Cortical spreading depression activates and upregulates MMP-9. *J of Clinical Investigations,* Vol. 113, n. 10, pp. 1447-1455. PMID: 15146242.

Hack GD, Hallgren RC (2004), Chronic headache relief after section of suboccipital muscle dural connections: a case report. *Headache,* Vol. 44, n. 1, pp. 84-89. PMID: 14979889.

__, Koritzer RT, Robinson WL, Hallgren RC, Greenman PE (1995), Anatomic relation between the rectus capitis posterior minor muscle and the dura mater. *Spine,* Vol. 20, n. 23, pp. 2484-2486. PMID: 8610241.

Hack, Richard (2001), *Hughes: The Private Diaries, Memos and Letters.* New Millennium Press, 444 pages.

Halbower AC, Janusz J, Brown M, Strain J, Friedman N, Accurso F, Smith PL (2012), Brain injury and cognitive deficits reverse with treatment of childhood obstructive sleep apnea. *American J of Respiratory Critical Care Medicine,* Vol. 185, A6722.

Hamilton, Richard (2013), Saving lives one click at a time: Seat belt use climbs to an all-time high. AAA *Motorist.* Vol. 60, n. 1, p 3.

Hammond, D Corydon (2007), *LENS: The Low Energy Neurofeedback System.* Routledge, 120 pp.

Harlow JM (1868), Recovery from the passage of an iron bar through the head. *Publications of the Massachusetts Medical Society,* Vol. 2, pp. 327-347.

Harlow JM (1848), Passage of an iron rod through the head. *Boston Medical and Surgical J,* Vol. 39, pp. 389-393. See also Hayden EC (2011), Neylan TC (1999), and Barker FG (1995).

Hayden EC (2011), Anatomy of a Brain Injury. *Nature,* January 11. Online: www.nature.com/news/2011/110111/full/news.2011.9.html. On Congresswoman Gabrielle Giffords.

Heitger MH, Jones RD, Macleod AD, Snell DL, Frampton CM, Anderson TJ (2009), Impaired eye movements in post-concussion syndrome indicate suboptimal brain function beyond the influence of depression, malingering or intellectual ability. *Brain,* Vol. 132 (Pt 10, pp. 2850-2870. PMID: 19617197 with free full text.

Hendrick, Bill (2011), Light Exposure May Cut Production of Melatonin: Study Shows Artificial Light Before Bedtime May Affect Quality of Sleep. *WebMD* (Jan 19).

http://www.webmd.com/sleep-disorders/news/20110119/light-exposure-may-cut-production-of-melatonin

Hodgson VR and Thomas LM (1971), *Comparison of Head Acceleration Injury Indices in Cadaver Skull Fractures*. Society of Automotive Engineers, SAE Technical Paper 710854. http://papers.sae.org/710854/.

Hoffman DA, Lubar JF, Thatcher RW, Sterman MB, Rosenfeld PJ, Striefel S, Trudeau D, Stockdale S (1999), Limitations of the American Academy of Neurology and American Clinical Neurophysiology Society paper on QEEG. *J of Neuropsychiatry and Clinical Neuroscience*, Vol. 11, n. 3, pp. 401-407. PMID: 10440020.

Hoge CW, Castro CA, Messer SC, McGurk D, Cotting DI, Koffman RL (2004), Combat duty in Iraq and Afghanistan, mental health problems, and barriers to care. *New England J of Medicine,* Vol 351, n. 1, pp. 13-22. PMID: 15229303.

Holtz RL (2013), Concussions on the Field, Repercussions in School: Research Focuses on How Brain Injuries Affect Normal Classwork. *The Wall Street Journal*, Aug 20, p. D1.

Howard, Johnette (2010) Chris Henry data sound football alarm: Is it possible that football is as dangerous to the brain as boxing? The results say yes. June 29, 2010, ESPN.com.

Hruby, Patrick (2012), Did Football Kill Austin Trenum? *Washingtonian* (August). Online: www.washingtonian.com/articles/people/did-football-kill-austin-trenum/

Hughes JR (1994), *EEG in Clinical Practice* (2nd Ed). Butterworth-Heinemann, 242 pp.

Ing C, DiMaggio C, Whitehouse A, Hegarty MK, Brady J, von Ungern-Sternberg JS, Davidson A, Wood AJJ, Li G and Sun LS (2012), Long-term differences in language and cognitive function after chldhood exposure to anesthesia. *Pediatrics*, Vol. 130, n. 3, e476-485. PMID: 22908104.

Jenkins, Sally (2013), Tackling the problem of kids' football. *The Washington Post,* Oct. 3, D1.

Johnson F, Semaan MT, Megerian CA (2008), Temporal bone fracture: evaluation and management in the modern era. *Otolaryngologic Clinics of North Americ*a, Vol. 41, n. 3, pp. 597-618. PMID: 18436001.

Jonas JB (2005), Tight necktie, intraocular pressure, and intracranial pressure. *British J of Ophthalmolo*gy, Vol. 89, n. 6, pp. 786–787. PMCID: PMC1772691 See also Talty P, O'Brien PD (2005).

Kahkeshani K, Ward PJ (2012), Connection between the spinal dura mater and suboccipital musculature: evidence for the myodural bridge and a route for its dissection—a review. *Clinical Anatomy*, Vol. 25, n. 4, pp. 415-422. PMID: 22488993.

Kahle W, Platzer, Werner (2004). *Color Atlas of Human Anatomy*, Vol 1: Locomotor system (5th ed.). Thieme, 435 pp.

Kaiser DA (2006), What is Quantitative EEG? *J of Neurotherapy*, Vol. 10, n. 4.

Kaplan MS, McFarland BH and Huguet N (2009), Firearm suicide among veternas in the general population: Findings from the National Violent Death Reporting System. *J of Trauma,* Vol. 67, n. 3, pp. 503-507. PMID: 19741391.

Katz JN, Harris MB (2008). Clinical practice. Lumbar spinal stenosis. *New England J of Medicine,* Vol. 358, n. 8, pp. 818–825. PMID 18287604.

Kay, Thomas (1986), *The Unseen Injury, Minor Head Trauma. An Introduction for Professionals*. National Head Injury Foundation, Inc., Washington DC.

Kays JL, Hurley RA, Taber KH (2012), The Dynamic Brain: Neuroplasticity and Mental Health. *J of Neuropsychiatry and Clinical Neuroscience*, Vol. 24, n. 2, pp. 118-124. PMID: 22772660.

Keating, Peter (2006), Doctor Yes. *ESPN.com*, October 28. Elliot Pellman, the NFL's top medical adviser, claims it's okay for players with concussions to get back in the game. Time for a second opinion. Online: www.sports.espn.go.com/espnmag/story?id=3644940

Keogh, Pamela Clarke (2004), *Elvis Presley: The Man, The Life, The Legend*. Atria Books, 272 pp.

Keyes, Daniel (1958 / 1966). *Flowers for Algernon*. Various publishers.

Keynes M (2005), The personality and health of King Henry VIII (1491-1547). *J of Medical Biography,* Vol. *3, pp.* 174-183. PMID: 16059531.

Khosla S, Melton III J, Dekutoski MB, Achenbach SJ, Oberg AL, Riggs BL (2003), Incidence of childhood distal forearm fractures over 30 years: A population-based study. *JAMA*, Vol. 290, n. 11, pp. 1479-1485. PMID: 13129988.

Kolla BP, Lovely JK, Mansukhani MP, Morgenthaler TI (2012), Zolpidem is independently associated with increased risk of inpatient falls. *J of Hospital Medicine*, Vol. 8, n. 1, pp. 1-6. PMID: 23165956.

Kontos AP, Dolese A, Elbin RJ, Covassin T, Warren BL (2011) Relationship of soccer heading to computerized neurocognitive performance and symptoms among female and male youth soccer players. *Brain Injury*, Vol. 25, n. 12, pp. 1234-1241. PMID: 21902552.

Koperer H, Deinsberger W, Jodicke A, and Boker DK (1999), Postoperative headache after the lateral suboccipital approach: craniotomy versus craniectomy. *Minimally Invasive Neurosurgery*, Vol. 42, n. 4, pp. 175-178. PMID: 10667820.

Kravitz HM, Esty ML, Katz, RS, Fawcett J (2006), Treatment of fibromyalgia syndrome using low-intensity neurofeedback with the Flexyx Neurotherapy System: A randomized controlled clinical trial. *J of Neurotherapy,* Vol. 10, n. 2/3, pp. 41-58.

Krawczyk M, Flinta I, Garncarek M, Jankowska EA, Banasiak W, Germany R, Javaheri S, Ponikowski P (2013). Sleep disordered breathing in patients with heart failure. *Cardiology J*, Vol. 20, n. 4, pp. 345-355. PMID: 23913452.

Kristman VL, Tator CH, Kreiger N, Richards D, Mainwaring L, Jaglal S, Tomlinson G, Comper P (2008), Does the apolipoprotein epsilon 4 allele predispose varsity athletes to concussion? A prospective cohort study. *Clinical J of Sport Medicine,* Vol. 18, n. 4, pp. 322-328. PMID: 18614883.

Kristof, Nicholas D (2012), Brain damage or PTSD? Many struggling veterans may be suffering from unseen injuries. *Pittsburgh Post-Gazette*, April 27, p. B-7.

Kuhn, Thomas (1962, 2012), *The Structure of Scientific Revolutions* (4th Ed). Univ. of Chicago Press, 264 pp.

Lambert GW, Reid C, Kaye DM, Jennings GL, Esler MD (2002), Effect of sunlight and season on serotonin turnover in the brain. *Lancet.* Vol. 360, n. 9348, pp. 1840-1842. PMID: 12480364.

Larson, Erik (2004) *The Devil in the White City: Murder, Magic, and Madness at the Fair that Changed America.* Vintage Books, 447 pp.

Lawrence Livermore National Laboratory (2010) A New Application for a Weapons Code. *Research Highlights* (March), pp. 14-17.

LeardMann CA, Powell TM, Smith TC, Bell MR, Smith B, Boyko EJ, Hooper TI, Gackstetter GD, Ghamsary M, Hoge CW (2013), Risk factors associated with suicide in current and former US military personnel. *JAMA*, Vol. 310, n. 5, pp. 496-506. PMID: 23925620.

Lehman EJ, Hein MJ, Baron SL, Gersic CM (2012), Neurodegenerative causes of death among retired National Football League players. *Neurology*, Vol. 79, n. 19, pp. 1970-1974. PMID: 22955124.

Lehrer, Jonah (2006), The Reinvention of Self. *Seed Magazine*, (Feb 22). Online: http://seedmagazine.com/content/print/the_reinvention_of_the_self/

Lehrer PM, Woolfok RL, and Sime WE (2008). *Principles and Practice of Stress Management,* Chapter 9. The Guilford Press, 734 pp.

Lévesque J, Beauregard M, Mensour B (2006), Effect of neurofeedback training on the neural substrates of selective attention in children with attention-deficit/hyperactivity disorder: a functional magnetic resonance imaging study. *Neuroscience Letters,* Vol. 394, n. 3, pp. 216-221. PMID: 16343769.

Levy AS, Smith RH (2000), Neurologic injuries in skiers and snowboarders. *Seminars in Neurology*, Vol. 20, n. 2, pp. 233-245. PMID: 10946744.

Lewis, Dorothy Otnow (1998), *Guilty by Reason of Insanity: A Psychiatrist Probes the Minds of Killers.* Fawcett, 301 pp.

Lezak MD, Howieson DB, and Loring DW, 2004). *Neuropsychological Assessment.* New York: Oxford, 1032 pp.

Life (1945), Peleliu: Tom Lea Paints Island Invasion. Jun 11, p. 65.

Lipscomb, Suzannah (2009a), *1536: The Year that Changed Henry VIII.* A Lion Book, Oxford, England, 240 pp.

__b, Suzannah (2009b), Henry VIII ascends to the throne of England. *History Today*, Vol. 59 n. 4.

See also http://www.historytoday.com/suzannah-lipscomb/henry-viii-ascends-throne-england.

Lustenberger T, Talving P, Barmparas G, Schnüriger B, Lam L, Inaba K, Demetriades D (2010), Skateboard-related injuries: not to be taken lightly. A National Trauma Databank Analysis. *J of Trauma*, Vol. 69, n. 4, pp. 924-927. PMID: 20065875.

Ma J, Huang S, Qin S, You C (2012), Progesterone for traumatic brain injury. *Cochrane Summaries*, Oct. 17. http://summaries.cochrane.org/CD008409/progesterone-for-traumatic-brain-injury. See PMID: 23076947.

Mancini T, Casanueva FF, Giustina A (2008). Hyperprolactinemia and prolactinomas. *Endocrinology & Metabolism Clinics of North America*, Vol. 37, n. 1, pp. 67-99. PMID 18226731.

Marsh, Dave (1999), *The Heart of Rock & Soul: The 1001 Greatest Singles Ever Made.* Da Capo, p. 430.

Martinell-Gispert-Saúch M, Gil-Saladié D, Delgado-González M (1997), [Aphasia in a polyglot: description and neuropsychological course: Article in Spanish]: *Revista de Neurologia,* Vol. 25, n. 140, pp. 562-565. PMID: 9172921.

Martinez-Conde, Susana and Macknik, Stephen L. (2013), What It Means To Be You. *Scientific American Mind*, Nov / Dec p. 4.

Maruish ME and Moses JA, Eds.(1996), *Clinical Neuropsychology: Theoretical Foundations for Practitioners.* New York: Lawrence Erlbaum Associates. Ch 7: Neuroimaging: Interface with clinical neuropsychology, by E. D. Bigler, S. S. Porter, C. M. Lowry.

Masferrer R, Masferrer M, Prendergast V, Harrington TR (2000), Grading Scale for Cerebral Concussions. *Barrow Quarterly*, Vol. 16, n. 1. Online: http://www.thebarrow.org/Education_And_Resources/Barrow_Quarterly/205077.

Matheron E and Kapoula Z (2011), Face Piercing (Body Art): Choosing Pleasure vs. Possible Pain and Posture Instability. *Frontiers in Physiology*, Vol 2, n. 64. PMCID: 21960975.

Max JE, Schachar RJ, Landis J, Bigler ED, Wilde EA, Saunders AE, Ewing-Cobbs L, Chapman SB, Dennis M, Hanten G, Levin HS (2013), Psychiatric disorders in children and adolescents in the first six months after mild traumatic brain injury. *J of Neuropsychiatry Clinical Neuroscience*, Vol. 25, n. 3, pp. 187-197. PMID: 24026712.

Mayers LB (2013), Outcomes of sport-related concussion among college athletes. *J of Neuropsychiatry and Clinical Neurosciences*, Vol. 25, n. 2, pp. 115-119. PMID: 23686028.

McCann M (1988), Stunt Injuries and Fatalities Increasing. *Arts Hazard News*, Center for Safety in the Arts, http://www.chicagoartistsresource.org/art-hazard-news-2-professions-theatre-tv-film-27/stunts.

McConnell WE, Howard RP, Van Poppel J, Krause R, Guzman HM, Bomar JB, Raddia JR, Benedict JY, Hatsell CP (1995), Human head and neck kinematics after low velocity rear-end impacts: Understanding "Whiplash". *SAE Technical Paper 952724*, pp. 215-238.

McGonigal, Jane (2009), *Avant Game: A Blog About Why Games Make Us Happy and Why They Can Change the World*. http://blog.avantgame.com/2009/09/super-better-or-how-to-turn-recovery.html.

McGrath, Ben (2011), The NFL and the concussion crisis. *The New Yorker*, January 31.
http://www.newyorker.com/reporting/2011/01/31/110131fa_fact_mcgrath

McGrath, Charles (2006), Commander of Sea, Myth and Tea Towel. *The New York Times*, Book Section, Jan 2. Review of *The Pursuit of Victory: The Life and Achievement of Horatio Nelson,* by Roger Knight, Basic Books, 874 pp. www.nytimes.com/2006/01/02/arts/02mcgr.html accessed 07/11/2012.

McKee AC (2012) quoted in Hruby, Patrick, *Washingtonian Magazine* (Jul 2012).
http://www.washingtonian.com/articles/people/did-football-kill-austin-trenum/index.php

McKee AC, Cantu RC, Nowinski CJ, Hedley-Whyte ET, Gavett BE, Budson AE, Santini VE, Lee HS, Kubilus CA, Stern RA (2009), Chronic Traumatic Encephalopathy in Athletes: Progressive Tauopathy following Repetitive Head Injury. *J of Neuropathology and Experimental Neurology*, Vol. 68, n. 7, pp. 709-735. PMID: 19535999.

McKenna PJ (1997). Schizophrenia and related syndromes. *Psychology Press,* p. 238.

Melnick, Meredith (2010), Study: Many Youth Offenders Have History of Traumatic Brain Injury. *Time*, Nov 11.

Meyers, Tom (2008), *Anatomy Trains*. Churchill Livingstone, 440 pp.

Milhoces, Gary (2007) NFL begins debate about concussions at summit. *USA Today,* Jun 20, Sports.
Online: www.usatoday.com/sports/football/nfl/2007-06-19-concussions-summit_N.htm. This meeting was the turning point in recognition of brain injury in professional football.

Miller BL, Cummings J, Mishkin F, Boone K, Prince F, Ponton M, Cotman C. (1998), Emergence of artistic talent in frontotemporal dementia. *Neurology*, Vol. 51, n. 4, pp. 978-982. PMID: 9781516.

Miller DB (1998), Low velocity impact, vehicular damage and passenger injury. *Cranio*, Vol. 16, n. 4, pp. 226-229. PMID: 10029749.

Miller MA, Croft LB, Belanger AR, Romero-Corral A, Somers VK, Roberts AJ, Goldman ME (2008), Prevalence of metabolic syndrome in retired National Football League players. *American J of Cardiology*, Vol. 101, n. 9, pp. 1281-1284. PMID: 18435958.

Millis SR and Volinsky CT (2001). Assessment of response bias in mild head injury: Beyond malingering tests. *J of of Clinical and Experimental Neuropsychology*, Vol. 23, n. 6, pp. 809-828. PMID: 11910546.

Mishra R and Kunkle F (2000), A 'Jekyll and Hyde' Personality; Md. Fugitive Alternates Between Charming and Violent. *The Washington Post*, (Mar 19, Section A-1).

Monastra VJ, Monastra DM, George S (2002), The effects of stimulant therapy, EEG biofeedback, and parenting style on the primary symptoms of attention-deficit/hyperactivity disorder. *Applied Psychophysiology and Biofeedback*, Vol. 27, n. 4, pp. 231-249. PMID: 12557451.

Moore, David Leon and Brady, Erik (2012) Junior Seau's final days plagued by sleepless nights. *USA Today*, May 31, Sports.

Moravec CS and McKee MG (2013), Psychophysiologic remodeling of the failing human heart. *Biofeedback*, Vol. 41, n. 1, pp. 7-12. See also PMID: 21972325.

Moseley GL, Parsons, TJ, and Spence C (2008), Visual distortion of a limb modulates the pain and swelling evoked by movement: *Current Biology*, Vol. 18, n. 22, R1047-R1048. PMID: 19036329.

Moss WC, King MJ, and Blackman EG (2009), Skull Flexure from Blast Waves: A New Mechanism for Brain Injury with Implications for Helmet Design. Lawrence Livermore National Laboratory, *Physical Review Letters*, Sep 4, Vol. 103, n. 10, p. 108702. PMID: 19792349.

Nakaguchi H, Fujimaki T, Ueki K, Takahashi M, Yoshida H, Kirino T (1999), Snowboard head injury: Prospective study in Chino, Nagano, for two seasons from 1995 to 1997. *J of Trauma*, Vol. 46, n. 6, pp. 1066-1069. PMID: 10372627.

Narayanan NS, Cavanagh JF, Frank MJ, Laubach M (2013), Common medial frontal mechanisms of adaptive control in humans and rodents. *Nature Neuroscience*. Oct 20. PMID: 24141310.

National Academy of Sciences, Institute of Medicine (2006), *Sleep Disorders and Sleep Deprivation*. See Colten HR and Altevogt BM (2006).

National Safety Council (2011), Injury Facts. NSC Press Product No. 02319-0000, 210 pp.

National Sleep Foundation (2012), Teens and Sleep. www.sleepfoundation.org/article/sleep-topics/teens-and-sleep, accessed Oct 4, 2012.

Nelson DV and Esty ML (2012), Neurotherapy of Traumatic Brain Injury/Post Traumatic Stress Symptoms in OEF/OIF Veterans. *J of Neuropsychiatry & Clinical Neurosciences*, Vol. 24, n. 2, pp. 237-240. PMID: 22772672.

__ and Esty ML (2009), Neurotherapy for pain in veterans with trauma spectrum disorders. *J of Pain,* Vol. 10, S18.

Newcomb, Douglas (2012), Why It Took Decades For a Female Crash Test Dummy to Debut: Automakers for years fought to use only crash dummies modeled after the average American male. *Exhaust Notes,* Aug 30, editorial: www.autos.msn.com.

New York City Department of Health and Mental Hygiene (2003), Certificate of Death No. 156-03-017846.

Neylan TC (1999), Frontal Lobe Function: Mr. Phineas Gage's Famous Injury. *J of Neuropsychiatry and Clinical Neurosciences*, Vol. 11, n. 2, pp. 280-281. PMID: 10334002.

Nowinski, Christopher (2012), www.SportsLegacy.com.

Nowinski, Christopher (2006), *Head Games*. Thought Leaders, LLC, 202 pp.

Nyad, Diana (2013), quoted in Alvarez, Lizette (2013), Sharks Absent, Swimmer, 64, Strokes From Cuba to Florida. *The New York Times*, Sept 2, Sports. Online: www.nytimes.com/2013/09/03/sports/nyad-completes-cuba-to-florida-swim.html?_r=0

Oliver M (2011), Alabama tornadoes: Deaths reveal helmets, car seats may boost chances. *The Birmingham News*, Sunday, Dec 04. http://blog.al.com/spotnews/2011/12/alabama_tornadoes_—_first_in.html

Omalu B, Bailes J, Hamilton RL, Kamboh MI, Hammers J, Case M, Fitzsimmons R (2011), Emerging histomorphologic phenotypes of chronic traumatic encephalopathy in American athletes. *Neurosurgery*, Vol. 69, n. 1, pp. 173-83. PMID: 21358359.

__, Hammers JL, Bailes J, Hamilton RL, Kamboh MI, Webster G, Fitzsimmons RP (2011), Chronic traumatic encephalopathy in an Iraqi war veteran with posttraumatic stress disorder who committed suicide. *Neurosurg Focus*, Nov, Vol. 31, n. 5, E3. PMID: 22044102.

__, DeKosky ST, Hamilton RL, Minster RL, Kamboh MI, Shakir AM, Wecht CH (2006), Chronic traumatic encephalopathy in a national football league player: Part II. *Neurosurgery*, Vol. 59, n. 5, pp. 1086-1092. PMID: 17143242. On the discovery of CTE in former Steeler's player Mike Webster.

__, DeKosky ST, Minster RL, Kamboh MI, Hamilton RL, Wecht CH (2005), Chronic traumatic encephalopathy in a National Football League player. *Neurosurgery*, Vol. 57, n. 1, pp. 128-134. PMID:15987548.

__, Fitzsimmons RP, Hammers J, Bailes J (2010), Chronic traumatic encephalopathy in a professional American wrestler. *J of Forensic Nursing*, Vol. 6, n. 3, pp. 130-136. PMID: 21175533. On Chris Benoit.

Pellegrino, Mark L (2001), From Whiplash to Fibromyalgia. ORC Publishing, 130 pp.

Pincus, Jonathan (2002), *Base Instincts: What Makes Killers Kill?* W. W. Norton & Company, 240 pp.

Ponikowski P, Javaheri S, Michalkiewicz D, Bart BA, Czarnecka D, Jastrzebski M, Kusiak A, Augostini R, Jagielski D, Witkowski T, Khayat RN, Oldenburg O, Gutleben KJ, Bitter T, Karim R, Iber C, Hasan A, Hibler K, Germany R, Abraham WT (2012), Transvenous phrenic nerve stimulation for the treatment of central sleep apnoea in heart failure. *European Heart J*, Vol. 33, n. 7, 889-894. PMID: 21856678.

Pontell ME, Scali F, Marshall E, Enix D (2013), The obliquus capitis inferior myodural bridge. *Clinical Anatomy*, Vol. 26, n. 4, pp. 450-454. PMID: 22836789.

Powell NB, Schechtman KB, Riley RW, Li K, Troell R, Guilleminault C (2001), The road to danger: the comparative risks of driving while sleepy. *Laryngoscope*, Vol. 111, n. 5, pp.887-893. PMID: 11359171.

Powner DJ, Boccalandro C, Alp MS, Vollmer DG (2006), Endocrine failure after traumatic brain injury in adults. *Neurocritical Care*, Vol. 5, n. 1, pp. 61-70. PMID: 16960299

Pryor Karen (2006), *Don't Shoot the Dog*. Ringpress Books, 202 pp.

Raines, Adrian (2013), *Anatomy of Violence: The Biological Roots of Crime*. Pantheon, 478 pp.

Reed, Tom (2012), A culture of head shots has seen plenty of change since last Cleveland Browns-Pittsburgh Steelers game. *The Plain Dealer,* Nov 24, Sports.

Reiner PB (2009), Meditation on Demand: New research reveals how meditation changes the brain. *Scientific American*, http://www.scientificamerican.com/article.cfm?id=meditation-on-demand

Resch J, Driscoll A, McCaffrey N, Brown C, Ferrara MS, Macciocchi S, Baumgartner T, Walpert K (2013), ImPact test-retest reliability: reliably unreliable? J Athletic Training, Vol. 48, n. 4, pp. 506-511.PMID: 23724770.

Resnick, Brian (2011), Chart: One Year of Prison Costs More Than One Year at Princeton. *The Atlantic*, Nov 1.

Resnick DK, Subach BR, Marion DW (1997), The Significance of Carotid Canal Involvement in Basilar Cranial Fracture. *Neurosurgery*, Vol. 40, n. 6, pp. 1177-1181. PMID: 9179890.

Riddick A, Marwitz J H, Kreutzer J S, and Zasler ND (2005), Evaluation of the Neurobehavioral Functioning Inventory as a Depression Screening Tool After Traumatic Brain Injury. *J Head Trauma Rehabilitation*, Vol. 20, n. 6, pp. 512-526. PMID: 16304488.

Robbins, Jim (2008), *A Symphony in the Brain: The Evolution of the New Brain Wave Biofeedback* (2nd Ed, 2008). Grove Press, Revised Edition, 272 pp.

Rogers, Dave (1982), *Rock 'n' Roll*. Routledge Kegan & Paul, 158 pp.

Rose SR, Auble BA (2012), Endocrine changes after pediatric traumatic brain injury. *Pituitary*, Vol. 15, n. 3, pp. 267-75. PMID: 22057966. See also Auble BA and Others (2013) on endocrine dysfunction in child abuse.

Ruff R and Riechers RG (2012), Effective treatment of traumatic brain injury: learning from experience. *JAMA*, Vol. 308, n. 19, pp. 2032-2033. PMID: 23168827.

Sacks, Oliver (2012), *Hallucinations*. Alfred A. Knopf, 352 pp.

Sanders MJ and McKenna K (2001), *Mosby's Paramedic Textbook*, 2nd revised Ed. Chapter 22, "Head and Facial Trauma." Mosby, 1532 pp.

Scali F, Pontell ME, Enix DE, Marshall E (2013), Histological analysis of the rectus capitis posterior major's myodural bridge. *Spine J*, Vol. 13, n. 5, pp. 558-563. PMID: 23406969.

Schoenberger NE, Shiflett SC, Esty ML, Ochs L, Matheis RJ (2001), Flexyx Neurotherapy System in the Treatment of Traumatic Brain Injury: An Initial Evaluation. *J of Head Trauma Rehabilitation,* Vol. 16, n. 3 (Jun), pp. 260-274. PMID: 11346448. Note: *Shiflett SC* is incorrectly cited in PubMed as *Shif SC*.

Schrotenboer, Brent (2009), Chris Mims: A fallen star's burnout. *U-T San Diego News,* June 7.

Schuenke M, Schulte E, Schumacher U, Ross LM, Lamperti ED, Voll M (2010), *Head and Neuroanatomy*, Thieme, 414 pp.

Schwarz, Alan (2009), New Sign of Brain Damage in N.F.L. *The New York Times*, Jan 27.

__ (2008), 12 Athletes Leaving Brains To Researchers. *The New York Times*, Sept 24.

__ (2007), Expert Ties Ex-Player's Suicide to Brain Damage. *The New York Times*, Jan 18.

Schwartz, Thomas F (1970), My Stay on Earth is Growing Very Short. *J of the Illinois Historical Society* (Spring), 5-33, p. 135. Quoted in Beidler AE (2009).

Serrador JM, Schlegel TT, Black FO, Wood SJ (2009). Vestibular effects on cerebral blood flow. *BMC Neuroscience*, Vol. 10 (Sep 23), p. 119. PMID: 19775430.

Shephard, Ben (2000), *A War of Nerves: Soldiers and Psychiatrists, 1914-1994*. London, Jonathan Cape.

Shifflett CM (2011), *Migraine Brains and Bodies. A Comprehensive Guide to Solving the Mystery of Your Migraines*. Round Earth Publishing, 296 pp.

Siever, D. (2003). Audio-visual entrainment: History and physiological mechanisms. *Biofeedback*, Vol. 31, n. 2, pp. 21-27.

Shimamura, Arthur P (2002), Muybridge in Motion: Travels in Art, Psychology and Neurology. *History of Photography*, Vol. 26, n. 4, pp. 341-350.

Shaver, Katherine (2012), Female dummy makes her mark on male-dominated crash tests. *The Washington Post*, March 25, Transportation. http://www.washingtonpost.com/local/trafficandcommuting/female-dummy-makes-her-mark-on-male-dominated-crash-tests/2012/03/07/gIQANBLjaS_story.html

Simons DG, Travell JG, Simons LS (1999), *Travell & Simons' Myofascial Pain and Dysfunction: The Trigger Point Manual (Vol 1. Upper Half of Body)*. Williams & Wilkins, 1038 pp.

Simpson D (2005), Phrenology and the neurosciences: Contributions of FJ Gall and JG Spurzheim. *ANZ J of Surgery*, Vol. 75, n. 6, p. 475-482. PMID: 15943741.

Society for Neuroscience (2005), Dialogues Between Neuroscience and Society. A presentation by the Dalai Lama.

Solms M (2000), Dreaming and REM sleep are controlled by different brain mechanisms. *The Behavioral and Brain Sciences*, Vol. 23, n. 6, pp. 843-850. PMID: 11515144.

__ (1995), New findings on the neurological organization of dreaming: implications for psychoanalysis. *Psychoanalytic Quarterly*, Vol. 64, n. 1, pp. 43-67. PMID: 7753944.

Soumekh B, Levine SC, Haines JJ, Wulf JA (1996), Retrospective study of postcraniotomy headaches in suboccipital approach: diagnosis and management. *American J of Otology,* Vol. 17, pp. 617-619. PMID: 8841709.

Stein DG (2013), A clinical/translational perspective: Can a developmental hormone play a role in the treatment of traumatic brain injury? *Hormones and Behavior*, Vol. 63, n. 2, pp. 291-300. PMID: 22626570.

__ and Macdonald MR (1978), Effects of central cortical EEG feedback training on incidence of poorly controlled seizures. *Epilepsia*, Vol. 19, n. 3, pp. 207-222. PMID: 354919

__, Wyrwicka W, and Roth SR (1969), Electrophysiological correlates and neural substrates of alimentary behavior in the cat. *Annals of the New York Academy of Sciences*, Vol. 157, n. 2, pp. 723-739.

__ and Wyrwicka W (1967), EEG correlates of sleep: Evidence for separate forebrain substrates. Brain Research, Vol. 6, n. 1, pp. 143-163. PMID: 6052533.

Suchoff IB, Ciuffreda KJ, Kapoor N (2001), *Visual & Vestibular Consequences of Acquired Brain Injury.* Optometric Extension Program, Santa Ana, CA, 244 pp.

Swanson, Kara L (1999), *I'll Carry the Fork! Recovering a Life After Brain Injury.* Rising Star Press, 205 pp.

Taber KH, Hurley RA (2009), PTSD and Combat-Related Injuries: Functional Neuroanatomy. *J of Neuropsychiatry and Clinical Neurosciences, Vol.* 21, n. 1, pp. 1-4. PMID: 19359445.

Talavage TM, Nauman EA, Breedlove EL, Yoruk U, Dye AE, Morigaki KE, Feuer H, Leverenz LJ (2013), Functionally-Detected Cognitive Impairment in High School Football Players Without Clinically-Diagnosed Concussion. *J of Neurotrauma,* Apr 11. PMID: 20883154.

Talty P, O'Brien PD (2005), Does extended wear of a tight necktie cause raised intraocular pressure? *J of Glaucoma.* Vol.14, n. 6, pp. 508-510. PMID: 16276286.

Tang-Schomer MD, Patel AR, Baas PW, Smith DH (2010), Mechanical breaking of microtubules in axons during dynamic stretch injury underlies delayed elasticity, microtubule disassembly, and axon degeneration. *FASEB Journal,* Vol. 24, n. 5, pp. 1401-1410. PMID: 20019243.

Tanriverdi F, Agha A, Aimaretti G, Casanueva FF, Kelestimur F, Klose M, Masel BE, Pereira AM, Popovic V, Schneider HJ. (2011), Manifesto for the current understanding and management of traumatic brain injury-induced hypopituitarism. *J of Endocrinol Investigations*, Vol. 34, n. 7, pp. 541-543. PMID: 21697650.

__, De Bellis A, Battaglia M, Bellastella G, Bizzarro A, Sinisi AA, Bellastella A, Unluhizarci K, Selcuklu A, Casanueva FF, Kelestimur F (2010), Investigation of antihypothalamus and antipituitary antibodies in amateur boxers: Is chronic repetitive head trauma-induced pituitary dysfunction associated with autoimmunity? *European J of Endocrinology*, Vol. 162, n. 5, pp. 861-867. PMID: 20176736.

__, Unluhizarci K, Karaca Z, Casanueva FF, Kelestimur F (2010), Hypopituitarism due to sports related head trauma and the effects of growth hormone replacement in retired amateur boxers. *Pituitary*, Vol. 13, n. 2, pp. 111-114. PMID: 19847653.

Taylor, Jill Bolte (2009), *My Stroke of Insight: A Brain Scientist's Personal Journey.* Plume, 224 pp. See her 2008 presentation at www.Ted.com/talks/jill_bolte_taylor_s_powerful_stroke_of_insight.html.

Teicher, Martin H (2002), Scars that won't heal: The neurobiology of child abuse. *Scientific American,* Vol. 286, n. 3, pp. 68-75.

Tennant, Forest (2013), Elvis Presley: Head Trauma, Autoimmunity, Pain, and Early Death. *Practical Pain Management*, Volume 13, n. 5. www.practicalpainmanagement.com/elvis-presley-head-trauma-autoimmunity-pain-early-death.

__ (2007), Howard Hughes and Pseudo-Addiction. *Practical Pain Management*, Vol. 7, n. 6. www.practicalpainmanagement.com/resources/howard-hughes-pseudoaddiction.

Terán-Santos J, Jiménez-Gómez A, Cordero-Guevara J (1999), The association between sleep apnea and the risk of traffic accidents. Cooperative Group Burgos-Santander. *New England J of Medicine*, Vol. 340, n. 11, pp. 847-851. PMID: 10080847.

Thatcher RW (2010), Validity and Reliability of Quantitative Electroencephalography. *J of Neurotherapy*, Vol. 14, n. 2, pp. 122-152.

__, North DM, Curtin RT, Walker RA, Biver CJ, Gomez JF, Salazar AM (2001), An EEG Severity Index of Traumatic Brain Injury. *J of Neuropsychiatry and Clinical Neurosciences*, Vol. 13, No. 1. [This study was done with veterans in the Defense and Veterans Head Injury Program.] PMID: 11207333.

Thomas, Katie (2012), N.F.L.'s Policy on Helmet-to-Helmet Hits Makes Highlights Distasteful. *The New York Times*, October 21, Sports. Additional information on injuries from helmet hits. Online: http://en.wikipedia.org/wiki/Helmet-to-helmet_collision.

Tierney RT, Mansell JL, Higgins M, McDevitt JK, Toone N, Gaughan JP, Mishra A, Krynetskiy E (2010), Apolipoprotein E genotype and concussion in college athletes. *Clinical J of Sport Medicine,* Vol. 20, n. 6, pp. 464-468. PMID: 21079443.

Tomoda A, Polcari A, Anderson CM, Teicher MH (2012), Reduced Visual Cortex Gray Matter Volume and Thickness in Young Adults Who Witnessed Domestic Violence during Childhood. *PLoS One, Vol.* 7, n. 12, e52528.

Turner, Justin G and Turner, Linda L (1972), *Mary Todd Lincoln — Her Life and Letters.* Knopf, 750 pp.

US Food and Drug Administration (2013), FDA permits marketing of first brain wave test to help assess children and teens for ADHD. Press release, Jul 15.

Van Horn JD, Irimia A, Torgerson CM, Chambers MC, Kikinis R, Toga AW (2012), Mapping Connectivity Damage in the Case of Phineas Gage. *PLoS ONE* , Vol. 7, n. 5.

Von Drehle, David (1995). *Among the Lowest of the Dead: The Culture on Death Row* Crown. 407 pp.

Walsh, Nancy (2013), Biomarkers Can Diagnose Mild Brain Injury. *MedPage Today*, Jun 20.

__ (2012), Afghan Tragedy Renews Focus on Head Trauma in Soldiers: *MedPage Today,* Mar 20.

Wasden CC, McIntosh SE, Keith DS, McCowan C (2009), An analysis of skiing and snowboarding injuries on Utah slopes. *J of Trauma*, Vol. 67, n. 5, pp. 1022-1026. PMID: 19901663.

Wasserman J, Feldman JS, and Koenigsberg RA (2012). Diffuse axonal injury. *Emedicine.com*. Retrieved 2012-07-10. Online: www.emedicine.medscape.com/article/339912-overview

Weiner MF, Hynan LS, Rossetti H, Falkowski J (2011), Luria's three-step test: What is it and what does it tell us? *International Psychogeriatrics*, Vol. 23, n. 10, pp. 1602–1606. PMCID: 21554794.

Weir, Alison (2008), *Henry VIII*. Ballantine Books, 642 pp.

White, Trumbull and Igleheart, William (1893), *The World's Columbian Exposition 1893*. International Publishing Co, Philadelphia and Chicago, 640 pp.

Wilde EA, Hunter JV, Newsome MR, Scheibel RS, Bigler ED, Johnson JL, Fearing MA, Cleavinger HB, Li X, Swank PR, Pedroza C, Roberson GS, Bachevalier J, Levin HS (2005) Frontal and temporal morphometric findings on MRI in children after moderate to severe traumatic brain injury. *J of Neurotrauma,* Vol. 22, n. 3, pp. 333-344. PMID: 15785229.

Wilkinson CW, Pagulayan KF, Petrie EC, Mayer CL, Colasurdo EA, Shofer JB, Hart KL, Hoff D, Tarabochia MA, Peskind ER (2012), High prevalence of chronic pituitary and target-organ hormone abnormalities after blast-related mild traumatic brain injury. *Frontiers in Neurology,* Vol. 7, n. 11. PMID: 22347210.

Williams WH, Cordan G, Mewse AJ, Tonks J, Burgess CN (2010), Self-reported traumatic brain injury in male young offenders: a risk factor for re-offending, poor mental health and violence? *Neuropsychol Rehabilitation*, Vol. 20, n. 6, pp. 801-812. PMID: 21069616.

Willis PF, Farrer TJ, Bigler ED (2011), Are Effort Measures Sensitive to Cognitive Impairment? *Military Medicine*, Vol. 176, n. 12, pp. 142 -1431. PMID: 22338360.

Wolff, Harold G (1948;1950), *Headache and Other Head Pain*. Oxford University Press, 648 pp.

World Health Organization (International Classification of Diseases and Related Health Problems ICD).

Wright DW, Kellermann AL, Hertzberg VS, Clark PL, Frankel M, Goldstein FC, Salomone JP, Dent LL, Harris OA, Ander DS, Lowery DW, Patel MM, Denson DD, Gordon AB, Wald MM, Gupta S, Hoffman SW, Stein DG (2007), ProTECT: a randomized clinical trial of progesterone for acute traumatic brain injury. *Annals of Emergency Medicine*, Vol. 49, n. 4, pp. 391-402. PMID: 17011666.

Wunderle K, Hoeger KM, Wasserman E, Bazarian JJ (2013), Menstrual Phase as Predictor of Outcome After Mild Traumatic Brain Injury in Women. *J of Head Trauma Rehabilitation,* Nov 20. PMID: 24220566.

Xiao G, Wei J, Yan W, Wang W, Lu Z (2008), Improved outcomes from the administration of progesterone for patients with acute severe traumatic brain injury: a randomized controlled trial. *Critical Care*. Vol.12, n. 2, p. R61. PMID:18447940.

Young T, Blustein J, Finn L, Palta M (1997), Sleep-disordered breathing and motor vehicle accidents in a population-based sample of employed adults. *Sleep*, Vol. 20, n. 8, pp. 608-613. PMID: 9351127.

Zafonte RD, Bagiella E, Ansel BM, Novack TA, Friedewald WT, Hesdorffer DC, Timmons SD, Jallo J, Eisenberg H, Hart T, Ricker JH, Diaz-Arrastia R, Merchant RE, Temkin NR, Melton S, Dikmen SS (2012), Effect of citicoline on functional and cognitive status among patients with traumatic brain injury: Citicoline Brain Injury Treatment Trial (COBRIT), *JAMA*, Vol. 308, n. 19, pp. 1993-2000. PMID: 23168823.

Zarembo, Alan (2013), War blasts may have hidden impact on weight gain, sex drive. *Los Angeles Times (Aug 1)*. Online: www.stripes.com/news/us/war-blasts-may-have-hidden-impact-on-weight-gain-sex-drive-1.233356

Ziejewski M (2013), New Developments in Understanding the Mechanism of Blast Related TBI. *North American Brain Injury Society*, 11th Annual Conference on Brain Injury, New Orleans, LA, Sept 20.

Index

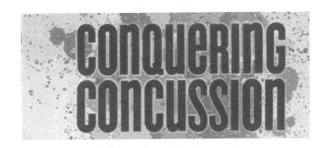

A novel look at concussion, traumatic brain injury (TBI), and healing the symptoms with neurofeedback. Written in plain language with clear graphics.

- **Part 1** Head injuries in history, from Henry VIII to Elvis Presley and the NFL. Learn what happens in concussion, the many symptoms that may appear, and the possibilities and limitations of standard tests.

- **Part 2** The origins, supporting research, and results of neurofeedback. Case histories of children, adults, and military veterans with memory problems, severe headache, insomnia and PTSD. Additional medical issues and how to avoid injury in the first place.

- **Part 3** The rest of the story: what happened to people never expected to work or function normally ever again. How they regained their skills, their jobs, their families and their lives.

"This book is impressive for a rare combination of expertise and readability. The historical perspective and excellent illustrations, both light and serious, make this as approachable as a serious medical book can be."

— E. James Lieberman, M.D., M.P.H

"An incredible resource. Chapters on symptoms and case histories create a one-stop resource for all aspects of concussion."

— Gilian Hotz Ph.D., Director, Concussion Program
Miller School of Medicine

"Even a 'small' concussion can have long-term effects and the symptoms can vary widely. The technology presented in this book abruptly ended our six months of misery and has turned my daughter's life around."

— Patty Whelpley

Softcover, 312 pages $24.95
Order your copy today from:

Round Earth Publishing
P. O. Box 157
Sewickley, PA 15143
(412) 741-7286 / sales@round-earth.com
For more information, see www.ConqueringConcussion.net

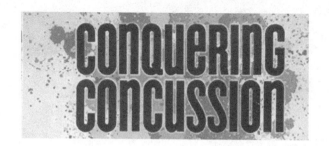

A novel look at concussion, traumatic brain injury (TBI), and healing the symptoms with neurofeedback. Written in plain language with clear graphics and detailed case histories.

Order Form	How Many?	Price	Total
Conquering Concussion Healing TBI Symptoms With Neurofeedback and Without Drugs		$24.95	$
Total:			$
US Shipping: Book Rate $4, Priority Mail $6			$
Tax: PA residents please add 7%:			$
TOTAL:			$
Shipping:			
Ship to Name (Please print):			
Ship to Address 1:			
Ship to Address 2:			
City: State: ZIP: Phone: ( )			
E-Mail:			
Credit Cards: __Visa __MasterCard __Discover			
Name as it appears on card (Please print):			
Billing Address:			
City: State: ZIP: Phone: ( )			
Expiration Date: / 3-digit code on back of card:_____			
Card Number: - - -			
Signature:			
Mail Check or Money Order to:			

Round Earth Publishing
P. O. Box 157
Sewickley, PA 15143
(412) 741-7286 / sales@round-earth.com
For more information, see www.ConqueringConcussion.net

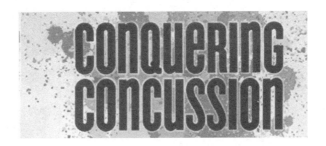

A novel look at concussion, traumatic brain injury (TBI), and healing the symptoms with neurofeedback. Written in plain language with clear graphics.

- **Part 1** Head injuries in history, from Henry VIII to Elvis Presley and the NFL. Learn what happens in concussion, the many symptoms that may appear, and the possibilities and limitations of standard tests.

- **Part 2** The origins, supporting research, and results of neurofeedback. Case histories of children, adults, and military veterans with memory problems, severe headache, insomnia and PTSD. Additional medical issues and how to avoid injury in the first place.

- **Part 3** The rest of the story: what happened to people never expected to work or function normally ever again. How they regained their skills, their jobs, their families and their lives.

—

Softcover, 312 pages $24.95
Order your copy today from:

Round Earth Publishing
P. O. Box 157
Sewickley, PA 15143
(412) 741-7286 / sales@round-earth.com
For more information, see www.ConqueringConcussion.net

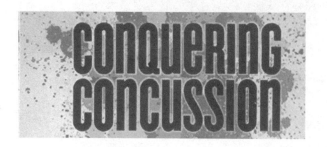

A novel look at concussion, traumatic brain injury (TBI), and healing the symptoms with neurofeedback. Written in plain language with clear graphics and detailed case histories.

Order Form	How Many?	Price	Total
Conquering Concussion Healing TBI Symptoms With Neurofeedback and Without Drugs		$24.95	$
Total:			$
US Shipping: Book Rate $4, Priority Mail $6			$
Tax: PA residents please add 7%:			$
TOTAL:			$
Shipping:			
Ship to Name (Please print):			
Ship to Address 1:			
Ship to Address 2:			
City: State: ZIP: Phone: ( )			
E-Mail:			
Credit Cards: __Visa __MasterCard __Discover			
Name as it appears on card (Please print):			
Billing Address:			
City: State: ZIP: Phone: ( )			
Expiration Date: / 3-digit code on back of card:_____			
Card Number: - - -			
Signature:			
Mail Check or Money Order to:			

Round Earth Publishing
P. O. Box 157
Sewickley, PA 15143
(412) 741-7286 / sales@round-earth.com
For more information, see www.ConqueringConcussion.net